Risk Factors and Prevention of Cardiovascular Diseases

Risk Factors and Prevention of Cardiovascular Diseases

Guest Editor

Małgorzata Poręba

MDPI

Basel • Beijing • Wuhan • Barcelona • Belgrade • Novi Sad • Cluj • Manchester

Guest Editor
Małgorzata Poręba
Department of Biological
Principles of Physical Activity
Wroclaw University of Health
and Sport Sciences
Wrocław
Poland

Editorial Office
MDPI AG
Grosspeteranlage 5
4052 Basel, Switzerland

This is a reprint of the Special Issue, published open access by the journal *Journal of Cardiovascular Development and Disease* (ISSN 2308-3425), freely accessible at: https://www.mdpi.com/journal/jcdd/special_issues/9565V8D9S4.

For citation purposes, cite each article independently as indicated on the article page online and as indicated below:

Lastname, A.A.; Lastname, B.B. Article Title. *Journal Name* **Year**, *Volume Number*, Page Range.

ISBN 978-3-7258-5503-2 (Hbk)
ISBN 978-3-7258-5504-9 (PDF)
https://doi.org/10.3390/books978-3-7258-5504-9

Contents

About the Editor

Małgorzata Poręba

Małgorzata Poręba works as an Associate Professor in the Department of Biological Principles of Physical Activity at Wroclaw University of Health and Sport Sciences in Poland. She is a physician with three specialties: cardiology, internal medicine, and balneology and physical medicine. In the last 25 years, she has participated in a variety of different research studies involving cardiovascular diseases, electrocardiography, and cardiovascular imaging, as well as the role of occupational and environmental medicine in treating cardiovascular complications. She is also interested in problems related to toxic elements in the human environment, participating in a number of projects in this field, and thus is not limited to topics relating to the circulatory system. In her early career, she worked in a hematology department, and her doctoral thesis and some of her other research focused on blood diseases including blood neoplasms. In her recent studies, she has concentrated on the relationships between physical activity and cardiovascular health and additionally on regeneration methods in sport. Her other area of interest is analyzing cardiovascular health status in seniors. Professor Poreba has taken part in numerous conferences and symposia, as well as medical courses, and as a researcher and physician possesses the ability to both work in a research laboratory and simultaneously apply typical diagnostic cardiological methods used in outpatient and inpatient circumstances.

Preface

It is a great pleasure to present this Reprint, which is a comprehensive compilation of reviews and research articles prepared by investigators from all over the world. There is still a constant need to evaluate the problem of cardiovascular diseases in the context of prevention and evaluate risk factors. Although treatment methods have improved greatly in recent decades, the importance of prevention cannot be underestimated. CVDs are the primary and leading causes of death in developed countries and are responsible for about one-third of global mortality.

Małgorzata Poręba
Guest Editor

Journal of
Cardiovascular
Development and Disease

MDPI

Review

Myocardial Late Gadolinium Enhancement (LGE) in Cardiac Magnetic Resonance Imaging (CMR)—An Important Risk Marker for Cardiac Disease

Claudia Meier [1,2], Michel Eisenblätter [2,3] and Stephan Gielen [1,2,*]

1 Universitätsklinik für Kardiologie, Angiologie und Internistische Intensivmedizin, Universitätsklinikum Ostwestfalen-Lippe, Campus Klinikum Lippe, D-32756 Detmold, Germany
2 Medizinische Fakultät, Universität Bielefeld, D-33615 Bielefeld, Germany
3 Universitätsinstitut für Diagnostische und Interventionelle Radiologie, Universitätsklinikum Ostwestfalen-Lippe, Campus Klinikum Lippe, D-32756 Detmold, Germany
* Correspondence: stephan.gielen@klinikum-lippe.de; Tel.: +49-5231-72-1181; Fax: +49-5231-72-1214

Abstract: Cardiovascular magnetic resonance (CMR) has significantly revolutionized the comprehension and diagnosis of cardiac diseases, particularly through the utilization of late gadolinium enhancement (LGE) imaging for tissue characterization. LGE enables the visualization of expanded extracellular spaces in conditions such as fibrosis, fibrofatty tissue, or edema. The growing recognition of LGE's prognostic capacity underscores its importance, evident in the increasing explicit recommendations within guidelines. Notably, the contemporary characterization of cardiomyopathies relies on LGE-based scar assessment by CMR to a large extent. This review describes the pattern and prognostic value of LGE in detail for various cardiac diseases. Despite its merits, establishing LGE as a reliable risk marker encounters challenges. Limitations arise from the fact that not all diseases show LGE, and it should always be analyzed in the context of all CMR sequences and the patient's medical history. In summary, LGE stands as a robust indicator of adverse outcomes in diverse cardiovascular diseases. Its further integration into routine practice is desirable, necessitating widespread availability and application to accumulate both individual and scientific experience.

Keywords: late gadolinium enhancement; cardiac magnetic resonance imaging; cardiomyopathy; myocardial vitality; risk stratification; review

1. Introduction

Cardiovascular magnetic resonance (CMR) has transformed the understanding and diagnostic pathway of various cardiac diseases, particularly with the use of late gadolinium enhancement (LGE) imaging for tissue characterization. In addition, the prognostic ability of LGE to predict outcome is becoming increasingly important, and that has been reflected by the growing numbers of explicit recommendations in the guidelines of the last years [1–3]. Furthermore, the new ESC guidelines for the management of cardiomyopathies [1] establish their new phenotypic description of cardiomyopathies on a LGE-based scar assessment by CMR. Especially in cardiomyopathies, traditional risk factors do not adequately predict outcome as there is no pathogenetic correlation. The presence, location, pattern, and extent of LGE has been shown to be a prospective and innovative risk marker for the development of a symptomatic phenotype and adverse events. The aim of this review is to highlight the role of LGE as a risk marker for various cardiovascular diseases.

When considering LGE as a "risk factor" for the development or exacerbation of heart disease, it should be noted that the presence of LGE itself does not cause the disease, but is a surrogate for certain physiological or anatomical characteristics, genetic predisposition or metabolic constellations that represent a risk. So, the term "risk marker" should be preferred. The use of the chelated paramagnetic contrast agent gadolinium within a CMR scan can visualize the widened extracellular space in, e.g., fibrosis, fibro-fatty tissue, or edema. This technique exploits differences in gadolinium washout kinetics and volume of distribution between scar or edematous tissue and normal myocardium. Gadolinium shows rapid washout from healthy myocardium. In contrast, it washes out more slowly from areas of fibrosis or edema where the extracellular space is enlarged. T1-weighted inversion recovery sequences, optimized to "null" the signal from healthy myocardium, reveal areas of, e.g., scar or edematous tissue as bright regions of high signal intensity by shortening T1 relaxation times.

2. LGE in Specific Phenotypes of Cardiovascular Disease

Different heart diseases cause a different pattern and a different extent of LGE, which is why the distribution pattern and the total burden of LGE as a risk marker must be considered separately for each disease and cannot be generalized. Furthermore, it must be noted that any change in interstitial space from any cause can be a potential origin of LGE. So, the common perception that LGE is synonymous with fibrosis and therefore dead tissue is too simplified.

It must be also emphasized that the interpretation of CMR images is only conclusive when all morpho-functional images (cine-imaging, perfusion-imaging) and all tissue-characterizing images (T1 weighted, T2 weighted, possibly multiparametric mapping, possibly T2 * weighted) are taken together and that the LGE cannot be interpreted on its own. Please note that the significance of the LGE was highlighted for this overview.

2.1. Ischemic Cardiomyopathy

Ischaemic cardiomyopathy (ICM) is a sub-entity of heart failure with reduced ejection fraction in which a mismatch between myocardial oxygen demand and vascular oxygen supply leads to reversible or irreversible myocardial damage. The majority of patients with ICM has experienced either a type I myocardial infarction following a plaque rupture and thrombus in epicardial conduction vessels or a type II myocardial infraction resulting from vasospasm, microvascular dysfunction, non-arteriosclerotic coronary dissection or regional non-obstructive relative ischemia. This is still the predominant cause of heart failure globally [4–6]. It typically results from a combination of irreversible loss of viable myocardial mass and a dysfunctional but still viable myocardium in the setting of chronically reduced myocardial blood flow.

The typical distribution of subendocardial LGE corresponding to a coronary artery territory identifies an ischemic scar, whereby the transmurality indicates the residual vitality [7] (Figures 1A,B and 2A,B). A transmural infarction affects all wall layers from the endocardium to the epicardium, whereas a non-transmural infarction originates from the endocardium and affects <100% of the wall thickness. The size of the infarction, evaluated through LGE-CMR, stands out as the most robust predictor of mortality and significant cardiac events. Not only the infarct transmurality, but also total scar mass, total scar as a percentage of LV volume, gray zone mass, and the peri-infarction-to-core infarction mass ratio are important for risk stratification [8]. So, CMR is also effective in assessing myocardial vitality through discrimination of the LGE extension and segmental kinesis and this can guide coronary revascularization [9]. There is a close relation between the percentage of the left ventricular wall thickness which is affected by the infarction scar and functional recovery after myocardial revascularization: wall segments with <25% LGE extension are more likely to regain contractility than segments with >50% LGE transmurality [10].

Guidelines recommend that CMR with LGE should be performed as soon as possible in patients with suspected MINOCA (Myocardial Infarction with Nonobstructive Coronary Arteries). The ischemic pattern in the absence of invasive stenosis reliably ensures the diagnosis [6,11,12]. In addition to its diagnostic value, the extent of LGE has been shown to have prognostic significance in MINOCA [13]. According to data from the SPINS registry, a greater extent of ischemic burden in ischaemic cardiomyopathy in general was associated with an increased risk of major cardiac events, including hospitalization for congestive heart failure [14,15]. In addition, the presence of transmural necrosis has been shown to correlate with responses to cardiac resynchronization therapy and the risk of arrhythmias [16–18]. In summary, LGE in ischemic cardiomyopathy is able to confirm the diagnosis, guide therapy, and predict outcome.

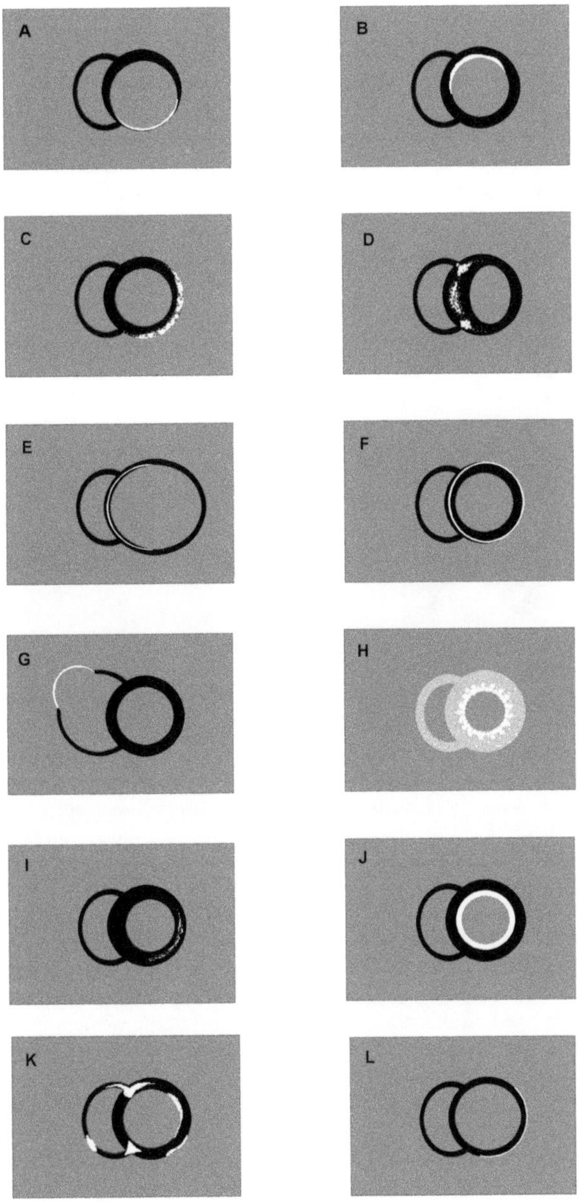

Figure 1. Scheme of typical LGE patterns in short axis view, T1-weighted inversion recovery sequence; black: myocardium without LGE, white: LGE. Please note: the distribution pattern may vary within certain limits and should only be assessed in the context of patient's history and the whole CMR examination. (**A**): Transmural ischemic scar with myocardial thinning as consequence of RCA-Infarction.

(**B**): Non-transmural ischemic scar as consequence of LAD-infarction. (**C**): Myocarditis with subepicardial inferolateral LGE. (**D**): Classical hypertrophic cardiomyopathy with LGE at the RV insertions and in the area of greatest hypertrophy. (**E**): Dilated cardiomyopathy with a fine line of intramural septal LGE. (**F**): Non-dilated cardiomyopathy with ring-like LGE and a septal intramural and lateral epicardial distribution. (**G**): Classical ARVC with right ventricular dilatation and aneurysms with LGE. (**H**): Cardiac amyloidosis with strong LGE originating from the subendocardium in the hypertrophied LV and RV myocardium. (**I**): Anderson–Fabry disease with mild intramural to subepicardial inferolateral LGE and hypertrophy. Note: relatively frequent, unspecific pattern, also possible with increasing pressure load or as post-inflammatory residual. Additional T1 mapping sequences required for differentiation. (**J**): Endomyocardial fibrosis with LGE in the thickened endocardium, here without thrombosis. (**K**): Cardiac sarcoidosis with patchy subendocardial, subepicardial or transmural distribution, anterior "Hook-sign" and inferior "Triangle sign" in place of the RV insertions. (**L**): Cardiac involvement in muscular dystrophy Duchenne with subepicardial lateral LGE in thinned myocardium. Note: also possible in DCM of other origin.

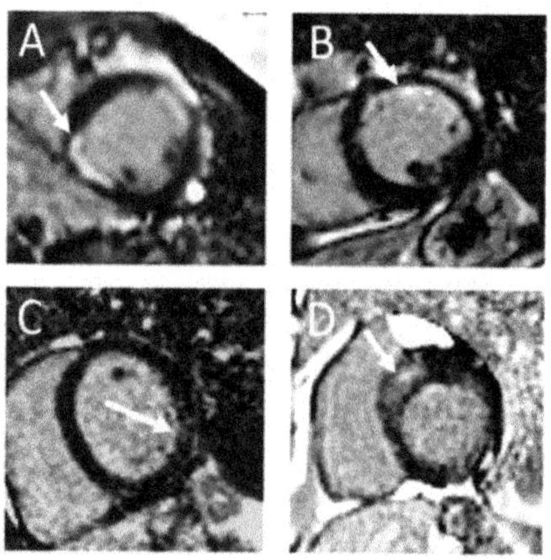

Figure 2. Illustrative examples of LGE in important cardiac diseases: (**A**): Patient with s/p ST-Elevation myocardial infarctions in anterior and inferolateral location with LGE >50% of myocardial wall thickness. (**B**): Patient with s/p non-ST-Elevation myocardial infarction in anterior location with subendocardial LGE < 50% of myocardial wall thickness. (**C**): Patient with viral myocarditis and patchy lateral LGE. (**D**): Patient with hypertrophic cardiomyopathy (HCM) and septal LGE in the area of greatest hypertrophy.

Central foci of low signal or hypoenhancement within the LGE of a myocardial infarction represent areas of microvascular obstruction (MVO) affecting vessels smaller than 200 μm, and are known angiographically as no-reflow zones. Typically, gadolinium penetrates slowly into the damaged capillaries, as evidenced by increasing whitening on very late sequences. This phenomenon is associated with a poor prognosis and serves as a marker for subsequent adverse left ventricular remodeling [19].

2.2. Myocarditis

Patients suspected of having myocarditis exhibit a diverse range of clinical presentations, making the diagnosis, monitoring, and prognosis challenging. While viruses are the primary cause of myocarditis, it can also be induced by factors such as drugs (e.g., checkpoint inhibitors [20]), toxic substances, or autoimmune conditions [21]. CMR diagnostics became particularly important in the time of COVID-19 associated myocarditis [22–24].

The first in 2009 published Lake Louise criteria (LLC) [25] for diagnosing acute myocarditis used specific tissue characteristics in CMR, including LGE imaging. The LCC have been updated recently [26] and now also include novel imaging techniques such as T1 and T2 mapping and ECV calculation. CMR has largely replaced endomyocardial biopsy, the gold standard of diagnosis, and extensive LGE has proven to increase the risk of adverse outcome [27]. In this context, LGE cannot be interpreted alone and especially T2 STIR sequences and T2 mapping are sensitive in detecting acute states of myocarditis by edematous water deposition in the extracellular space. It could even be shown that CMR was able to change the initial suspected diagnosis of acute myocarditis (which was created according to the 2013 European Society of Cardiology position statement criteria for clinically suspected myocarditis [28]) to another diagnosis in almost 20% of cases [29].

Myocarditis often shows a subepicardial patchy pattern of LGE, predominantly in the basal inferolateral wall, although other locations do not exclude this diagnosis (Figures 1C and 2C). In the acute phase of inflammation, the extent of the LGE is greater than in the healed residual and may even disappear completely. This is because acute oedema is also a cause of extracellular space expansion and not just irreversible cell damage. In the case of pronounced myocarditis, a CMR follow-up is recommended after approx. 3–6 months to assess whether the acute reaction has subsided and to evaluate the final extent of the scar burden [30]. The extent of LGE has been shown to be negatively correlated with left ventricular function and could predict improvement in follow-up [31]. In addition, LGE has been shown to be a tool for predicting outcome in myocarditis [31,32].

2.3. Hypertrophic Cardiomyopathy

CMR significantly helps to distinguish the different subtypes of the heterogeneous group of diseases with a hypertrophic phenotype, which previously could only be clarified by biopsy. The classic phenotype of hypertrophic cardiomyopathy (HCM) is an asymmetric, septal hypertrophy with (HOCM) or without obstruction of the outflow tract, caused by an autosomal dominant mutation in the sarcomere genes with a prevalence of about 1:350 [33]. CMR is especially important in the detection of midventricular or apical variants of HCM, in which echocardiographic evaluation has limitations [34]. In addition, CMR can detect myocardial crypts [35] and papillary muscle abnormalities [36], which may be a subclinical marker of HCM, and depict apical aneurysms with and without thrombus formation, which is considered a major risk factor in the American College of Cardiology/American Heart Association (ACC/AHA) [37] and ESC [2] guidelines, leading to recommendations for implantable cardioverter-defibrillator (ICD) implantation.

LGE in HCM signifies replacement fibrosis, and its prognostic significance is well-established. It is detected in over 50% of HCM patients, typically manifesting as a mid-mural pattern within the most hypertrophied segments [38] and on right ventricular insertion points (Figures 1D and 2D). In the advanced stages of the disease, LGE with transmural extension may be observed, carrying a poorer prognosis, because the extent of LGE consistently correlates with an increased incidence of sudden cardiac death [39]. In a pivotal multicenter study, the presence of LGE exceeding 15% of the left ventricular (LV) mass was associated with a more than two-fold risk of SCD in patients initially classified as low risk by conventional tools, compared to patients without LGE [38]. Consequently, the presence of "extensive LGE" ($\geq$15% of total LV mass) is considered a high-risk parameter and it has been incorporated in both guidelines mentioned above. Recent findings indicate that HCM patients exhibiting non-extensive LGE, the involvement of subendocardium, rather than the extent of LGE, is linked to unfavorable outcomes [40]. For HCM patients without a defibrillator, CMR should be repeated every 3–5 years to monitor the progression of LGE and reassess strategies for preventing SCD [37].

2.4. Dilated Cardiomyopathy

Dilated cardiomyopathy (DCM) is the phenotypic description for a group of heart diseases associated with increased enddiastolic volume, reduced ejection fraction and usually increased filling pressures. The causes are very diverse and can be genetic, inflammatory, toxic, autoimmune, metabolic, or associated with neuromuscular diseases or congenital heart defects. The dilated form of ischemic cardiomyopathy should not be referred as DCM. The dilatation itself may reflect the final stage of a previously non-dilated cardiomyopathy, which makes identification using LGE at early stages particularly important. The new entity-term "non-dilated left ventricular cardiomyopathy" is discussed separately below.

LGE in DCM is often located in the mid-wall of the basoseptal segments of the heart but can have a variety of patterns (Figure 1E). The presence of LGE in DCM patients varies from 21% to 70%, and showed an averaged occurrence of 44% in a large meta-analysis [41]. The so called "ring-like" pattern especially is gaining in importance lately [42,43] (Figure 1F), because the distribution allows conclusions about the etiology and therefore leads to risk stratification.

LGE is able to identify fibrosis and the microstructure of fibrosis has been observed to influence electrical reentry [44]. Understanding these pathomechanism can enhance risk stratification and inform decisions regarding treatment. LGE has been related to adverse clinical outcomes in a large number of patients with DCM [41,45–48]. T1 mapping and ECV may have limited value in DCM, attributing this limitation to reduced accuracy caused by myocardial thinning [49].

2.5. Non-Dilated Left Ventricular Cardiomyopathy

The self-titled "major innovation" of the ESC guideline for cardiomyopathies [1] is the implementation of tissue characterization by LGE in CMR. For the new recognized phenotype, the term non-dilated left ventricular cardiomyopathy (NDLVC) is used, "defined as the presence of non-ischaemic LV scarring or fatty replacement regardless of the presence of global or regional wall motion abnormalities, or isolated global LV hypokinesia without scarring" [1].

CMR with LGE is the only way to presume a specific NDLVC, except for genetic testing, which is generally not carried out in previously asymptomatic or less symptomatic individuals. The prognostic significance varies with the underlying etiology. Some specific genotypes are associated with an increased risk of life-threatening arrythmias, e.g., LMNA mutation [50]. The LGE pattern cannot be used to draw absolutely certain conclusions about the underlying mutation, but it can help to guide genetic diagnostics and identify patients at high risk at an early stage. As mentioned above, the ring-like or nearly ring-like pattern gains special importance (Figure 1F): For example, mutations in the gen of filamin C, desmoplakin and phospholamban frequently show a subepicardial, ring-like pattern. Titin, laminin A/C and genotypes of Duchenne muscular dystrophy often show less or even no scar, with a more septal or inferolateral localized pattern and a more severe kinetic dysfunction [1,43]. It becomes clear that the total burden of LGE must be considered in relation to the underlying disease in order to assess the risk.

2.6. Arrhythmogenic Cardiomyopathy

Arrhythmogenic cardiomyopathy (ARVC) is a genetic disorder characterized by replacement of myocardium by fatty and fibrous tissue, frequent right ventricular enlargement, dyskinetic aneurysms and occurrence of ventricular arrhythmias. The International Task Force published the updated diagnostic criteria, called the Padua-criteria in 2020, which take the possible involvement of the left ventricle and the role of CMR more into account [51]. The ESC guidelines do not recommend the recently used term arrhythmogenic cardiomyopathy (ARC), as it lacks a morphological or functional definition [1]. It has to be mentioned that fatty replacement is not specific for ARVC, and diagnosis cannot be made only by CMR. Right ventricular ejection fraction measured by CMR is the only influencing factor in the ARVC calculator (ARVC Risk Calculator) until now.

Depending on the affected area, LGE can present with a patchy distribution pattern, especially in areas of dyskinesis and thinning (Figure 1G). Previously, the so-called "triangle of dysplasia" (RV outflow tract, RV cardiac apex, subtricuspid region of the free RV wall) was assumed to be the predilection site. Today we know from CMR studies that up to 76% of ARVC subjects have left ventricular involvement [52]. The LGE usually affect the inferior and lateral walls of the LV without abnormal wall motion. Although the presence and extent of LGE has been shown to be associated with poor prognosis [52–54], because LGE reflects the arrhythmogenic substrate of ventricular arrhythmia, is not yet fully established as a risk marker.

2.7. Cardiac Amyloidosis

In cardiac amyloidosis (CA) there is an expansion of the intercellular space due to deposition of amyloid fibrils, mainly Transthyretin (ATTR) or immunoglobulin-derived light chains (AL), which lead to pseudo-hypertrophy of the myocardium [55,56]. Hypertrophy often extends to the right ventricle, the atria and the interatrial septum, including thickening of the valves. This leads to a predominant diastolic dysfunction with typical symptoms of venous congestion.

Corresponding to hypertrophy, patients show a very characteristic pattern of LGE, which begins diffuse subendocardial in all affected parts of the heart (Figure 1H). In many patients a typical so-called zebra pattern of LGE distribution can be found with a subendocardial and an epicardial hyperintense line separated by a mid-myocardial hypointense zone. A transmural, strong enhancement occurs in advanced stages, what makes it difficult to null the myocardium in the T1-weighted inversion recovery sequences for LGE and simultaneously utilize this special phenomenon for diagnosis [57]. The extent of LGE correlates with the burden of disease, so LGE is a risk marker of disease progression [58]. Because LGE burden as a visual parameter is difficult to assess in small changes, CMR techniques such as pre-/post-contrast T1-mapping with subsequent ECV calculation, which is based on the extent of Gadolinium uptake, is more sensitive to monitor CA [59,60]. CMR has becoming increasingly important in diagnostics [55]. Risk stratification based on LGE/T1/ECV values is not yet a standardized clinical tool, but it is still used in individual cases to monitor follow-up and decide on therapy in expert centers. Several studies found a strong correlation between mortality and gadolinium uptake [61–63].

2.8. Fabry Disease

Fabry disease is an X-linked lysosomal storage disorder with a hypertrophic phenotype, which arises from the accumulation of glycosphingolipids and the hypertrophy of myocytes [64]. The early stage of the disease typically shows reduced T1 mapping values, which distinguishes Fabry disease from the most other hypertrophic phenotypes. In the course of the disease, increasing fibrosis can lead to a pseudo-normalization of the values.

LGE is often located in the inferolateral segments of the LV basis with a mid-mural to subepicardial deposition [39] (Figure 1I). The LGE can even be there in mutation carriers without the presence of hypertrophy. It is a risk marker for poor response to enzyme replacement therapy with alpha-galactosidase and associated with adverse outcome [64].

2.9. Endomyocardial Fibrosis

Endomyocardial fibrosis (EMF) shows an apical hypertrophy due to thickening of the endocardium by deposition of fibrous tissue. EMF is not sufficiently recognized in western countries, because it is predominant in tropical regions [65]. The causes are divers, e.g., expose to toxic agents or inflammation, such as Löffler endocarditis, the cardiac involvement in hypereosinophilia syndrome. This leads to reduced end-diastolic volume with symptoms of diastolic dysfunction.

CMR with LGE is considered the gold standard for evaluating EMF, particularly for the localization, characterization, and quantification of fibrous tissue. LGE lies in the thickened subendocardial layer, apically emphasized (Figure 1J). An apical thrombus is often present. LGE strongly correlates with histopathological findings, and the extent of LGE is associated with an increased risk of mortality [66].

2.10. Cardiac Sarcoidosis

Sarcoidosis is a special case of inflammation, which has to discussed separately. It is an inflammatory, granuloma-forming disease of unknown origin, which is mainly characterized by involvement of the lungs and mediastinal lymph nodes. Cardiac involvement is found in 10–25% of all sarcoidosis patients and can also occur in isolation in individual cases. Involvement of the left ventricular myocardium and the conduction system is predominant, so that affected patients often present clinically with cardiac arrhythmias and/or heart failure symptoms [67,68]. In addition to clinical, laboratory and nuclear examinations, CMR has a special role.

LGE often shows a typically multifocal, patchy pattern, which can lead to the visual diagnosis of cardiac sarcoidosis (Figure 1K). The LGE cannot be assigned to any coronary area, occurs subendocardially, subepicardially, and also transmurally, and often shows an impressive intensity, which contrasts with an often preserved function. The basal septum or the anteroseptal wall with affection to the RV (sometimes called "hook sign"), the basal inferolateral wall and the inferior RV insertion ("triangle sign") are predicating sites [68]. Cardiac involvement has significant prognostic importance. According to the guidelines, primary prophylactic implantation of an ICD should be considered if there is a pronounced scar on CMR, regardless of the LVEF [69].

2.11. Neuromuscular Diseases with Cardiac Involvement

Neuromuscular diseases present with symptoms affecting the skeletal muscle and show a varying prevalence of cardiac involvement, which significantly affects mortality. Phenotypically, a DCM or NDLVD may be present.

LGE with subepicardial involvement of the LV lateral free wall was found to be the most frequent pattern in muscular dystrophy [70] (Figure 1L). Mitochondriopathies show a completely different pattern, for example in MELAS (Mitochondrial encephalopathy, lactic acidosis, and stroke-like episodes) LGE is focally accentuated and diffusely distributed [71]. The presence of LGE indicates individuals who are at risk of developing progressive left ventricular dysfunction and was also linked to a heightened risk of mortality [72].

2.12. LGE for Further Cardiac Diseases

The presence of LGE has been recognized in several other cardiological conditions. It has been used in some cases for diagnostic and prognostic purposes, but so far it has been of secondary importance or not fully understood. For example, congenital heart disease or acquired valve disorders may develop fibrosis due to abnormal filling pressures or surgical scars. LGE was a powerful predictor of all-cause mortality in patients with aortic stenosis [73], but this does not currently play a major role in the evaluation of patients. Non-compaction cardiomyopathy usually shows no or few LGE but small studies suggest the value of LGE risk stratification in this patients [74], although a lower sensitivity must also be assumed here with thinner myocardium. Takotsubo syndrome usually shows no or rapidly transient LGE. Takotsubo or myocarditis illustrates that in reversible damage of the myocardium, LGE or a part of the full extent of LGE is transient. The prognostic significance of the transient detection of LGE has not yet been sufficiently researched.

3. Discussion

CMR is characterized by its ability to provide precise anatomy and functional evaluation. In addition, it enables early detection and differentiation of various cardiomyopathies through high spatial resolution and tissue characterization capabilities, implemented by differently weighted sequence types and the use of the MRI contrast agent gadolinium. LGE imaging has proven to be a valuable marker for risk stratification in various heart diseases. LGE should not be considered in isolation, as other CMR techniques are of great importance, such as cine-imaging as the gold standard for right and left ventricular ejection fraction assessment, native and post-contrast T1 mapping for quantification of even subclinical tissue alteration, T2-weighted images to assess oedema, or stress perfusion imaging as a CMR-guided selection strategy for revascularization.

The patient evaluation should include the medical history, family history, physical examination, electrocardiographic patterns, and transthoracic echocardiography (TTE) as the gold standard of cardiological imaging prior to CMR. It must be emphasized that a comprehensive medical history including extracardiac symptoms is essential for the correct interpretation of CMR images. TTE is widely available, easy to use and is primarily used for anatomical and functional assessment. In some cases, e.g., evaluation of valve stenosis and assessment of diastolic dysfunction, it is superior to CMR. TTE plays an important role in the initial assessment and in raising diagnostic suspicions, but its utility becomes limited when establishing differential diagnosis, based on tissue characterization.

There are some difficulties in establishing LGE as a risk marker, using HCM as an example: first, observational studies have identified several risk factors for sudden cardiac death in HCM but individually, these factors exhibit a low positive predictive value [2]. Efforts to establish the prognostic significance of LGE for sudden cardiac death in HCM patients have been hampered by similar problems, namely the relatively low event rates [75]. The prevalence of LGE is much higher, than the rate of adverse events. Therefore, relatively small study populations do not have sufficient statistical power. At least a meta-analysis of nearly 3000 patients showed that LGE is associated with a 2,3-fold increased risk of SCD [76], so LGE has been suggested to improve risk stratification [37]. Now it is recommended in the ESC guidelines for patients who are in the low to intermediate risk category (by first using the HCM risk calculator) to improve decision-making about prophylactic ICD-implantation [1,2] (IIa/B [2], IIb/B [1]). Second, several studies observed that maximum wall thickness was significantly higher in patients with LGE compared to those without LGE [77,78]. Consequently, all patients with a wall thickness exceeding 30 mm, an established risk factor for sudden death, were exclusively present in the LGE groups in those studies. So, whether LGE is an epiphenomenon of advanced cardiac remodeling that correlates with existing prognostic markers (e.g., myocardial mass) and is thereby confounded, or whether it has independent prognostic significance, is not yet fully understood. Third, there can be another confounder, namely the technical method of interpretation because LGE quantification dependents on CMR acquisition, type, and amount of contrast. In clinical routine LGE is assessed visually, which clearly depends on subjective judgement and personal experience but is not inferior to quantitative measurement when assessed by an experienced physician. To quantify LGE, the 2-standard deviation technique is the only one validated against histological examination [79]. A generally accepted, standardized method for the quantification of fibrosis in CMR has not yet been established.

Prior problems of CMR have been solved in current times: nephrogenic systemic fibrosis as a rare complication of linear unstable gadolinium chelates of the first generation in patients with severe renal impairment. It is practically not reported with the use of newer, macrocyclic gadolinium contrasts. Modern Gadolinium-based contrast agents can be safely utilized for patients with an estimated glomerular filtration rate $> 30\ mL/min/1.73m^2$. Depending on the urgency and under strict precautions, the use of gadolinium based contrast agent is possible even in patients requiring dialysis [80–82]. In addition, there have been limitations in imaging patients with cardiac implantable electrical devices (CIEDs) due to safety concerns and image artefacts. Today, there are solutions to reduce the artefacts, such as wideband sequences for LGE imaging, so CMR is possible even in patients with a large subcutaneous implantable cardioverter defibrillator [83]. In addition, MR-conditional devices have been available for around 10 years and data on formally non-conditional CIEDs are comprehensive and still growing [84].

The upgrading of the CMR in the guidelines is certainly to be encouraged. However, this also means that non-implementation of a CMR will increasingly have to be regarded as non-compliance with the guideline. In reality, access to CMR in many regions is often limited by cost and reimbursement, as well as by the qualifications of the assessing physicians and the lack of training centers. For this reason, widespread availability and broad application would be desirable to gather individual and scientific experience.

However, again in a large meta-analysis with almost 8000 patients and a heterogenous spectrum of cardiovascular diseases LGE was strongly correlated with various adverse outcomes, including all-cause mortality (HR 2.96, 95% CI: 2.37, 3.70, $p < 0.001$), cardiovascular mortality (HR 3.27, 95% CI: 2.05, 5.22, $p < 0.001$) and ventricular arrhythmia/sudden cardiac death (HR 3.76, 95% CI: 3.14, 4.52, $p < 0.001$) [85]. In addition, LGE was associated with mortality in both, left ventricular ejection fraction under and over 35%, and this in individuals with nonischemic and ischemic cardiomyopathy. In conclusion, CMR has proven as robust marker of adverse outcome in cardiovascular disease of different origin.

4. Limitations

It should be noted that LGE accumulation is not typical for all cardiac diseases. Typically, channelopathies show no conspicuous features in the CMR, including no LGE. CMR has proven as an outstanding screening and therapy monitoring tool for cardiac iron overload, showing characteristically lowered T1 and T2 * values [86], but LGE imaging is not relevant here.

There is limited diagnostic specificity concerning LGE alone: similar distribution patterns can indicate very different diseases (e.g., basal, subepicardial, inferolateral LGE in muscular dystrophy Duchenne or myocarditis). A great deal of experience and the overall medical context are therefore important for the interpretation of the images.

The sensitivity of the method is also limited because it depends on the severity of the disease, i.e., the degree of cell destruction or replacement. So, the absence of visible LGE does not exclude the diagnosis. Multi-parametric CMR, especially the more sensitive T1 mapping, is recommended to overcome this problem. However, this method is not available in all centers due to a lack of software solutions and has not yet been sufficiently validated for all diseases.

5. Conclusions

LGE in CMR has proven as a valuable tool for diagnosis and beyond that as a reliable risk marker of adverse outcome in cardiovascular disease of different origin. Compared to the pre-CMR era, risk acquisition and stratification needs to be rethought nowadays. CMR with LGE should be offered in every initial assessment of cardiomyopathy, as recommended in the guidelines. As a result, early diagnosis, correct risk assessment, and targeted therapy will have an impact on survival rates.

6. Future Directions

Instead of considering CMR as a reserve diagnostic for special cases, it will be necessary to integrate it more into everyday life. Widespread availability and application would be desirable to gain individual and scientific experience.

Author Contributions: Conceptualization, C.M. and S.G.; methodology, C.M.; investigation, C.M.; writing—original draft preparation, C.M.; writing—review and editing, M.E. and S.G.; visualization, C.M.; supervision, S.G.; project administration, S.G. All authors have read and agreed to the published version of the manuscript.

Funding: This research received no external funding.

Institutional Review Board Statement: This review did not require ethical approval.

Informed Consent Statement: Patient consent was obtained in the cited studies where necessary.

Data Availability Statement: Publicly available datasets were analyzed in this study. This data can be found here: https://pubmed.ncbi.nlm.nih.gov/ (accessed on 1 December 2023).

Conflicts of Interest: The authors declare no conflicts of interest.

References

1. Arbelo, E.; Protonotarios, A.; Gimeno, J.R.; Arbustini, E.; Barriales-Villa, R.; Basso, C.; Bezzina, C.R.; Biagini, E.; Blom, N.A.; de Boer, R.A.; et al. 2023 ESC Guidelines for the Management of Cardiomyopathies. *Eur. Heart J.* **2023**, *44*, 3503–3626. [CrossRef] [PubMed]
2. Zeppenfeld, K.; Tfelt-Hansen, J.; de Riva, M.; Winkel, B.G.; Behr, E.R.; Blom, N.A.; Charron, P.; Corrado, D.; Dagres, N.; de Chillou, C.; et al. 2022 ESC Guidelines for the Management of Patients with Ventricular Arrhythmias and the Prevention of Sudden Cardiac Death: Developed by the Task Force for the Management of Patients with Ventricular Arrhythmias and the Prevention of Sudden Cardiac Death of the European Society of Cardiology (ESC) Endorsed by the Association for European Paediatric and Congenital Cardiology (AEPC). *Eur. Heart J.* **2022**, *43*, 3997–4126. [CrossRef] [PubMed]
3. von Knobelsdorff-Brenkenhoff, F.; Schulz-Menger, J. Cardiovascular Magnetic Resonance in the Guidelines of the European Society of Cardiology: A Comprehensive Summary and Update. *J. Cardiovasc. Magn. Reson.* **2023**, *25*, 42. [CrossRef] [PubMed]
4. Del Buono, M.G.; Moroni, F.; Montone, R.A.; Azzalini, L.; Sanna, T.; Abbate, A. Ischemic Cardiomyopathy and Heart Failure After Acute Myocardial Infarction. *Curr. Cardiol. Rep.* **2022**, *24*, 1505–1515. [CrossRef] [PubMed]
5. Cleland, J.G.; McGowan, J. Heart Failure Due to Ischaemic Heart Disease: Epidemiology, Pathophysiology and Progression. *J. Cardiovasc. Pharmacol.* **1999**, *33* (Suppl. S3), S17–S29. [CrossRef] [PubMed]
6. Thygesen, K.; Alpert, J.S.; Jaffe, A.S.; Chaitman, B.R.; Bax, J.J.; Morrow, D.A.; White, H.D. Executive Group on behalf of the Joint European Society of Cardiology (ESC)/American College of Cardiology (ACC)/American Heart Association (AHA)/World Heart Federation (WHF) Task Force for the Universal Definition of Myocardial Infarction Fourth Universal Definition of Myocardial Infarction (2018). *Circulation* **2018**, *138*, e618–e651. [CrossRef] [PubMed]
7. Eichstaedt, H.W.; Felix, R.; Danne, O.; Dougherty, F.C.; Schmutzler, H. Imaging of Acute Myocardial Infarction by Magnetic Resonance Tomography (MRT) Using the Paramagnetic Relaxation Substance Gadolinium-DTPA. *Cardiovasc. Drugs Ther.* **1989**, *3*, 779–788. [CrossRef]
8. Disertori, M.; Rigoni, M.; Pace, N.; Casolo, G.; Masè, M.; Gonzini, L.; Lucci, D.; Nollo, G.; Ravelli, F. Myocardial Fibrosis Assessment by LGE Is a Powerful Predictor of Ventricular Tachyarrhythmias in Ischemic and Nonischemic LV Dysfunction: A Meta-Analysis. *JACC Cardiovasc. Imaging* **2016**, *9*, 1046–1055. [CrossRef]
9. Kim, R.J.; Wu, E.; Rafael, A.; Chen, E.L.; Parker, M.A.; Simonetti, O.; Klocke, F.J.; Bonow, R.O.; Judd, R.M. The Use of Contrast-Enhanced Magnetic Resonance Imaging to Identify Reversible Myocardial Dysfunction. *N. Engl. J. Med.* **2000**, *343*, 1445–1453. [CrossRef]
10. Bergamaschi, L.; Pavon, A.G.; Angeli, F.; Tuttolomondo, D.; Belmonte, M.; Armillotta, M.; Sansonetti, A.; Foà, A.; Paolisso, P.; Baggiano, A.; et al. The Role of Non-Invasive Multimodality Imaging in Chronic Coronary Syndrome: Anatomical and Functional Pathways. *Diagnostics* **2023**, *13*, 2083. [CrossRef]
11. Sykes, R.; Doherty, D.; Mangion, K.; Morrow, A.; Berry, C. What an Interventionalist Needs to Know About MI with Non-Obstructive Coronary Arteries. *Interv. Cardiol.* **2021**, *16*, e10. [CrossRef]
12. Collet, J.-P.; Thiele, H.; Barbato, E.; Barthélémy, O.; Bauersachs, J.; Bhatt, D.L.; Dendale, P.; Dorobantu, M.; Edvardsen, T.; Folliguet, T.; et al. 2020 ESC Guidelines for the Management of Acute Coronary Syndromes in Patients Presenting without Persistent ST-Segment Elevation. *Eur. Heart J.* **2021**, *42*, 1289–1367. [CrossRef] [PubMed]
13. Bergamaschi, L.; Foà, A.; Paolisso, P.; Renzulli, M.; Angeli, F.; Fabrizio, M.; Bartoli, L.; Armillotta, M.; Sansonetti, A.; Amicone, S.; et al. Prognostic Role of Early Cardiac Magnetic Resonance in Myocardial Infarction With Nonobstructive Coronary Arteries. *JACC Cardiovasc. Imaging* **2023**, in press. [CrossRef]
14. Ge, Y.; Antiochos, P.; Steel, K.; Bingham, S.; Abdullah, S.; Chen, Y.-Y.; Mikolich, J.R.; Arai, A.E.; Bandettini, W.P.; Shanbhag, S.M.; et al. Prognostic Value of Stress CMR Perfusion Imaging in Patients With Reduced Left Ventricular Function. *JACC Cardiovasc. Imaging* **2020**, *13*, 2132–2145. [CrossRef] [PubMed]
15. Patel, A.R.; Salerno, M.; Kwong, R.Y.; Singh, A.; Heydari, B.; Kramer, C.M. Stress Cardiac Magnetic Resonance Myocardial Perfusion Imaging: JACC Review Topic of the Week. *J. Am. Coll. Cardiol.* **2021**, *78*, 1655–1668. [CrossRef] [PubMed]
16. Alexandre, J.; Saloux, E.; Dugué, A.E.; Lebon, A.; Lemaitre, A.; Roule, V.; Labombarda, F.; Provost, N.; Gomes, S.; Scanu, P.; et al. Scar Extent Evaluated by Late Gadolinium Enhancement CMR: A Powerful Predictor of Long Term Appropriate ICD Therapy in Patients with Coronary Artery Disease. *J. Cardiovasc. Magn. Reson.* **2013**, *15*, 12. [CrossRef]
17. Scott, P.A.; Rosengarten, J.A.; Murday, D.C.; Peebles, C.R.; Harden, S.P.; Curzen, N.P.; Morgan, J.M. Left Ventricular Scar Burden Specifies the Potential for Ventricular Arrhythmogenesis: An LGE-CMR Study. *J. Cardiovasc. Electrophysiol.* **2013**, *24*, 430–436. [CrossRef]
18. Chalil, S.; Foley, P.W.X.; Muyhaldeen, S.A.; Patel, K.C.R.; Yousef, Z.R.; Smith, R.E.A.; Frenneaux, M.P.; Leyva, F. Late Gadolinium Enhancement-Cardiovascular Magnetic Resonance as a Predictor of Response to Cardiac Resynchronization Therapy in Patients with Ischaemic Cardiomyopathy. *Europace* **2007**, *9*, 1031–1037. [CrossRef] [PubMed]
19. Wu, K.C. CMR of Microvascular Obstruction and Hemorrhage in Myocardial Infarction. *J. Cardiovasc. Magn. Reson.* **2012**, *14*, 68. [CrossRef]
20. Chatzantonis, G.; Evers, G.; Meier, C.; Bietenbeck, M.; Florian, A.; Klingel, K.; Bleckmann, A.; Yilmaz, A. Immune Checkpoint Inhibitor-Associated Myocarditis: A Run of Bad Luck or Rather Deficient-Monitoring Protocol? *JACC Case Rep.* **2020**, *2*, 630–635. [CrossRef]

21. Bietenbeck, M.; Florian, A.; Shomanova, Z.; Klingel, K.; Yilmaz, A. Novel CMR Techniques Enable Detection of Even Mild Autoimmune Myocarditis in a Patient with Systemic Lupus Erythematosus. *Clin. Res. Cardiol.* **2017**, *106*, 560–563. [CrossRef]
22. Meier, C.; Korthals, D.; Bietenbeck, M.; Chamling, B.; Drakos, S.; Vehof, V.; Stalling, P.; Yilmaz, A. Serial Cardiovascular Magnetic Resonance Studies Prior to and After mRNA-Based COVID-19 Booster Vaccination to Assess Booster-Associated Cardiac Effects. *Front. Cardiovasc. Med.* **2022**, *9*, 877183. [CrossRef]
23. Drakos, S.; Chatzantonis, G.; Bietenbeck, M.; Evers, G.; Schulze, A.B.; Mohr, M.; Fonfara, H.; Meier, C.; Yilmaz, A. A Cardiovascular Magnetic Resonance Imaging-Based Pilot Study to Assess Coronary Microvascular Disease in COVID-19 Patients. *Sci. Rep.* **2021**, *11*, 15667. [CrossRef]
24. Chamling, B.; Vehof, V.; Drakos, S.; Weil, M.; Stalling, P.; Vahlhaus, C.; Mueller, P.; Bietenbeck, M.; Reinecke, H.; Meier, C.; et al. Occurrence of Acute Infarct-like Myocarditis Following COVID-19 Vaccination: Just an Accidental Co-Incidence or Rather Vaccination-Associated Autoimmune Myocarditis? *Clin. Res. Cardiol.* **2021**, *110*, 1850–1854. [CrossRef]
25. Friedrich, M.G.; Sechtem, U.; Schulz-Menger, J.; Holmvang, G.; Alakija, P.; Cooper, L.T.; White, J.A.; Abdel-Aty, H.; Gutberlet, M.; Prasad, S.; et al. Cardiovascular Magnetic Resonance in Myocarditis: A JACC White Paper. *J. Am. Coll. Cardiol.* **2009**, *53*, 1475–1487. [CrossRef] [PubMed]
26. Ferreira, V.M.; Schulz-Menger, J.; Holmvang, G.; Kramer, C.M.; Carbone, I.; Sechtem, U.; Kindermann, I.; Gutberlet, M.; Cooper, L.T.; Liu, P.; et al. Cardiovascular Magnetic Resonance in Nonischemic Myocardial Inflammation: Expert Recommendations. *J. Am. Coll. Cardiol.* **2018**, *72*, 3158–3176. [CrossRef] [PubMed]
27. Gräni, C.; Eichhorn, C.; Bière, L.; Murthy, V.L.; Agarwal, V.; Kaneko, K.; Cuddy, S.; Aghayev, A.; Steigner, M.; Blankstein, R.; et al. Prognostic Value of Cardiac Magnetic Resonance Tissue Characterization in Risk Stratifying Patients with Suspected Myocarditis. *J. Am. Coll. Cardiol.* **2017**, *70*, 1964–1976. [CrossRef] [PubMed]
28. Caforio, A.L.P.; Pankuweit, S.; Arbustini, E.; Basso, C.; Gimeno-Blanes, J.; Felix, S.B.; Fu, M.; Heliö, T.; Heymans, S.; Jahns, R.; et al. Current State of Knowledge on Aetiology, Diagnosis, Management, and Therapy of Myocarditis: A Position Statement of the European Society of Cardiology Working Group on Myocardial and Pericardial Diseases. *Eur. Heart J.* **2013**, *34*, 2636–2648. [CrossRef] [PubMed]
29. Biesbroek, P.S.; Hirsch, A.; Zweerink, A.; van de Ven, P.M.; Beek, A.M.; Groenink, M.; Windhausen, F.; Planken, R.N.; van Rossum, A.C.; Nijveldt, R. Additional Diagnostic Value of CMR to the European Society of Cardiology (ESC) Position Statement Criteria in a Large Clinical Population of Patients with Suspected Myocarditis. *Eur. Heart J.-Cardiovasc. Imaging* **2018**, *19*, 1397–1407. [CrossRef] [PubMed]
30. Aquaro, G.D.; Ghebru Habtemicael, Y.; Camastra, G.; Monti, L.; Dellegrottaglie, S.; Moro, C.; Lanzillo, C.; Scatteia, A.; Di Roma, M.; Pontone, G.; et al. Prognostic Value of Repeating Cardiac Magnetic Resonance in Patients with Acute Myocarditis. *J. Am. Coll. Cardiol.* **2019**, *74*, 2439–2448. [CrossRef] [PubMed]
31. Jiang, L.; Zuo, H.; Liu, J.; Wang, J.; Zhang, K.; Zhang, C.; Peng, X.; Liu, Y.; Wang, D.; Li, H.; et al. The Pattern of Late Gadolinium Enhancement by Cardiac MRI in Fulminant Myocarditis and Its Prognostic Implication: A Two-Year Follow-up Study. *Front. Cardiovasc. Med.* **2023**, *10*, 1144469. [CrossRef]
32. Barone-Rochette, G.; Augier, C.; Rodière, M.; Quesada, J.-L.; Foote, A.; Bouvaist, H.; Marlière, S.; Fagret, D.; Baguet, J.P.; Vanzetto, G. Potentially Simple Score of Late Gadolinium Enhancement Cardiac MR in Acute Myocarditis Outcome. *J. Magn. Reson. Imaging* **2014**, *40*, 1347–1354. [CrossRef]
33. Maron, B.J.; Desai, M.Y.; Nishimura, R.A.; Spirito, P.; Rakowski, H.; Towbin, J.A.; Rowin, E.J.; Maron, M.S.; Sherrid, M.V. Diagnosis and Evaluation of Hypertrophic Cardiomyopathy: JACC State-of-the-Art Review. *J. Am. Coll. Cardiol.* **2022**, *79*, 372–389. [CrossRef] [PubMed]
34. Nagueh, S.F.; Phelan, D.; Abraham, T.; Armour, A.; Desai, M.Y.; Dragulescu, A.; Gilliland, Y.; Lester, S.J.; Maldonado, Y.; Mohiddin, S.; et al. Recommendations for Multimodality Cardiovascular Imaging of Patients with Hypertrophic Cardiomyopathy: An Update from the American Society of Echocardiography, in Collaboration with the American Society of Nuclear Cardiology, the Society for Cardiovascular Magnetic Resonance, and the Society of Cardiovascular Computed Tomography. *J. Am. Soc. Echocardiogr.* **2022**, *35*, 533–569. [CrossRef] [PubMed]
35. Maron, M.S.; Rowin, E.J.; Lin, D.; Appelbaum, E.; Chan, R.H.; Gibson, C.M.; Lesser, J.R.; Lindberg, J.; Haas, T.S.; Udelson, J.E.; et al. Prevalence and Clinical Profile of Myocardial Crypts in Hypertrophic Cardiomyopathy. *Circ. Cardiovasc. Imaging* **2012**, *5*, 441–447. [CrossRef] [PubMed]
36. Tao, J.; Duan, F.; Long, J.; Meng, Q.; Zhang, B.; Zhu, Z.; Wang, H. The Role of the Submitral Apparatus in Hypertrophic Obstructive Cardiomyopathy. *J. Am. Soc. Echocardiogr.* **2023**, *36*, 133–145. [CrossRef] [PubMed]
37. Writing Committee Members; Ommen, S.R.; Mital, S.; Burke, M.A.; Day, S.M.; Deswal, A.; Elliott, P.; Evanovich, L.L.; Hung, J.; Joglar, J.A.; et al. 2020 AHA/ACC Guideline for the Diagnosis and Treatment of Patients with Hypertrophic Cardiomyopathy: A Report of the American College of Cardiology/American Heart Association Joint Committee on Clinical Practice Guidelines. *J. Thorac. Cardiovasc. Surg.* **2021**, *162*, e23–e106. [CrossRef] [PubMed]
38. Chan, R.H.; Maron, B.J.; Olivotto, I.; Pencina, M.J.; Assenza, G.E.; Haas, T.; Lesser, J.R.; Gruner, C.; Crean, A.M.; Rakowski, H.; et al. Prognostic Value of Quantitative Contrast-Enhanced Cardiovascular Magnetic Resonance for the Evaluation of Sudden Death Risk in Patients with Hypertrophic Cardiomyopathy. *Circulation* **2014**, *130*, 484–495. [CrossRef]
39. Casas, G.; Rodríguez-Palomares, J.F. Multimodality Cardiac Imaging in Cardiomyopathies: From Diagnosis to Prognosis. *J. Clin. Med.* **2022**, *11*, 578. [CrossRef]

40. Yang, S.; Zhao, K.; Yang, K.; Song, J.; Yu, S.; Wang, J.; Dong, Z.; Ma, X.; Yin, G.; Li, J.; et al. Subendocardial Involvement as an Underrecognized LGE Subtype Related to Adverse Outcomes in Hypertrophic Cardiomyopathy. *JACC Cardiovasc. Imaging* **2023**, *16*, 1163–1177. [CrossRef]
41. Di Marco, A.; Anguera, I.; Schmitt, M.; Klem, I.; Neilan, T.G.; White, J.A.; Sramko, M.; Masci, P.G.; Barison, A.; Mckenna, P.; et al. Late Gadolinium Enhancement and the Risk for Ventricular Arrhythmias or Sudden Death in Dilated Cardiomyopathy: Systematic Review and Meta-Analysis. *JACC Heart Fail.* **2017**, *5*, 28–38. [CrossRef]
42. Chen, W.; Qian, W.; Zhang, X.; Li, D.; Qian, Z.; Xu, H.; Liao, S.; Chen, X.; Wang, Y.; Hou, X.; et al. Ring-like Late Gadolinium Enhancement for Predicting Ventricular Tachyarrhythmias in Non-Ischaemic Dilated Cardiomyopathy. *Eur. Heart J. Cardiovasc. Imaging* **2021**, *22*, 1130–1138. [CrossRef] [PubMed]
43. Bietenbeck, M.; Meier, C.; Korthals, D.; Theofanidou, M.; Stalling, P.; Dittmann, S.; Schulze-Bahr, E.; Eckardt, L.; Yilmaz, A. Possible Causes and Clinical Relevance of a "Ring-Like" Late Gadolinium Enhancement Pattern. *JACC Cardiovasc. Imaging* **2023**, *17*, 104–106. [CrossRef] [PubMed]
44. Balaban, G.; Halliday, B.P.; Mendonca Costa, C.; Bai, W.; Porter, B.; Rinaldi, C.A.; Plank, G.; Rueckert, D.; Prasad, S.K.; Bishop, M.J. Fibrosis Microstructure Modulates Reentry in Non-Ischemic Dilated Cardiomyopathy: Insights from Imaged Guided 2D Computational Modeling. *Front. Physiol.* **2018**, *9*, 1832. [CrossRef] [PubMed]
45. Assomull, R.G.; Prasad, S.K.; Lyne, J.; Smith, G.; Burman, E.D.; Khan, M.; Sheppard, M.N.; Poole-Wilson, P.A.; Pennell, D.J. Cardiovascular Magnetic Resonance, Fibrosis, and Prognosis in Dilated Cardiomyopathy. *J. Am. Coll. Cardiol.* **2006**, *48*, 1977–1985. [CrossRef] [PubMed]
46. Gulati, A.; Jabbour, A.; Ismail, T.F.; Guha, K.; Khwaja, J.; Raza, S.; Morarji, K.; Brown, T.D.H.; Ismail, N.A.; Dweck, M.R.; et al. Association of Fibrosis with Mortality and Sudden Cardiac Death in Patients with Nonischemic Dilated Cardiomyopathy. *JAMA* **2013**, *309*, 896–908. [CrossRef] [PubMed]
47. Anagnostopoulos, I.; Kousta, M.; Kossyvakis, C.; Lakka, E.; Paraskevaidis, N.T.; Schizas, N.; Alexopoulos, N.; Deftereos, S.; Giannopoulos, G. The Prognostic Role of Late Gadolinium Enhancement on Cardiac Magnetic Resonance in Patients with Nonischemic Cardiomyopathy and Reduced Ejection Fraction, Implanted with Cardioverter Defibrillators for Primary Prevention. A Systematic Review and Meta-Analysis. *J. Interv. Card. Electrophysiol.* **2022**, *63*, 523–530. [CrossRef] [PubMed]
48. Dang, Y.; Hou, Y. The Prognostic Value of Late Gadolinium Enhancement in Heart Diseases: An Umbrella Review of Meta-Analyses of Observational Studies. *Eur. Radiol.* **2021**, *31*, 4528–4537. [CrossRef] [PubMed]
49. Halliday, B.P. State of the Art: Multimodality Imaging in Dilated Cardiomyopathy. *Heart* **2022**, *108*, 1910–1917. [CrossRef]
50. Schulze-Bahr, E.; Klaassen, S.; Gerull, B.; Von Kodolitsch, Y.; Landmesser, U.; Rieß, O.; Meder, B.; Schunkert, H. Gendiagnostik bei kardiovaskulären Erkrankungen: Konsensuspapier der Deutschen Gesellschaft für Kardiologie (DGK), der Gesellschaft für Humangenetik (GfH) und der Deutschen Gesellschaft für Pädiatrische Kardiologie (DGPK). *Kardiologie* **2023**, *17*, 300–349. [CrossRef]
51. Corrado, D.; Perazzolo Marra, M.; Zorzi, A.; Beffagna, G.; Cipriani, A.; Lazzari, M.D.; Migliore, F.; Pilichou, K.; Rampazzo, A.; Rigato, I.; et al. Diagnosis of Arrhythmogenic Cardiomyopathy: The Padua Criteria. *Int. J. Cardiol.* **2020**, *319*, 106–114. [CrossRef]
52. Liu, Y.; Yu, J.; Liu, J.; Wu, B.; Cui, Q.; Shen, W.; Xia, S. Prognostic Value of Late Gadolinium Enhancement in Arrhythmogenic Right Ventricular Cardiomyopathy: A Meta-Analysis. *Clin. Radiol.* **2021**, *76*, 628.e9–628.e15. [CrossRef]
53. Tandri, H.; Saranathan, M.; Rodriguez, E.R.; Martinez, C.; Bomma, C.; Nasir, K.; Rosen, B.; Lima, J.A.C.; Calkins, H.; Bluemke, D.A. Noninvasive Detection of Myocardial Fibrosis in Arrhythmogenic Right Ventricular Cardiomyopathy Using Delayed-Enhancement Magnetic Resonance Imaging. *J. Am. Coll. Cardiol.* **2005**, *45*, 98–103. [CrossRef] [PubMed]
54. Zhang, N.; Song, Y.; Hua, W.; Hu, Y.; Chen, L.; Cai, M.; Niu, H.; Cai, C.; Gu, M.; Zhao, S.; et al. Left Ventricular Involvement Assessed by LGE-CMR in Predicting the Risk of Adverse Outcomes of Arrhythmogenic Cardiomyopathy with ICDs. *Int. J. Cardiol.* **2021**, *337*, 79–85. [CrossRef] [PubMed]
55. Yilmaz, A.; Bauersachs, J.; Bengel, F.; Büchel, R.; Kindermann, I.; Klingel, K.; Knebel, F.; Meder, B.; Morbach, C.; Nagel, E.; et al. Diagnosis and Treatment of Cardiac Amyloidosis: Position Statement of the German Cardiac Society (DGK). *Clin. Res. Cardiol.* **2021**, *110*, 479–506. [CrossRef]
56. Meier, C.; Yilmaz, A. Diagnostics of cardiac amyloidosis. *Inn. Med.* **2023**, *64*, 830–841. [CrossRef]
57. Garcia-Pavia, P.; Rapezzi, C.; Adler, Y.; Arad, M.; Basso, C.; Brucato, A.; Burazor, I.; Caforio, A.L.P.; Damy, T.; Eriksson, U.; et al. Diagnosis and Treatment of Cardiac Amyloidosis: A Position Statement of the ESC Working Group on Myocardial and Pericardial Diseases. *Eur. Heart J.* **2021**, *42*, 1554–1568. [CrossRef]
58. Chamling, B.; Bietenbeck, M.; Korthals, D.; Drakos, S.; Vehof, V.; Stalling, P.; Meier, C.; Yilmaz, A. Therapeutic Value of Tafamidis in Patients with Wild-Type Transthyretin Amyloidosis (ATTRwt) with Cardiomyopathy Based on Cardiovascular Magnetic Resonance (CMR) Imaging. *Clin. Res. Cardiol.* **2022**, *112*, 353–362. [CrossRef] [PubMed]
59. Korthals, D.; Chatzantonis, G.; Bietenbeck, M.; Meier, C.; Stalling, P.; Yilmaz, A. CMR-Based T1-Mapping Offers Superior Diagnostic Value Compared to Longitudinal Strain-Based Assessment of Relative Apical Sparing in Cardiac Amyloidosis. *Sci. Rep.* **2021**, *11*, 15521. [CrossRef]
60. Chatzantonis, G.; Bietenbeck, M.; Elsanhoury, A.; Tschöpe, C.; Pieske, B.; Tauscher, G.; Vietheer, J.; Shomanova, Z.; Mahrholdt, H.; Rolf, A.; et al. Diagnostic Value of Cardiovascular Magnetic Resonance in Comparison to Endomyocardial Biopsy in Cardiac Amyloidosis: A Multi-Centre Study. *Clin. Res. Cardiol.* **2021**, *110*, 555–568. [CrossRef]

61. Mekinian, A.; Lions, C.; Leleu, X.; Duhamel, A.; Lamblin, N.; Coiteux, V.; De Groote, P.; Hatron, P.-Y.; Facon, T.; Beregi, J.-P.; et al. Prognosis Assessment of Cardiac Involvement in Systemic AL Amyloidosis by Magnetic Resonance Imaging. *Am. J. Med.* **2010**, *123*, 864–868. [CrossRef] [PubMed]
62. Fontana, M.; Pica, S.; Reant, P.; Abdel-Gadir, A.; Treibel, T.A.; Banypersad, S.M.; Maestrini, V.; Barcella, W.; Rosmini, S.; Bulluck, H.; et al. Prognostic Value of Late Gadolinium Enhancement Cardiovascular Magnetic Resonance in Cardiac Amyloidosis. *Circulation* **2015**, *132*, 1570–1579. [CrossRef] [PubMed]
63. Austin, B.A.; Tang, W.H.W.; Rodriguez, E.R.; Tan, C.; Flamm, S.D.; Taylor, D.O.; Starling, R.C.; Desai, M.Y. Delayed Hyper-Enhancement Magnetic Resonance Imaging Provides Incremental Diagnostic and Prognostic Utility in Suspected Cardiac Amyloidosis. *JACC Cardiovasc. Imaging* **2009**, *2*, 1369–1377. [CrossRef] [PubMed]
64. Pieroni, M.; Moon, J.C.; Arbustini, E.; Barriales-Villa, R.; Camporeale, A.; Vujkovac, A.C.; Elliott, P.M.; Hagege, A.; Kuusisto, J.; Linhart, A.; et al. Cardiac Involvement in Fabry Disease: JACC Review Topic of the Week. *J. Am. Coll. Cardiol.* **2021**, *77*, 922–936. [CrossRef] [PubMed]
65. Duraes, A.R.; de Souza Lima Bitar, Y.; Roever, L.; Neto, M.G. Endomyocardial Fibrosis: Past, Present, and Future. *Heart Fail. Rev.* **2020**, *25*, 725–730. [CrossRef] [PubMed]
66. Salemi, V.M.C.; Rochitte, C.E.; Shiozaki, A.A.; Andrade, J.M.; Parga, J.R.; de Ávila, L.F.; Benvenuti, L.A.; Cestari, I.N.; Picard, M.H.; Kim, R.J.; et al. Late Gadolinium Enhancement Magnetic Resonance Imaging in the Diagnosis and Prognosis of Endomyocardial Fibrosis Patients. *Circ. Cardiovasc. Imaging* **2011**, *4*, 304–311. [CrossRef]
67. Chatzantonis, G.; Meier, C.; Yilmaz, A. Diagnostik und Therapie der kardialen Sarkoidose. *Kardiol. Up2date* **2020**, *16*, 111–126. [CrossRef]
68. Yilmaz, A.; Meier, C. Kardiale Beteiligung bei Sarkoidose. In *Klinische Kardiologie: Krankheiten des Herzens, des Kreislaufs und der Herznahen Gefäße*; Marx, N., Erdmann, E., Eds.; Springer Reference Medizin; Springer: Berlin/Heidelberg, Germany, 2022; pp. 1–14. ISBN 978-3-662-62939-0.
69. Al-Khatib, S.M.; Stevenson, W.G.; Ackerman, M.J.; Bryant, W.J.; Callans, D.J.; Curtis, A.B.; Deal, B.J.; Dickfeld, T.; Field, M.E.; Fonarow, G.C.; et al. 2017 AHA/ACC/HRS Guideline for Management of Patients With Ventricular Arrhythmias and the Prevention of Sudden Cardiac Death: A Report of the American College of Cardiology/American Heart Association Task Force on Clinical Practice Guidelines and the Heart Rhythm Society. *Circulation* **2018**, *138*, e272–e391. [CrossRef]
70. Florian, A.; Rösch, S.; Bietenbeck, M.; Engelen, M.; Stypmann, J.; Waltenberger, J.; Sechtem, U.; Yilmaz, A. Cardiac Involvement in Female Duchenne and Becker Muscular Dystrophy Carriers in Comparison to Their First-Degree Male Relatives: A Comparative Cardiovascular Magnetic Resonance Study. *Eur. Heart J. Cardiovasc. Imaging* **2016**, *17*, 326–333. [CrossRef]
71. Florian, A.; Ludwig, A.; Stubbe-Dräger, B.; Boentert, M.; Young, P.; Waltenberger, J.; Rösch, S.; Sechtem, U.; Yilmaz, A. Characteristic Cardiac Phenotypes Are Detected by Cardiovascular Magnetic Resonance in Patients with Different Clinical Phenotypes and Genotypes of Mitochondrial Myopathy. *J. Cardiovasc. Magn. Reson.* **2015**, *17*, 40. [CrossRef]
72. Tandon, A.; Villa, C.R.; Hor, K.N.; Jefferies, J.L.; Gao, Z.; Towbin, J.A.; Wong, B.L.; Mazur, W.; Fleck, R.J.; Sticka, J.J.; et al. Myocardial Fibrosis Burden Predicts Left Ventricular Ejection Fraction and Is Associated with Age and Steroid Treatment Duration in Duchenne Muscular Dystrophy. *J. Am. Heart Assoc.* **2015**, *4*, e001338. [CrossRef]
73. Papanastasiou, C.A.; Kokkinidis, D.G.; Kampaktsis, P.N.; Bikakis, I.; Cunha, D.K.; Oikonomou, E.K.; Greenwood, J.P.; Garcia, M.J.; Karamitsos, T.D. The Prognostic Role of Late Gadolinium Enhancement in Aortic Stenosis: A Systematic Review and Meta-Analysis. *JACC Cardiovasc. Imaging* **2020**, *13*, 385–392. [CrossRef]
74. Huang, W.; Sun, R.; Liu, W.; Xu, R.; Zhou, Z.; Bai, W.; Hou, R.; Xu, H.; Guo, Y.; Yu, L.; et al. Prognostic Value of Late Gadolinium Enhancement in Left Ventricular Noncompaction: A Multicenter Study. *Diagnostics* **2022**, *12*, 2457. [CrossRef] [PubMed]
75. Rubinshtein, R.; Glockner, J.F.; Ommen, S.R.; Araoz, P.A.; Ackerman, M.J.; Sorajja, P.; Bos, J.M.; Tajik, A.J.; Valeti, U.S.; Nishimura, R.A.; et al. Characteristics and Clinical Significance of Late Gadolinium Enhancement by Contrast-Enhanced Magnetic Resonance Imaging in Patients with Hypertrophic Cardiomyopathy. *Circ. Heart Fail.* **2010**, *3*, 51–58. [CrossRef] [PubMed]
76. Kamp, N.J.; Chery, G.; Kosinski, A.S.; Desai, M.Y.; Wazni, O.; Schmidler, G.S.; Patel, M.; Lopes, R.D.; Morin, D.P.; Al-Khatib, S.M. Risk Stratification Using Late Gadolinium Enhancement on Cardiac Magnetic Resonance Imaging in Patients with Hypertrophic Cardiomyopathy: A Systematic Review and Meta-Analysis. *Prog. Cardiovasc. Dis.* **2021**, *66*, 10–16. [CrossRef] [PubMed]
77. O'Hanlon, R.; Grasso, A.; Roughton, M.; Moon, J.C.; Clark, S.; Wage, R.; Webb, J.; Kulkarni, M.; Dawson, D.; Sulaibeekh, L.; et al. Prognostic Significance of Myocardial Fibrosis in Hypertrophic Cardiomyopathy. *J. Am. Coll. Cardiol.* **2010**, *56*, 867–874. [CrossRef]
78. Bruder, O.; Wagner, A.; Jensen, C.J.; Schneider, S.; Ong, P.; Kispert, E.-M.; Nassenstein, K.; Schlosser, T.; Sabin, G.V.; Sechtem, U.; et al. Myocardial Scar Visualized by Cardiovascular Magnetic Resonance Imaging Predicts Major Adverse Events in Patients with Hypertrophic Cardiomyopathy. *J. Am. Coll. Cardiol.* **2010**, *56*, 875–887. [CrossRef]
79. Moon, J.C.C.; Reed, E.; Sheppard, M.N.; Elkington, A.G.; Ho, S.Y.; Burke, M.; Petrou, M.; Pennell, D.J. The Histologic Basis of Late Gadolinium Enhancement Cardiovascular Magnetic Resonance in Hypertrophic Cardiomyopathy. *J. Am. Coll. Cardiol.* **2004**, *43*, 2260–2264. [CrossRef]
80. Weinreb, J.C.; Rodby, R.A.; Yee, J.; Wang, C.L.; Fine, D.; McDonald, R.J.; Perazella, M.A.; Dillman, J.R.; Davenport, M.S. Use of Intravenous Gadolinium-Based Contrast Media in Patients with Kidney Disease: Consensus Statements from the American College of Radiology and the National Kidney Foundation. *Radiology* **2021**, *298*, 28–35. [CrossRef]

81. Woolen, S.A.; Shankar, P.R.; Gagnier, J.J.; MacEachern, M.P.; Singer, L.; Davenport, M.S. Risk of Nephrogenic Systemic Fibrosis in Patients with Stage 4 or 5 Chronic Kidney Disease Receiving a Group II Gadolinium-Based Contrast Agent: A Systematic Review and Meta-Analysis. *JAMA Intern. Med.* **2020**, *180*, 223–230. [CrossRef]
82. Uhlig, J.; Lücke, C.; Vliegenthart, R.; Loewe, C.; Grothoff, M.; Schuster, A.; Lurz, P.; Jacquier, A.; Francone, M.; Zapf, A.; et al. Acute Adverse Events in Cardiac MR Imaging with Gadolinium-Based Contrast Agents: Results from the European Society of Cardiovascular Radiology (ESCR) MRCT Registry in 72,839 Patients. *Eur. Radiol.* **2019**, *29*, 3686–3695. [CrossRef]
83. Holtstiege, V.; Meier, C.; Bietenbeck, M.; Chatzantonis, G.; Florian, A.; Köbe, J.; Reinke, F.; Eckardt, L.; Yilamz, A. Clinical Experience Regarding Safety and Diagnostic Value of Cardiovascular Magnetic Resonance in Patients with a Subcutaneous Implantable Cardioverter/Defibrillator (S-ICD) at 1.5 T. *JCMR J. Cardiovasc. Magn. Reson.* **2020**, *22*, 35. [CrossRef]
84. Munawar, D.A.; Chan, J.E.Z.; Emami, M.; Kadhim, K.; Khokhar, K.; O'Shea, C.; Iwai, S.; Pitman, B.; Linz, D.; Munawar, M.; et al. Magnetic Resonance Imaging in Non-Conditional Pacemakers and Implantable Cardioverter-Defibrillators: A Systematic Review and Meta-Analysis. *Europace* **2020**, *22*, 288–298. [CrossRef] [PubMed]
85. Ganesan, A.N.; Gunton, J.; Nucifora, G.; McGavigan, A.D.; Selvanayagam, J.B. Impact of Late Gadolinium Enhancement on Mortality, Sudden Death and Major Adverse Cardiovascular Events in Ischemic and Nonischemic Cardiomyopathy: A Systematic Review and Meta-Analysis. *Int. J. Cardiol.* **2018**, *254*, 230–237. [CrossRef] [PubMed]
86. Cadour, F.; Ernst, O.; Dacher, J.-N. Can Cardiac Magnetic Resonance Imaging Be Used as a Screening Tool for Iron Overload? *Diagn. Interv. Imaging* **2023**, *104*, 519–520. [CrossRef] [PubMed]

Journal of
Cardiovascular Development and Disease

MDPI

Systematic Review

The Relationship between Subclinical Hypothyroidism and Carotid Intima-Media Thickness as a Potential Marker of Cardiovascular Risk: A Systematic Review and a Meta-Analysis

Oana-Maria Isailă [1,*], Victor Eduard Stoian [2,*], Iuliu Fulga [3], Alin-Ionut Piraianu [3] and Sorin Hostiuc [1]

1 Department of Legal Medicine and Bioethics, Faculty of Dentistry, "Carol Davila" University of Medicine and Pharmacy, 020021 Bucharest, Romania; sorin.hostiuc@umfcd.ro
2 Department of Legal Medicine, Legal Medicine Service Dâmbovița, 130083 Târgoviște, Romania
3 Department of Legal Medicine, Dunărea de Jos University, 800201 Galați, Romania
* Correspondence: oana-maria.isaila@umfcd.ro (O.-M.I.); victoreduard14@gmail.com (V.E.S.)

Abstract: Background and Objectives: Thyroid dysfunction is known to have significant consequences on the cardiovascular system. The correlation between carotid intima-media thickness (CIMT) and subclinical hypothyroidism (SCH) has been frequently evaluated in clinical studies in recent years. This study aimed to evaluate the significance of this association through a meta-analysis. Methods: We conducted a systematic search of PubMed, MedLine, Scopus, and Web of Science databases using the keywords 'subclinical hypothyroidism and carotid intima-media thickness', from the beginning of each database until January 2023. We established the inclusion and exclusion criteria and considered studies that met the inclusion criteria. We used Jamovi for statistical analysis of the data. Results: We identified 39 observational studies that met the inclusion criteria, with 3430 subjects: 1545 SCH and 1885 EU. Compared to euthyroid subjects (EU), subjects with subclinical hypothyroidism (SCH) had significantly increased carotid intima-media thickness (CIMT) values; the estimated average mean difference was 0.08 (95% CI 0.05 to 0.10), $p < 0.01$, $I^2 = 93.82\%$. After the sensitivity analysis, a total of 19 from the 39 abovementioned studies were analyzed, with most studies showing a positive association between SCH and thickening of the carotid wall; the estimated average mean difference was 0.04 (95% CI 0.02 to 0.07), $p = 0.03$, $I^2 = 77.7$. In addition, female sex, advanced age, and high cholesterol levels statistically significantly influenced this association. Conclusions: Our meta-analysis indicates a significant positive association between SCH and increased CIMT, but with some limitations.

Keywords: carotid intima-media thickness; subclinical hypothyroidism; cardiovascular risk; screening

1. Introduction

Subclinical hypothyroidism (SCH) is characterized by elevated serum thyroid-stimulating hormone (TSH) levels (above normal) and normal FT4 levels [1]. In most cases, this biohumoral alteration is insidious and is usually discovered incidentally, leading to a high variability of the reported prevalence, from 5.6% to 20.42%, depending on the population being subjected to analysis [2–5].

Carotid intima-media thickness (CIMT) is a measure of the thickness of the innermost layers of the carotid artery walls. It is used to determine the early stages of subclinical atherosclerosis, a condition in which the arteries become narrowed and hardened due to the buildup of plaque. CIMT is measured using ultrasound technology to analyze the thickness of the intima and the mean wall of the carotid artery. The relationship between CIMT and cardiovascular disease has been established, indicating the importance of this analysis. The factors responsible for atherosclerosis can lead to an increase in CIMT through hypertrophy of the intimal or medial carotid layers [6]. The use of CIMT in medical practice provides a noninvasive, reproducible, and cost-effective analysis with minimal risk to patients [7].

Multiple studies have shown an association between SCH and atherosclerotic cardiovascular disease. One of the early studies in this area was conducted by Hak et al. in the Rotterdam study to show a connection between subclinical hypothyroidism, aortic atherosclerosis, and myocardial pathology in elderly women with an autoimmune thyroid component. In addition, the study found that thyroid autoimmunity itself was not linked to carotid atherosclerosis or myocardial infarction [8]. In the Whickham survey, during 20 years of follow-up, a positive association was revealed between mortality following myocardial ischemic pathology and subclinical hypothyroidism [9].

Based on these findings, numerous recent studies have analyzed the association between SCH and increased CIMT as a cardiovascular risk factor, and the results have sometimes been discordant. The underlying mechanism of the positive association between subclinical hypothyroidism and vascular atheromatosis consists of a predisposition to endothelial dysfunction caused by TSH level by decreasing the endothelial response to vascular stimuli [10]; increasing inflammation and oxidative stress [11]; and through total cholesterol, triglycerides, and LDL cholesterol [12,13].

The purpose of this meta-analysis was to perform an updated analysis of the correlation between SCH and CIMT as a cardiovascular risk marker: an easy, noninvasive, and accessible marker that could constitute a good screening method for the prevention of cardiovascular pathology.

2. Materials and Methods

We undertook a study in adherence with the PRISMA guidelines for reporting systematic literature reviews and meta-analyses of observational studies [14].

2.1. Search Method

We conducted a systematized search in the PubMed, MedLine, Scopus, and Web of Science databases using the following keywords: "subclinical hypothyroidism and carotid intima-media thickness", from the beginning of each database until January 2023. The baseline list of each study was reviewed for inclusion in the meta-analysis. We imported the references and summaries into the Mendeley Desktop software v1.19.8.

2.2. Selection Criteria

Inclusion criteria: Studies meeting the following inclusion criteria were included: (1) studies that analyzed the association between subclinical hypothyroidism and CIMT or from which this association could be investigated; (2) case-control studies; (3) persons in the control group had normal thyroid function with TSH values within the normal reference range; (4) CIMT value reported both for persons in the study group, with subclinical hypothyroidism, and for persons in the control group, with thyroid function in the normal reference range; (5) studies that also reported T4 value; (6) studies that reported 95% confidence interval.

In the case of studies analyzing the effectiveness of levothyroxine therapy, we used only the data presented for the subjects before initiating this treatment.

The following were excluded: (1) studies that did not provide any relevant information to obtain the necessary data; (2) series of cases/case presentations; (3) studies that analyzed persons with overt hypothyroidism or hyperthyroidism; (4) studies involving persons already undergoing treatment, reporting only drug therapy values; (5) non-control studies, animal studies, reviews; (6) studies that did not provide the mean value, standard deviation, or median parameters of interest.

2.3. Data Collection and Analysis

For each study, we conducted database research, extracted the data, and included it in Excel datasheets. The following information was obtained: author names, year, geographic region, TSH cut-off value, number of subjects, mean age, sex, BMI, TSH, CIMT, and lipidic profile.

In the case of studies that showed the mean value of the left CIMT and the mean value of the right CIMT separately, we calculated the common mean value by applying the formula for combined groups:

$$\text{mean of total group} = (n1 \times X1 + n2 \times X2)/(n1 + n2)$$

$$\text{variance of total group} = n1 \times (S1^2 + d1^2) + n2 \times (S2^2 + d2^2)/(n1 + n2)$$

where n1 = No. of observations in 'region 1', n2 = No. of observations in 'region 2', X1 = mean of region 1, X2 = mean of region 2, $S1^2$ = variance of region 1, $S2^2$ = variance of region 2 [15].

For studies reporting the median, we calculated the mean value based on the estimation method proposed by Luo et al. [16] and the standard deviation using the method proposed by Wan et al. [17,18].

For the studies that did not calculate the body mass index (BMI) using the classic method, the reported BMI value was not taken into account, being discordant with those from the rest of the included studies.

2.4. Quality Assessment

The methodological quality of each study was assessed according to the Newcastle–Ottawa scale (NOS) [19]. The scoring system consisted of three sections (case selection, comparability, and exposure) and the assessment included scores from 0 to 8 (Table 1). The closer the NOS score was to 8, the more methodologically qualitative the study was.

Table 1. Studies included in meta-analysis.

Author	Year	Country	TSH Cut off Value (mUI/mL)	Participants (SCH/EU)	Age (SCH/EU)	NOS
Monzani [20]	2004	Italy	>3.6	45/32	37 ± 1/35 ± 1	8
Cikim [21]	2004	Turkey	>4.20	25/23	32.2 ±9.6/35.8 ± 7.9	7
Duman [22]	2007	Turkey	>4.2	40/20	37 ± 12.6/36.7 ± 12.2	7
de Almeida [23]	2007	Brazil	>4	30/27	43 ± 9.7/43.1 ± 8.3	8
Kim [24]	2009	Korea	>5.5	36/32	36 ± 6.2/36.1 ± 5.4	7
Kebapcilar [25]	2010	Turkey	>5	38/19	49.7 ± 10/49.9 ± 8.1	8
Velkoska [26]	2011	Macedonia	>4.2	67/30	42.4 ± 16.2/43.6 ± 12.8	7
Gunduz [27]	2012	Turkey	>4	16/20	40.8 ± 11.8/32.8 ± 5.7	7
Asik [28]	2013	Turkey	>5.49	33/32	38.1 ± 15/39.4 ± 9.7	8
Knapp [29]	2013	Poland	–	40/15	34.8 ± 4.1/31.6 ± 9.3	4
Varim [30]	2013	Turkey	>4.5	50/50	29.5 ± 8.9/29.8 ± 7.6	7
Kilic [31]	2013	Turkey	>4.2	32/29	41.5 ± 12/38.1 ± 11.4	5
Unsal [32]	2014	Turkey	>4.2	56/46	41.3 ± 14.4/36 ± 10.5	7
Akkoca [33]	2014	Turkey	>4.2	20/20	34.4 ± 1.4/35.2 ± 2.2	7
Gunes [34]	2014	Turkey	>4.2	39/29	40.4 ± 15.3/41 ± 13.8	8
Akbaba [35]	2015	Turkey	>4	51/43	36.9 ± 10/34.9 ± 8.4	8
Zha [36]	2015	China	>4.5	10/10	53.2 ± 5.4/52 ± 5.7	7
Tudoran [37]	2015	Romania	>4.2	15/15	36.7 ± 5.2/42.1 ± 6.8	4
Yazici [38]	2015	Turkey	>4	43/30	35.2 ± 1/34.5 ± 8.2	8
Niknam [39]	2016	Iran	>4	25/25	35.9 ± 7.6/37.5 ± 7.3	8
Fraca [40]	2016	Brazil	>4.5	16/15	39.6 ± 10.1/45 ± 7.4	5

Table 1. *Cont.*

Author	Year	Country	TSH Cut off Value (mUI/mL)	Participants (SCH/EU)	Age (SCH/EU)	NOS
Cerbone [41]	2016	Italy	>4.2	39/39	9.1 ± 3.5/9.4 ± 3.6	8
Isik-Balci [42]	2016	Turkey	NA	53/31	9.2 ± 4.2/7.1 ± 5.1	4
Rahman [43]	2016	Bangladesh	>5	26/30	30 ± 7.4/32 ± 8.7	8
Altay [44]	2017	Turkey	NA	35/30	34.4 ± 10.3/32.5 ± 7.5	5
Yadav [45]	2017	India	>7.5	27/20	10.9 ± 2.3/10.8 ± 2.4	8
Tanaka [46]	2018	Japan	>4.5	55/674	60.1 ± 7/56.1 ± 9.4	5
Saif [47]	2018	Egypt	>4.8	30/40	34 ± 8/36 ± 4.8	8
Yasar [48]	2018	Turkey	>5.6	160/86	39.5 ± 14.8/40.4 ± 10.0	7
Vijayan [49]	2018	India	>4.2	30/30	33.9 ± 10.6/37.9 ± 9.7	8
Tan [50]	2019	Turkey	>4.94	40/40	32 ± 27/28 ± 19	8
Farghaly [51]	2019	Egypt	>4	32/32	13.6 ± 2.4/13.2 ± 2.1	8
Dogan [52]	2019	Turkey	>4.2	50/37	35.3 ± 9.5/35.6 ± 1.9	6
Soto-Garcia [53]	2020	Mexic	>4	18/18	37 ± 12.9/36.8 ± 12.7	8
Asoglu [54]	2021	Turkey	>4.2	80/43	44.0 ± 13.1/46.7 ± 8.3	7
El Hini [55]	2021	Egypt	>4.5	36/36	40.2 ± 8.6/35.6 ± 9.9	6
Gonulalaln [56]	2021	Turkey	>4	30/52	35 ± 13.6/38.7 ± 10.4	7
Sahu [57]	2022	India	>5	42/50	10.3 ± 3.7/10.1 ± 3.1	7
Sharma [58]	2022	India	>4.2	35/35	46.2 ± 10/41.1 ± 11.1	6

2.5. Statistical Analysis and Risk of Bias

Statistical analysis of data was carried out using Jamovi 2.3.21. The differences between the study and control groups were rendered as standardized mean difference (SMD) and 95% confidence interval for continuous-type variables. Differences were considered statistically significant at $p < 0.05$.

For the age difference mediator, we applied the formula

$$\text{Ls\_age\_mean} - \text{Lc\_age\_mean}$$

For the sex difference mediator, we applied the formula

$$(\text{Ls\_female}/(\text{Ls\_female} + \text{Ls\_male}) - \text{Lc\_female}/(\text{Lc\_female} + \text{Lc\_male})) \times 100$$

For the body mass index (BMI) moderator, we applied the formula

$$\text{Ls\_BMI\_mean} - \text{Lc\_BMI\_mean}$$

For the Cholesterol moderator, we applied the formula

$$\text{Ls\_Cho\_mean} - \text{Lc\_Cho\_mean}$$

For the LDL moderator, we applied the formula

$$\text{Ls\_LDL\_mean} - \text{Lc\_LDL\_mean}$$

For the HDL moderator, we applied the formula

$$\text{Ls\_HDL\_mean} - \text{Lc\_HDL\_mean}$$

For the Triglycerides moderator, we applied the formula

$$Ls\_Trygliceridcs\_mean - Lc\_Tryglicerides\_mean$$

where Ls = study group, Lc = control group.

The analysis was performed using the mean difference as the outcome measure. A random effects model was used to fit the data. The amount of heterogeneity (tau^2) was estimated using the DerSimonian–Laird estimator [59]. In addition, the Q-test of heterogeneity [60] and I^2 statistics were analyzed, where $I^2 > 50\%$ indicated significant heterogeneity and $I^2 < 25\%$ was most likely not significant heterogeneity.

For publication bias analysis, we visually analyzed the symmetry of the funnel diagram, the rank correlation test, and the regression test using the standard error of the observed outcomes as predictors.

3. Results

3.1. Study Selection

Following the initial analysis of the database, we obtained 949 articles. After excluding duplicates and irrelevant studies, we finally included 39 studies for further evaluation. (Figure 1, Tables 2–4).

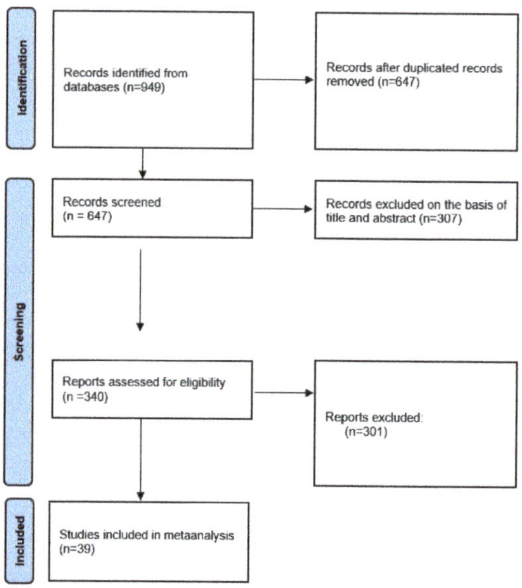

Figure 1. Search synthesis. Prisma flow diagram [14].

Table 2. CIMT and TSH assessment in analyzed studies.

Authors	Year	CIMT Assay	TSH Assay
Monzani [20]	2004	High-resolution ultrasonography using multiple equipment types and 7.5 MHz linear transducer—multiple measurements of both carotid arteries and internal carotid arteries	Ultrasensitive immunoradiometric assay (IRMA) method
Cikim [21]	2004	High-resolution ultrasound imaging (Vingmed System Five, 10 mH linear probe)—both common carotid arteries; three measurements from each subject	Autoanalyzer Roche/Hitachi Modular System—method not specified

Table 2. *Cont.*

Authors	Year	CIMT Assay	TSH Assay
Duman [22]	2007	High-resolution ultrasonography with a 7.5 MHz linear array transducer using a vascular ultrasound system (ATL-3500-HDI; Philips Medical Systems, Andover, MA, USA)—multiple measurements of both common carotid arteries	Roche/Hitachi modular analytics SWA—immunoassay
de Almeida [23]	2007	High-resolution ultrasound with Acusson Aspem Advanced and 10 MHz linear transducer—multiple measurements of both common carotid arteries and bifurcation	Imunometric measurement (IMMULITE DPC®)
Kim [24]	2009	High-resolution ultrasonographic system (Prosound α10) with 10.0 MHz linear transducer—multiple measurements in the mid and distal portion of the common carotid arteries	Chemiluminescent immunometric assay
Kebapcilar [25]	2010	High-definition ultrasonography (Philips HDI 5000) with L12-5 linear wide-band probe—two measurements, one proximal and one distal for each common carotid artery	Chemiluminescent immunometric assay (Immulite 2000)
Velkoska [26]	2011	Ultrasound system HP Agilent S4500 with 7.5–10.0 MHz linear transducer—two measurements of the right carotid artery	Immulite 2000 chemiluminescent analyzer
Gunduz [27]	2012	Gray-scale high-resolution color Doppler ultrasound (Prosound SSD—3500 SV ALOKA)—one measurement for each common carotid artery	Immulite 2000 chemiluminescent analyzer
Asik [28]	2013	Echocardiography machine VIVID 3 equipped with linear-array imaging probe—one measurement 10 mm proximal to the right carotid artery bifurcation	Chemiluminometric method (ADVIA Centaur analyzer
Knapp [29]	2013	Ultrasound imaging (Philips iE33) with 1–5 MHz sector transducer and 3–11 MHz linear-array high-resolution transducer—two measurements for each common carotid artery	Method not specified
Varim [30]	2013	Ultrasound with Siemens Sonoline Ultrasound using a 10 MHz linear probe—three measurements for each common carotid artery	Method not specified
Kilic [31]	2013	Ultrasound imaging (Vivid 7 dimensions) with 12 MHz linear array transducer—two measurements for each common carotid artery	Immunochemiluminescence method (Cobalt 6000 analyzer)
Unsal [32]	2014	High-resolution ultrasonography (Hitachi EUB 7000 HV) with 13 MHz probe—three measurements for each common carotid artery	Chemiluminescence assay (Advia Centaur) and specific electrochemiluminescence immunoassay (Elecsys 2010 Cobas)
Akkoca [33]	2014	Gray-scale, high-resolution color Doppler ultrasound (Siemens) with 13 MHz linear transducer—one measurement for each carotid artery	Chemiluminescence method (Immulite 2000)
Gunes [34]	2014	Ultrasound imaging (VIVID 3 machine) with 2.5 MHz linear-array probe—three measurements approximately 10 mm proximal of the carotid bifurcation for the right common carotid artery	Electro-chemiluminescence immunoassay "ECLIA" (Roche Cobas E601 analyzer)

Table 2. *Cont.*

Authors	Year	CIMT Assay	TSH Assay
Akbaba [35]	2015	High-resolution B-mode ultrasound (Loqic 3 device) with 11 MHz linear array transducer—three measurements for each common carotid artery	Chemiluminescence micro-particle immunoassay (Abbot Architect 2000)
Zha [36]	2015	Color ultrasound (Toshiba Aplio 500) with 9 Mhz linear-array transducer—three measurements for each common carotid artery	Chemiluminescence procedure (Roche Cobas E610)
Tudoran [37]	2015	Echocardiography device (Aloka CV Prosound SSD-4000 SV) with 10 MHz linear transducer—five measurements for each carotid artery beginning from carotid bulb dilation	Method not specified
Yazici [38]	2015	Ultrasound imaging (GE Vingmed) with 10 MHz broadband linear probe—number of measurements and sites not specified	Method not specified
Nikna [39]	2015	Sonogram B-mode imaging—number of measurements and sites not specified	Method not specified
França [40]	2016	Ultrasound imaging with 7.5 MHz multifrequency linear array probe (device not specified)—three measurements of the common carotid artery	Electrochemiluminescence immunoassay (Roche Diagnostics kits)
Cerbone [41]	2016	Ultrasound imaging (GE Vivid I) with 7.0 MHz—multiple measurements above the carotid sinus for both common carotid arteries	Chemiluminescence method (Immulite 2000)
Isik-Balci [42]	2016	Ultrasound imaging (Logiq E9 ultrasound) with a 6–15 MHz linear array probe—three measurements 20 mm proximal to the carotid bifurcation	Electrochemiluminescence (Roche Cobas 6000)
Rahman [43]	2016	Ultrasound imaging (DC-7 scanner) with 7.5–10 MHz linear transducer—one measurement 1.5 cm superior to the carotid bifurcation for each carotid artery	Immunoradiometric assay
Altay [44]	2017	Ultrasound imaging (General Electric Logic 5 Pro) with 12 MHz—five measurements for each common carotid artery, 1 cm distal to the main carotid artery bulb	Method not specified
Yadav [45]	2017	B-mode ultrasound imaging (Siemens) with 10 MHz linear transducer—number of measurements and sites not specified	Chemiluminescence immunoassay (IMMULITE 1000)
Tanaka [46]	2018	High-resolution B-mode ultrasonography (UF-4300R) with 7.5 MHz linear array probe—unspecified number of measurements for both common carotid arteries 20 mm proximal to the carotid bulb	CLIA immunoassay
Saif [47]	2018	High-resolution color-codded Doppler ultrasonography (ALT HDI) with 12 MHz linear array probe—four measurements for both common carotid arteries	Method not specified
Yasar [48]	2018	Ultrasound imaging (Toshiba Aplio 300) with 9–13 MHz linear probe—unspecified number of measurements 2 cm proximal to the carotid bulb	Chemiluminescent method (Immulite 2000)

Table 2. *Cont.*

Authors	Year	CIMT Assay	TSH Assay
Vijayan [49]	2018	Ultrasound imaging (Mindray DC-8) with 7 MHz linear transducer—unspecified number of measurements 10 mm proximal to the right common carotid artery	Chemiluminescent immunometric assay
Tan [50]	2019	B-mode ultrasonography with 7.5–13.5 MHz multifrequency linear array probe—three measurements for each common carotid artery	Electrochemiluminescence method (Abbot Aeroset kit)
Farghaly [51]	2019	Color duplex flow imaging (Acuson 128 XP)—three measurements at 1–2 cm proximal to the carotid bulb for each common carotid artery	Ultrasensitive immunometric assay (Immulite 2000 Third Generation)
Dogan [52]	2019	Ultrasonography (Aloka Prosound SSD 5000) with 7.5 MHz linear probe—unspecified number of measurements 10 mm proximal to the bifurcation for each common carotid artery	Electrochemiluminescence assay
Soto-Garcia [53]	2020	B-mode ultrasonography with 7.5–13.5 MHz multifrequency linear array probe—three measurements for each common carotid artery	Method not specified
Asoglu [54]	2021	Unspecified equipment and number of measurements 1–2 cm proximal to the carotid artery bifurcation	Chemiluminescence methods
El Hini [55]	2021	Method not specified	Enzyme-linked fluorescence immunoassay (BioMerieux Mini Vidas)
Gonulalaln [56]	2021	B-mode ultrasonography (LOGIQ P5)—three measurements 1 cm proximal to the bifurcation for each common carotid artery	Method not specified
Sahu [57]	2022	Color duplex flow imaging (Samsung HS 70 A) with 7 MHz probe—unspecified number of measurements for both common carotid arteries	Electrochemiluminescence assay (Roche Cobas 411)
Sharma [58]	2022	Unspecified equipment and number of measurements 1 cm proximal to the carotid artery bifurcation	Method not specified

Table 3. Carotid intima-media thickness (CIMT) and body mass index (BMI) in subclinical hypothyroidism (SCH) versus euthyroidism (EU) in the analyzed studies.

Authors	SCH_BMI	EU_BMI	SCH_CIMT	EU_CIMT
Monzani [20]	24.7 ± 3.5	24.2 ± 3.7	0.75 ± 0.13	0.63 ± 0.07
Cikim [21]	26.03 ± 6.21	27.04 ± 4.95	0.55 ± 0.14	0.54 ± 0.14
Duman [22]	25.1 ± 4.3	24.7 ± 2.5	0.66 ± 0.16	0.54 ± 0.10
de Almeida [23]	27.3 ± 4.6	25.41 ± 4.38	0.57 ± 0.70	0.57 ± 0.68
Kim [24]	23.1 ± 2.8	23.3 ± 3.1	0.66 ± 0.10	0.57 ± 0.08
Kebapcilar [25]	28.58 ± 5.81	28.45 ± 5.25	0.64 ± 0.13	0.57 ± 0.08
Velkoska [26]	27.8 ± 5.6	25.4 ± 5.1	0.61 ± 0.1	056 ± 0.1
Gunduz [27]	26.72 ± 2.32	24.34 ± 2.43	0.61 ± 0.11	0.53 ± 0.08
Asik [28]	30.37 ± 7.67	27.79 ± 3.64	0.54 ± 0.14	0.51 ± 0.11
Knapp [29]	24.43 ± 4.3	21.8 ± 1.48	0.61 ± 0.14	0.32 ± 0.1
Varim [30]	25.7 ± 4	25.66 ± 4.24	0.4 ± 0.2	0.4 ± 0.1
Kilic [31]	28.6 ± 5.9	24.9 ± 6.5	0.05 ± 0.01	0.06 ± 0.01

Table 3. *Cont.*

Authors	SCH_BMI	EU_BMI	SCH_CIMT	EU_CIMT
Unsal [32]	-	-	0.53 ± 0.11	0.5 ± 0.86
Akkoca [33]	28.42 ± 1.86	27.97 ± 4.15	0.74 ± 0.8	0.38 ± 0.74
Gunes [34]	28.79 ± 6.6	27.46 ± 5.35	0.65 ± 0.13	0.55 ± 0.11
Akbaba [35]	26.1 ± 5.5	25.7 ± 4.2	0.74 ± 0.3	0.47 ± 0.5
Zha [36]	24.4 ± 1.8	24 ± 1.6	0.82 ± 0.14	0.75 ± 0.09
Tudoran [37]	26.24 ± 2.7	27.5 ± 6.71	0.72 ± 0.14	0.62 ± 0.31
Yazici [38]	25.1 ± 5.6	25.0 ± 4.1	0.50 ± 0.09	0.48 ± 0.04
Niknam [39]	26 ± 2	25.82 ± 2	0.56 ± 0.09	0.58 ± 0.08
França [40]	26.5 ± 4.4	24.6 ± 2.98	0.62 ± 0.11	0.66 ± 0.14
Cerbone [41]	-	-	0.44 ± 0.08	0.44 ± 0.06
Isik-Balci [42]	17.56 ± 3.61	17.56 ± 2.47	0.5 ± 0.09	0.43 ± 0.03
Rahman [43]	25.6 ± 4.7	-	0.08 ± 0.05	0.6 ± 0.05
Altay [44]	27.6 ± 5.9	23.7 ± 3.9	0.63 ± 0.10	0.55 ± 0.05
Yadav [45]	17.79 ± 4.11	15.99 ± 1.69	0.48 ± 0.07	0.47 ± 0.08
Tanaka [46]	22.1 ± 2.7	22.1 ± 3.1	0.59 ± 0.12	0.57 ± 0.1
Saif [47]	26 ± 3.6	24 ± 2.3	0.6 ± 0.2	0.45 ± 0.07
Yasar [48]	30.22 ± 5.71	29.6 ± 6.12	0.55 ± 0.13	0.43 ± 0.19
Vijayan [49]	24.66 ± 4.13	22.86 ± 3.01	0.55 ± 0.10	0.47 ± 0.06
Tan [50]	23.67 ± 5.37	21.39 ± 3.52	0.5 ± 0.27	0.5 ± 0.16
Farghaly [51]	-	-	0.44 ± 0.08	0.44 ± 0.06
Dogan [52]	25.2 ± 3.8	31.4 ± 44.9	0.59 ± 0.12	0.43 ± 0.8
Soto-Garcia [53]	26.8 ± 4.7	29.6 ± 3.6	0.49 ± 0.12	0.42 ± 0.07
Asoglu [54]	26.5 ± 2.4	26.2 ± 2.4	0.8 ± 0.3	0.5 ± 0.2
El Hini [55]	26.7 ± 2	23.3 ± 0.84	0.56 ± 0.09	0.51 ± 0.06
Gonulalaln [56]	29.87 ± 5.09	29.12 ± 5.83	0.61 ± 0.11	0.35 ± 0.12
Sahu [57]	20.39 ± 2.51	18.81 ± 3.13	0.52 ± 0.12	0.49 ± 0.08
Sharma [58]	23.76 ± 1.77	23.12 ± 1.73	0.68 ± 0.14	0.59 ± 0.17

Table 4. CIMT in SCH vs. EU depending on TSH cut-off values.

Author	Year	TSH Cut off Value (mUI/mL)	SCH_CIMT	EU_CIMT
Monzani [20]	2004	>3.6	0.75 ± 0.13	0.63 ± 0.07
Cikim [21]	2004	>4.20	0.55 ± 0.14	0.54 ± 0.14
Duman [22]	2007	>4.2	0.66 ± 0.16	0.54 ± 0.10
de Almeida [23]	2007	>4	0.57 ± 0.70	0.57 ± 0.68
Kim [24]	2009	>5.5	0.66 ± 0.10	0.57 ± 0.08
Kebapcilar [25]	2010	>5	0.64 ± 0.13	0.57 ± 0.08
Velkoska [26]	2011	>4.2	0.61 ± 0.1	056 ± 0.1
Gunduz [27]	2012	>4	0.61 ± 0.11	0.53 ± 0.08
Asik [28]	2013	>5.49	0.54 ± 0.14	0.51 ± 0.11
Knapp [29]	2013	–	0.61 ± 0.14	0.32 ± 0.1

Table 4. *Cont.*

Author	Year	TSH Cut off Value (mUI/mL)	SCH_CIMT	EU_CIMT
Varim [30]	2013	>4.5	0.4 ± 0.2	0.4 ± 0.1
Kilic [31]	2013	>4.2	0.05 ± 0.01	0.06 ± 0.01
Unsal [32]	2014	>4.2	0.53 ± 0.11	0.5 ± 0.86
Akkoca [33]	2014	>4.2	0.74 ± 0.8	.0.38 ± 0.74
Gunes [34]	2014	>4.2	0.65 ± 0.13	0.55 ± 0.11
Akbaba [35]	2015	>4	0.74 ± 0.3	0.47 ± 0.5
Zha [36]	2015	>4.5	0.82 ± 0.14	0.75 ± 0.09
Tudoran [37]	2015	>4.2	0.72 ± 0.14	0.62 ± 0.31
Yazici [38]	2015	>4	0.50 ± 0.09	0.48 ± 0.04
Niknam [39]	2016	>4	0.56 ± 0.09	0.58 ± 0.08
Franca [40]	2016	>4.5	0.62 ± 0.11	0.66 ± 0.14
Cerbone [41]	2016	>4.2	0.44 ± 0.08	0.44 ± 0.06
Isik-Balci [42]	2016	NA	0.5 ± 0.09	0.43 ± 0.03
Rahman [43]	2016	>5	0.08 ± 0.05	0.6 ± 0.05
Altay [44]	2017	NA	0.63 ± 0.10	0.55 ± 0.05
Yadav [45]	2017	>7.5	0.48 ± 0.07	0.47 ± 0.08
Tanaka [46]	2018	>4.5	0.59 ± 0.12	0.57 ± 0.1
Saif [47]	2018	>4.8	0.6 ± 0.2	0.45 ± 0.07
Yasar [48]	2018	>5.6	0.55 ± 0.13	0.43 ± 0.19
Vijayan [49]	2018	>4.2	0.55 ± 0.10	0.47 ± 0.06
Tan [50]	2019	>4.94	0.5 ± 0.27	0.5 ± 0.16
Farghaly [51]	2019	>4	0.44 ± 0.08	0.44 ± 0.06
Dogan [52]	2019	>4.2	0.59 ± 0.12	0.43 ± 0.8
Soto-Garcia [53]	2020	>4	0.49 ± 0.12	0.42 ± 0.07
Asoglu [54]	2021	>4.2	0.8 ± 0.3	0.5 ± 0.2
El Hini [55]	2021	>4.5	0.56 ± 0.09	0.51 ± 0.06
Gonulalaln [56]	2021	>4	0.61 ± 0.11	0.35 ± 0.12
Sahu [57]	2022	>5	0.52 ± 0.12	0.49 ± 0.08
Sharma [58]	2022	>4.2	0.68 ± 0.14	0.59 ± 0.17

3.2. CIMT in SCH Versus EU

A total of 39 studies with 3430 subjects were analyzed, comprising 1545 SCH and 1885 EU. The observed mean difference ranged from −0.04 to 0.36, with most studies showing a positive association between SCH and the thickening of the carotid wall (79%). The estimated average mean difference between SCH and EU was 0.08 [0.05–0.10], statistically significant, $p < 0.01$ (Figure 2). The heterogeneity of the studies was high ($I^2 = 93.82\%$).

The publication bias was not statistically significant; neither the rank correlation nor the regression test indicated any funnel plot asymmetry ($p = 0.96$ and $p = 0.060$, respectively), with most cases distributed at the top of the funnel plot (Figure 3).

By using the sex ratio, age ratio, BMI ratio, LDL ratio, HDL ratio, and triglycerides ratio as moderators, the statistical significance of the study was not modified.

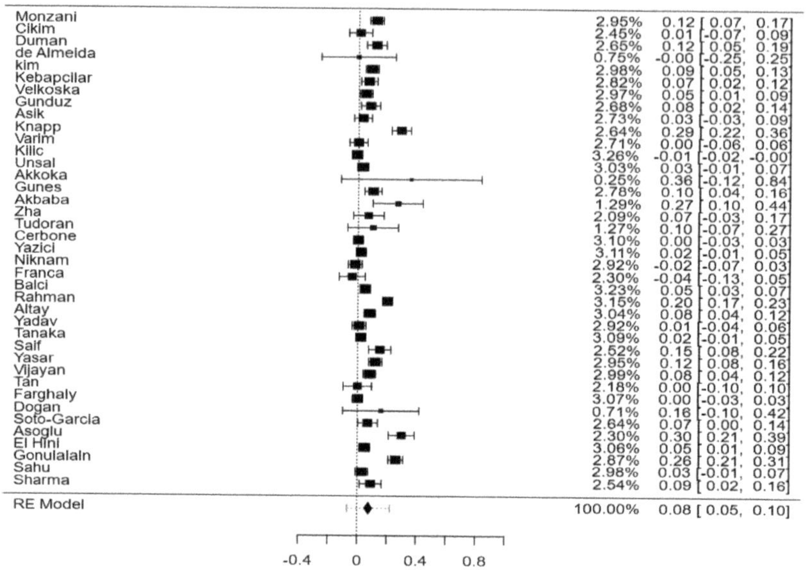

Figure 2. CIMT in SCH versus EU in the 39 included studies.

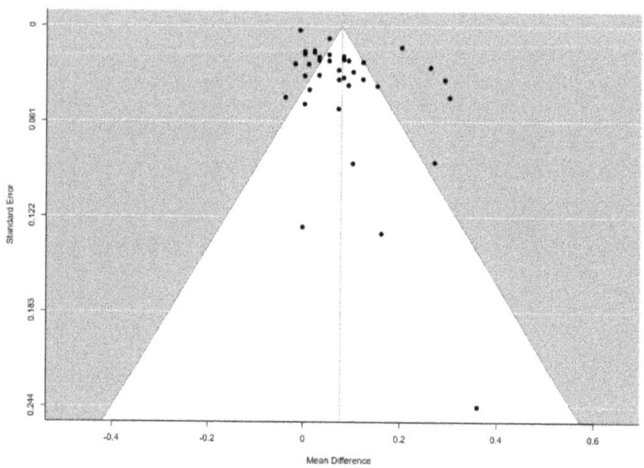

Figure 3. Funnel plot for the 39 studies included in the analysis.

We conducted a sensitivity analysis by excluding single studies and performing additional analysis for each study excluded. None of the excluded studies had a significant effect on the overall results of the meta-analysis. To ensure the accuracy of the results, we excluded studies that did not provide information about how CIMT and/or TSH were assessed, studies that utilized outdated or less accurate ultrasound devices to measure CIMT, studies that did not specify the cut-off value for TSH, studies that reported CIMT values well below the lower limit of the normal range, studies that included pediatric populations, studies that did not report BMI values or did not provide a clear explanation of how BMI values were calculated, and studies that showed significant numerical differences between the control group and the study group. After conducting further analysis of the excluded categories, it was observed that there was no significant impact on the overall statistical significance of the meta-analysis. The level of heterogeneity remained highly significant, and the moderators, including sex, age, LDL, HDL, triglycerides, and BMI ratio, did not alter the statistical significance of the results.

After excluding all the abovementioned study categories once, except for the studies on pediatric populations, a total of 19 studies were analyzed. The observed mean difference ranged from −0.04 to 0.36, with most studies showing a positive association between SCH and the thickening of the carotid wall (68%). The estimated average mean difference between SCH and Eu was 0.04 [0.02–0.07], statistically significant, $p = 0.03$ (Figure 4). The heterogeneity of the studies was most likely substantial ($I^2 = 77.7\%$).

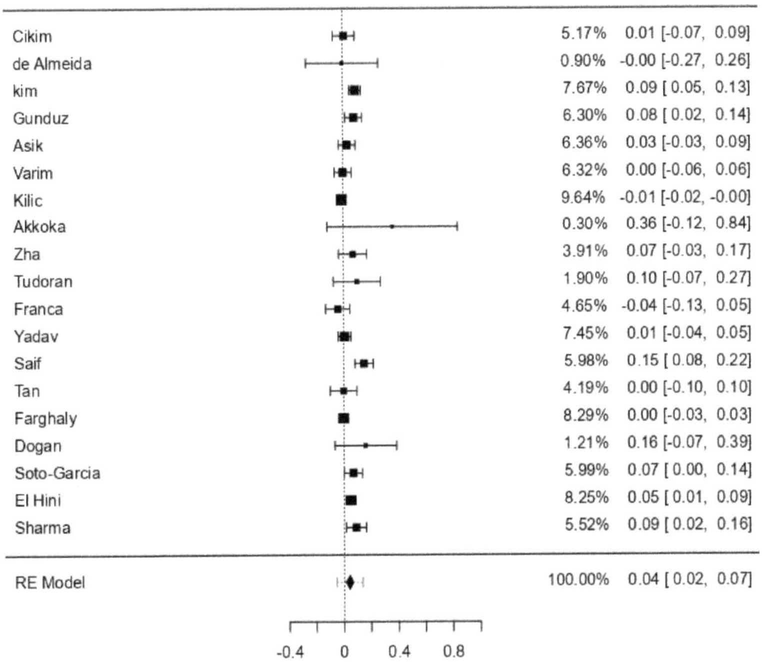

Figure 4. CIMT in SCH versus EU in the 19 analyzed studies.

After performing the sensitivity analysis, no significant statistical changes were observed in the overall effect, indicating that the meta-analysis was stable.

For the 19 studies that remained after applying the abovementioned exclusion criteria, the publication bias was not statistically significant; neither the rank correlation nor the regression test indicated any funnel plot asymmetry ($p = 0.89$ and $p = 0.10$, respectively), with most cases distributed at the top of the funnel plot (Figure 5).

By using the age ratio as a moderator for the abovementioned 19 studies, the statistical significance of the meta-analysis was changed, $p = 0.07$ [0.01–0.06]. The heterogeneity of the studies was most likely substantial ($I^2 = 76.7\%$). Advanced age was a confounding factor in the studied correlation (Figure 6).

By also using sex ratio as a moderator for the abovementioned 19 studies, the statistical significance of the meta-analysis was changed, $p = 0.06$ [0.01–0.07]. The heterogeneity of the studies was most likely substantial ($I^2 = 74.03\%$). The SCH–CIMT correlation was influenced by the sex of the subjects, female sex being a confounding factor in this regard (Figure 7).

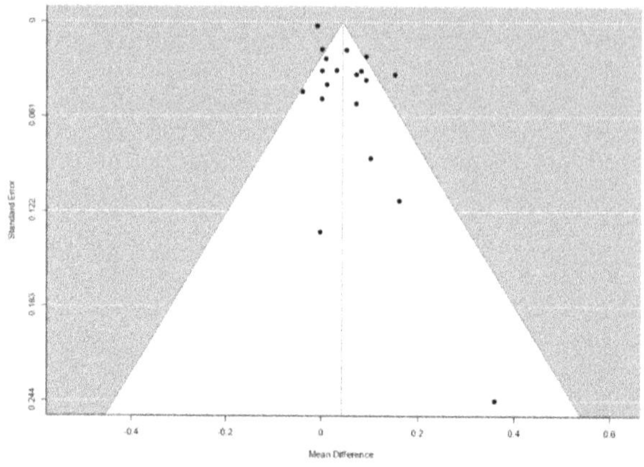

Figure 5. Funnel plot for the 19 analyzed studies.

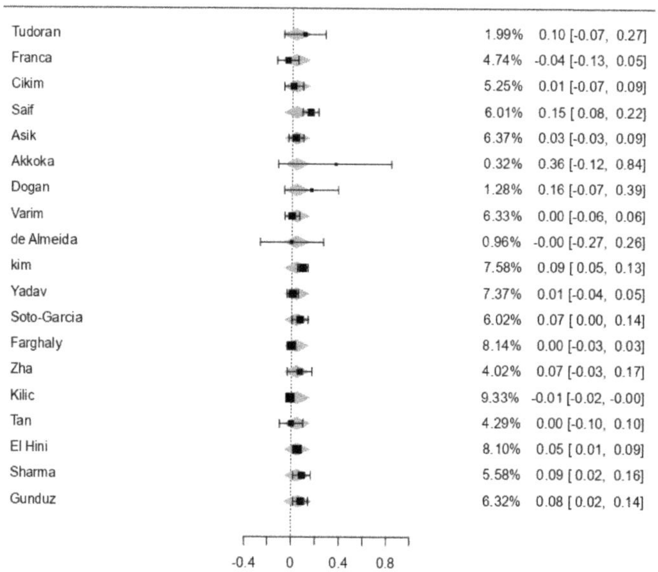

Figure 6. CIMT in SCH versus EU in the 19 included studies, using age ratio as a moderator.

Regarding the lipidic profile, using cholesterol ratio as a moderator for the above-mentioned 19 studies that exposed this metabolic parameter (16 studies), the statistical significance of the meta-analysis was changed, $p = 0.08$ [0.01–0.06]. The heterogeneity of the studies was reduced ($I^2 = 54.43\%$). The SCH–CIMT correlation was influenced by high cholesterol levels (Figure 8).

Using BMI ratio, LDL ratio, HDL ratio, and triglycerides ratio as moderators, the statistical significance of the study was not modified and the heterogeneity of the studies was most likely substantial.

By filtering the studies depending on the cut-off value for TSH, with a threshold of 4.2, the statistical significance of the study was not modified, $p = 0.04$ [0–0.08], with substantial heterogeneity ($I^2 = 68.85\%$).

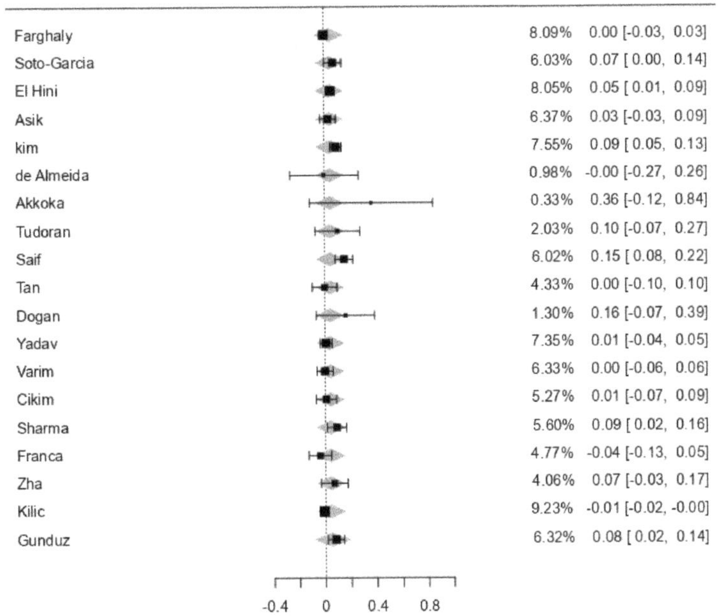

Figure 7. CIMT in SCH versus EU in the 19 included studies, using sex ratio as a moderator.

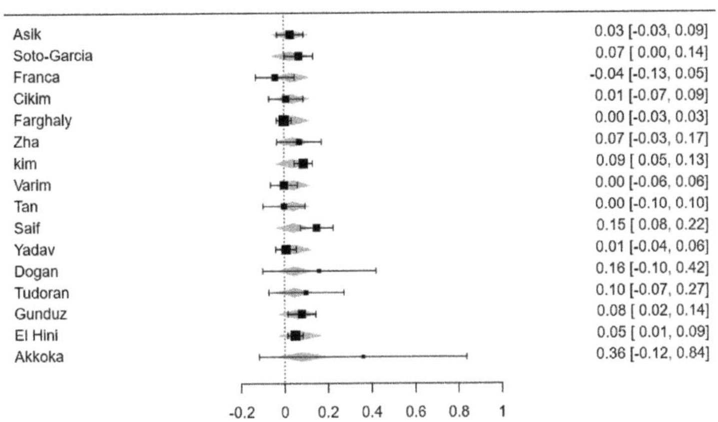

Figure 8. CIMT in SCH versus EU in the 16 included studies, using cholesterol ratio as a moderator.

4. Discussion

This meta-analysis indicates a significant positive correlation between SCH and increased CIMT, with some limitations. Additionally, female sex, advanced age, and high cholesterol levels significantly influenced this correlation.

A previous meta-analysis on this topic, conducted by Gao et al. approximately 10 years ago within eight studies, obtained similar results [61]. Yao et al., in a meta-analysis that included 27 case-control studies in which they analyzed potential non-invasive markers for cardiovascular risk in people with subclinical hypothyroidism, found a significantly positive association between SCH and the thickening of the arterial wall, with increased risk of cardiovascular pathologies [62]. CIMT may also be a predictor for the risk of ischemic stroke. Sahoo et al. measured CIMT at the level of the common carotid artery among patients with ischemic stroke and found them to have an average of 0.798 mm CIMT, while in the control group the mean CIMT was 0.6 mm, a statistically significant difference [63]. CIMT at the level of the common carotid artery is a factor that helps predict cardiovascular risks, and the evaluation of this parameter at the level of the internal carotid artery improves its classification [64]. A recently conducted joint study of 9020 U.S. adults, by Inoue et al., found that cardiovascular disease mediated the association between subclinical hypothyroidism and all-cause mortality, especially among women and the elderly [65]. According to a study conducted by Vaya et al., patients with SCH show an increased risk of cardiovascular disease when compared to those with EU. This is characterized by higher levels of plasma viscosity, fibrinogen, homocysteine, and erythrocyte distribution [66]. In postmenopausal women, SCH has been associated with increased levels of inflammatory markers such as CRP, homocysteine, uric acid, and TNFα [67].

From a pathophysiological standpoint, the mechanisms of these changes are derived from the role of the thyroid hormones on metabolic parameters, including lipoprotein metabolism [68]. With an increase in TSH levels, there was an increase in cholesterol, triglycerides, and LDL-c, and a decrease in HDL-c levels; this association has a linear character [69]. People with subclinical hypothyroidism have a higher increased risk compared to euthyroid patients of developing hypercholesterolemia, increased levels of LDL-c and CRP, and elevated diastolic blood pressure [70]. The major cardiovascular risk factors are diabetes, central obesity, dyslipidemia, elevated LDL-c levels, and high blood pressure [71], which entails an increased risk of atheromatosis and myocardial ischemia. However, the etiology of hypothyroidism does not seem to influence these cardio-vascular metabolic parameters. For example, antithyroid peroxidase antibodies have not been positively associated with cardiovascular risk in patients with subclinical hypothyroidism [72].

Subclinical hypothyroidism is common in medical practice, and its diagnosis should consider demographics relative to the TSH reference range in the healthy population. According to the literature, in a considerable proportion of patients, subclinical hypothyroidism can be physiologically reversible, without any medication in this regard, but there are also persistent, progressive forms, mainly against the background of chronic autoimmune thyroiditis. Once subclinical hypothyroidism is detected, the patient requires periodic medical evaluations to allow risk stratification [73,74].

Studies that examined the evolution of pre-existing cardiac pathology in people with newly diagnosed SCH found a worsening of the cardiac pathology prognosis compared to that of euthyroid patients, during the follow-up period of less than 5 years observed in patients with SCH, including the need for ventricular stimulation and heart transplantation, or even death [74–76]. Corona et al. suggest that subclinical hypothyroidism affects cardiovascular risk factors, but its effects are mediated by the pre-existence/coexistence of these risk factors, instead of terminating a specific pathophysiological mechanism [77].

Regarding effective treatment to minimize cardiovascular consequences, meta-analyses have revealed the positive effect of levothyroxine administration, which led to a decrease in CIMT [78,79]. In a meta-analysis of 119 clinical trials [80], it was seen that following a decrease in CIMT progression, cardiovascular risks decreased. In contrast, in a randomized study of 185 elderly patients, administration of levothyroxine treatment for one year did not reduce the progression of CIMT compared to the placebo group [81].

According to the last ETA guideline issued 10 years ago for the treatment of subclin-ical hypothyroidism, treatment suggestions take into account the patient's age and serum TSH, with a reference age of 70 years and a TSH level of 10 mUI/mL. LT4 therapy is considered per primam only if TSH has values greater than or equal to 10 mUI/mL. For people under 70 years of age, it is recommended that LT4 be administered, and in people over 70 years of age, LT4 is recommended only if there are clear symptoms of hypothyroidism or increased cardiovascular risk [82]. These indications are derived from studies that demonstrated the effectiveness of LT4 treatment in subclinical hypothyroidism in people under 70 years of age, whereas no decrease in ischemic cardiac events was observed in persons above this age limit [83]. One explanation for these results could be the etiology of subclinical hypothyroidism, which in young people has a more frequent autoimmune etiology, while in the elderly it was found that it can also be a change without pathological significance but was rather physiological, as revealed by the study of Surks and Hollowell, who concluded that TSH levels increase progressively, physiologically, with age [84].

The applicability of this research in clinical medical practice could lie in its potential for non-invasive screening to predict cardiovascular risk in patients with subclinical hypothyroidism, as well as the prompt analysis of optimal therapy. At the same time, the positive association between SCH and atheromatosis could be a potential indication for thyroid function testing in patients with cardio-vascular pathology.

The limitations of this meta-analysis were: the different cut-off values of TSH between studies and the lack of uniformity in the evaluation of the THS value; some studies did not specify the TSH assessment method; the lack of metabolic profile analysis in some studies; the low number of persons in the analyzed studies; the different number of persons in the study group versus the control group in some studies; studies limited to certain age groups; the narrow geographical distribution of the studies- out of the 39 studies included in the meta-analysis, the majority (19 original studies) took place in Turkey, leading to an absence of evidence from Western developed countries.

The small number of randomized clinical trials and cohort studies on this topic, often considered more adequate at establishing cause–effect relationships compared to case-control studies, represents another study limitation.

Also as a limitation, the absence in the included studies of a normal value, threshold of CIMT, and additional data regarding classic cardiovascular risk factors, such as menopause, smoking, alcohol consumption, blood pressure, diabetes mellitus, and diet, should be considered as potential confounding factors. In addition, in the studies on this topic, no data were found to attest to the pathological role of subclinical hypothyroidism per se in terms of clinical cardiovascular complications due to subclinical hypothyroidism.

As another limitation, the significant heterogeneity among studies was very important. Even if we could not identify all the studies that were the sources of this heterogeneity, the stability of the outcomes was confirmed after adjusting for potential publication bias.

5. Conclusions

These research findings suggest, with some limitations, a statistically significant positive association between SCH and increased CIMT. There are necessary large-scale, prospective studies to be conducted on substantial populations, taking into account traditional cardiovascular risk factors and incorporating long-term follow-up for accurate risk stratification and optimal therapeutic indication.

Author Contributions: Conceptualization, O.-M.I.; methodology, O.-M.I., S.H.; software, O.-M.I., S.H.; validation, O.-M.I., S.H., V.E.S.; formal analysis, O.-M.I., S.H., V.E.S.; investigation, O.-M.I., S.H., V.E.S.; resources, O.-M.I., S.H., I.F., A.-I.P., V.E.S.; data curation, O.-M.I., S.H., V.E.S., I.F., A.-I.P.; writing—original draft preparation, O.-M.I.; writing—review and editing O.-M.I., V.E.S.; visualization, O.-M.I., S.H., V.E.S., I.F., A.-I.P.; supervision, O.-M.I., S.H.; project administration, O.-M.I.; funding acquisition, O.-M.I. All authors have read and agreed to the published version of the manuscript.

Funding: This research was financially supported by "Carol Davila" University of Medicine and Pharmacy Bucharest, Romania, through Contract no. 33PFE/30.12.2021, funded by the Ministry of Research and Innovation within PNCDI III, Program 1—Development of the National RD system, Subprogram 1.2—Institutional Performance—RDI excellence funding projects.

Institutional Review Board Statement: Not applicable.

Informed Consent Statement: Not applicable.

Data Availability Statement: The original data presented in the study are openly available in PubMed, MedLine, Scopus, and Web of Science databases.

Conflicts of Interest: The authors declare no conflicts of interest. The funders had no role in the design of the study; in the collection, analyses, or interpretation of data; in the writing of the manuscript; or in the decision to publish the results.

References

1. Cooper, D.S. Clinical Practice. Subclinical hypothyroidism. *N. Engl. J. Med.* **2001**, *345*, 260–265. [CrossRef]
2. Al Eidan, E.; Rahman, S.U.; Al Qahtani, S.; Al Farhan, A.I.; Abdulmajeed, I. Prevalence of subclinical hypothyroidism in adults visiting primary health-care setting in Riyadh. *J. Community Hosp. Intern. Med. Perspect.* **2018**, *8*, 11–15. [CrossRef]
3. Rohil, V.; Mishra, A.K.; Shrewastawa, M.K.; Mehta, K.D.; Lamsal, M.; Baral, N.; Majhi, S. Subclinical hypothyroidism in eastern Nepal: A hospital based study. *Kathmandu Univ. Med. J. (KUMJ)* **2010**, *8*, 231–237. [CrossRef] [PubMed]
4. Risal, P.; Adhikari, B.; Shrestha, R.; Manandhar, S.; Bhatt, R.D.; Hada, M. Analysis of Factors Associated with Thyroid Dysfunction: A Hospital Based Study. *Kathmandu Univ. Med. J. (KUMJ)* **2019**, *17*, 88–92. [PubMed]
5. Abu-Helalah, M.; Alshraideh, H.A.; Al-Sarayreh, S.A.; Al Shawabkeh, A.H.K.; Nesheiwat, A.; Younes, N.; Al-Hader, A. A Cross-Sectional Study to Assess the Prevalence of Adult Thyroid Dysfunction Disorders in Jordan. *Thyroid* **2019**, *29*, 1052–1059. [CrossRef] [PubMed]
6. Stein, J.H.; Korcarz, C.E.; Hurst, R.T.; Lonn, E.; Kendall, C.B.; Mohler, E.R.; Najjar, S.S.; Rembold, C.M.; Post, W.S. Use of carotid ultrasound to identify subclinical vascular disease and evaluate cardiovascular disease risk: A consensus statement from the American Society of Echocardiography Carotid Intima-Media Thickness Task Force. Endorsed by the Society for Vascular Medicine. *J. Am. Soc. Echocardiogr.* **2008**, *21*, 93–111. [CrossRef] [PubMed]
7. Cobble, M.; Bale, B. Carotid intima-media thickness: Knowledge and application to everyday practice. *Postgrad. Med.* **2010**, *122*, 10–18. [CrossRef] [PubMed]
8. Hak, A.E.; Pols, H.A.; Visser, T.J.; Drexhage, H.A.; Hofman, A.; Witteman, J.C. Subclinical hypothyroidism is an independent risk factor for atherosclerosis and myocardial infarction in elderly women: The Rotterdam Study. *Ann. Intern. Med.* **2000**, *132*, 270–278. [CrossRef]
9. Razvi, S.; Weaver, J.U.; Vanderpump, M.P.; Pearce, S.H.S. The incidence of ischemic heart disease and mortality in people with subclinical hypothyroidism: Reanalysis of the Whickham Survey cohort. *J. Clin. Endocrinol. Metab.* **2010**, *95*, 1734–1740. [CrossRef]
10. Türemen, E.E.; Çetinarslan, B.; Sahin, T.; Cantürk, Z.; Tarkun, I. Endothelial dysfunction and low grade chronic inflammation in subclinical hypothyroidism due to autoimmune thyroiditis. *Endocr. J.* **2011**, *58*, 349–354. [CrossRef]
11. Dardano, A.; Ghiadoni, L.; Plantinga, Y.; Caraccio, N.; Bemi, A.; Duranti, E.; Taddei, S.; Ferrannini, E.; Salvetti, A.; Monzani, F. Recombinant human thyrotropin reduces endothelium-dependent vasodilation in patients monitored for differentiated thyroid carcinoma. *J. Clin. Endocrinol. Metab.* **2006**, *91*, 4175–4178. [CrossRef] [PubMed]
12. Lai, Y.; Wang, J.; Jiang, F.; Wang, B.; Chen, Y.; Li, M.; Liu, H.; Li, C.; Xue, H.; Li, N.; et al. The relationship between serum thyrotropin and components of metabolic syndrome. *Endocr. J.* **2011**, *58*, 23–30. [CrossRef] [PubMed]
13. Lu, M.; Yang, C.-B.; Gao, L.; Zhao, J.-J. Mechanism of subclinical hypothyroidism accelerating endothelial dysfunction (Review). *Exp. Ther. Med.* **2015**, *9*, 3–10. [CrossRef] [PubMed]
14. Page, M.J.; McKenzie, J.E.; Bossuyt, P.M.; Boutron, I.; Hoffmann, T.C.; Mulrow, C.D.; Shamseer, L.; Tetzlaff, J.M.; Akl, E.A.; Brennan, S.E.; et al. The PRISMA 2020 statement: An updated guideline for reporting systematic reviews. *BMJ* **2021**, *372*, n71. Available online: https://www.bmj.com/content/372/bmj.n71 (accessed on 18 December 2022). [CrossRef] [PubMed]
15. Higgins, J.P.T.; Thomas, J.; Chandler, J.; Cumpston, M.; Li, T.; Page, M.J.; Welch, V.A. Cochrane Handbook for Systematic Reviews of Interventions Version 6.4 (Updated August 2023). Cochrane. 2023. Available online: www.training.cochrane.org/handbook (accessed on 3 December 2023).
16. Luo, D.; Wan, X.; Liu, J.; Tong, T. Optimally estimating the sample mean from the sample size, median, mid-range, and/or mid-quartile range. *Stat. Methods Med. Res.* **2018**, *27*, 1785–1805. [CrossRef] [PubMed]
17. Wan, X.; Wang, W.; Liu, J.; Tong, T. Estimating the sample mean and standard deviation from the sample size, median, range and/or interquartile range. *BMC Med. Res. Methodol.* **2014**, *14*, 135. [CrossRef]
18. HKBU-Math, Estimating the Sample Mean and Standard Deviation (SD) from the Five-Number Summary and Its Application in Meta-Analysis. Available online: https://www.math.hkbu.edu.hk/~tongt/papers/median2mean.html (accessed on 20 January 2023).
19. Wells, G.A.; Shea, B.; O'Connell, D.; Peterson, J.; Welch, V.; Losos, M.; Tugwell, P. The Newcastle-Ottawa Scale (NOS) for Assessing the Quality of Nonrandomised Studies in Meta-Analyses. Available online: https://www.ohri.ca/programs/clinical_epidemiology/oxford.asp (accessed on 10 January 2023).
20. Monzani, F.; Caraccio, N.; Kozàkowà, M.; Dardano, A.; Vittone, F.; Virdis, A.; Taddei, S.; Palombo, C.; Ferrannini, E. Effect of levothyroxine replacement on lipid profile and intima-media thickness in subclinical hypothyroidism: A double-blind, placebo-controlled study. *J. Clin. Endocrinol. Metab.* **2004**, *89*, 2099–2106. [CrossRef]
21. Cikim, A.S.; Oflaz, H.; Ozbey, N.; Cikim, K.; Umman, S.; Meric, M.; Sencer, E.; Molvalilar, S. Evaluation of Endothelial Function in Subclinical Hypothyroidism and Subclinical Hyperthyroidism. *Thyroid* **2004**, *14*, 605–609. [CrossRef]
22. Duman, D.; Demirtunc, R.; Sahin, S.; Esertas, K. The effects of simvastatin and levothyroxine on intima-media thickness of the carotid artery in female normolipemic patients with subclinical hypothyroidism: A prospective, randomized-controlled study. *J. Cardiovasc. Med.* **2007**, *8*, 1007–1011. [CrossRef]
23. Almeida, C.A.d.; Teixeira, P.d.F.d.S.; Soares, D.V.; Cabral, M.D.; Costa, S.M.d.; Salles, E.F.d.; Silva, N.A.d.O.e.; de Morais, F.F.; Buescu, A.; Henriques, J.M.; et al. Espessura íntima-média carotídea como marcador de risco cardiovascular em pacientes com hipotireoidismo subclínico. *Arq. Bras. Endocrinol. Metabol.* **2007**, *51*, 472–477. [CrossRef]
24. Kim, S.-K.; Kim, S.-H.; Park, K.-S.; Park, S.-W.; Cho, Y.-W. Regression of the increased common carotid artery-intima media thickness in subclinical hypothyroidism after thyroid hormone replacement. *Endocr. J.* **2009**, *56*, 753–758. [CrossRef]

25. Kebapcilar, L.; Comlekci, A.; Tuncel, P.; Solak, A.; Secil, M.; Gencel, O.; Sahin, M.; Sari, I.; Yeşil, S. Effect of levothyroxine replacement therapy on paraoxonase-1 and carotid intima-media thickness in subclinical hypothyroidism. *Med. Sci. Monit.* **2010**, *16*, 47.
26. Valentina, V.N.; Marijan, B.; Chedo, D.; Branka, K. Subclinical hypothyroidism and risk to carotid atherosclerosis. *Arq. Bras. Endocrinol. Metabol.* **2011**, *55*, 475–480. [CrossRef] [PubMed]
27. Gunduz, M.; Gunduz, E.; Kircelli, F.; Okur, N.; Ozkaya, M. Role of surrogate markers of atherosclerosis in clinical and subclinical thyroidism. *Int. J. Endocrinol.* **2012**, *2012*, 109797. [CrossRef]
28. Asik, M.; Sahin, S.; Ozkul, F.; Anaforoglu, I.; Ayhan, S.; Karagol, S.; Gunes, F.; Algun, E. Evaluation of epicardial fat tissue thickness in patients with Hashimoto thyroiditis. *Clin. Endocrinol.* **2013**, *79*, 571–576. [CrossRef] [PubMed]
29. Knapp, M.; Lisowska, A.; Sobkowicz, B.; Tycińska, A.; Sawicki, R.; Musiał, W.J. Myocardial perfusion and intima-media thickness in patients with subclinical hypothyroidism. *Adv. Med. Sci.* **2013**, *58*, 44–49. [CrossRef] [PubMed]
30. Varim, C.; Yldiz, M. Assessment of carotid artery intima media thicknes in patients with subclinical hypothyroidism. *Ortadogu Med. J.* **2013**, *5*, 6–12.
31. Kilic, I.D.; Tanriverdi, H.; Fenkci, S.; Akin, F.; Uslu, S.; Kaftan, A. Noninvasive indicators of atherosclerosis in subclinical hypothyroidism. *Indian J. Endocrinol. Metab.* **2013**, *17*, 271–275. [CrossRef]
32. Unsal, I.O.; Topaloglu, O.; Cakir, E.; Bozkurt, N.C.; Karbek, B.; Gungunes, A.; Arslan, M.S.; Akkaymak, E.T.; Ucan, B.; Demirci, T.; et al. Effect of L-thyroxin therapy on thyroid volume and carotid artery Intima-media thickness in the patients with subclinical hypothyroidism. *J. Med. Disord.* **2014**, *2*, 1. [CrossRef]
33. Akkoca, A.N.; Özdemir, Z.T.; Özler, G.S.; Karabulut, L. The evaluation of carotid intima thickness in clinical and subclinical hypothyroidism and effects of thyroid hormone treatment. *Am. J. Clin. Exp. Med.* **2014**, *2*, 59–63.
34. Gunes, F.; Asik, M.; Temiz, A.; Vural, A.; Sen, H.; Binnetoglu, E.; Bozkurt, N.; Tekeli, Z.; Erbag, G.; Ukinc, K.; et al. Serum H-FABP levels in patients with hypothyroidism. *Wien. Klin. Wochenschr.* **2014**, *126*, 727–733. [CrossRef]
35. Akbaba, G.; Berker, D.; Isık, S.; Tuna, M.M.; Koparal, S.; Vural, M.; Yılmaz, F.M.; Topcuoglu, C.; Guler, S. Changes in the before and after thyroxine treatment levels of adipose tissue, leptin, and resistin in subclinical hypothyroid patients. *Wien. Klin. Wochenschr.* **2016**, *128*, 579–585. [CrossRef] [PubMed]
36. Zha, K.; Zuo, C.; Wang, A.; Zhang, B.; Zhang, Y.; Wang, B.; Wang, Y.; Zhao, J.; Gao, L.; Xu, C. LDL in patients with subclinical hypothyroidism shows increased lipid peroxidation. *Lipids Health Dis.* **2015**, *14*, 95. [CrossRef] [PubMed]
37. Tudoran, M.; Tudoran, C. Particularities of endothelial dysfunction in hypothyroid patients. *Kardiol. Pol.* **2015**, *73*, 337–343. [CrossRef]
38. Yazıcı, D.; Özben, B.; Toprak, A.; Yavuz, D.; Aydın, H.; Tarçın, Ö.; Deyneli, O.; Akalın, S. Effects of restoration of the euthyroid state on epicardial adipose tissue and carotid intima media thickness in subclinical hypothyroid patients. *Endocrine* **2015**, *48*, 909–915. [CrossRef] [PubMed]
39. Niknam, N.; Khalili, N.; Khosravi, E.; Nourbakhsh, M. Endothelial dysfunction in patients with subclinical hypothyroidism and the effects of treatment with levothyroxine. *Adv. Biomed. Res.* **2016**, *5*, 38. [CrossRef]
40. França, M.M.; Nogueira, C.R.; Hueb, J.C.; Mendes, A.L.; Padovani, C.R.; Mazeto, G.M.F.d.S. Higher Carotid Intima-Media Thickness in Subclinical Hypothyroidism Associated with the Metabolic Syndrome. *Metab. Syndr. Relat. Disord.* **2016**, *14*, 381–385. [CrossRef] [PubMed]
41. Cerbone, M.; Capalbo, D.; Wasniewska, M.; Alfano, S.; Raso, G.M.; Oliviero, U.; Cittadini, A.; De Luca, F.; Salerno, M. Effects of L-thyroxine treatment on early markers of atherosclerotic disease in children with subclinical hypothyroidism. *Eur. J. Endocrinol.* **2016**, *175*, 11–19. [CrossRef] [PubMed]
42. Isik-Balci, Y.; Agladioglu, S.; Agladioglu, K.; Kilic-Toprak, E.; Kilic-Erkek, O.; Ozhan, B.; Polat, A.; Bor-Kucukatay, M. Impaired Hemorheological Parameters and Increased Carotid Intima-Media Thickness in Children with Subclinical Hypothyroidism. *Horm. Res. Paediatr.* **2016**, *85*, 250–256. [CrossRef]
43. Rahman, F.; Haque, F.S.; Biswas, S.K.; Begum, R.; Hossain, S.; Sharmin, S.; Rahman, M.; Hossain, S.; Nahar, K. Evaluation of Carotid Intima-Medica Thickness in Sub-clinical Hypothyroid Patients. *Bangladesh J. Nucl. Med.* **2016**, *19*, 123–127. [CrossRef]
44. Altay, M.; Karakoç, M.A.; Çakır, N.; Demirtaş, C.Y.; Cerit, E.T.; Aktürk, M.; Ateş, İ.; Bukan, N.; Arslan, M. Serum Total Sialic Acid Level is Elevated in Hypothyroid Patients as an Atherosclerotic Risk Factor. *J. Clin. Lab. Anal.* **2017**, *31*, e22034. [CrossRef]
45. Yadav, Y.; Saikia, U.K.; Sarma, D.; Hazarika, M. Cardiovascular Risk Factors in Children and Adolescents with Subclinical Hypothyroidism. *Indian J. Endocrinol. Metab.* **2017**, *21*, 823–829. [CrossRef]
46. Tanaka, Y.; Furusyo, N.; Kato, Y.; Ueyama, T.; Yamasaki, S.; Ikezaki, H.; Murata, M.; Hayashi, J. Correlation between Thyroid Stimulating Hormone and Renal Function in Euthyroid Residents of Japan: Results from the Kyushu and Okinawa Population Study (KOPS). *J. Atheroscler. Thromb.* **2018**, *25*, 335–343. [CrossRef] [PubMed]
47. Saif, A.; Mousa, S.; Assem, M.; Tharwat, N.; Abdelhamid, A. Endothelial dysfunction and the risk of atherosclerosis in overt and subclinical hypothyroidism. *Endocr. Connect.* **2018**, *7*, 1075–1080. [CrossRef]
48. Yasar, H.Y.; Demirpence, M.; Colak, A.; Yurdakul, L.; Zeytinli, M.; Turkon, H.; Ekinci, F.; Günaslan, A.; Yasar, E. Serum irisin and apelin levels and markers of atherosclerosis in patients with subclinical hypothyroidism. *Arch. Endocrinol. Metab.* **2019**, *63*, 16–21. [CrossRef] [PubMed]
49. Vijayan, V.; Jayasingh, K.; Jayaraman, G.; Green, S.R.; Deyagarasan, E. Assessment of carotid intima-media thickness in hypothyroidism and the effect of thyroid replacement therapy. *Int. J. Adv. Med.* **2018**, *5*, 281–288. [CrossRef]

50. Tan, M.; Korkmaz, H.; Aydin, H.; Doğuç, D.K. FABP4 levels in hypothyroidism and its relationship with subclinical atherosclerosis. *Turk. J. Med. Sci.* **2019**, *49*, 1490–1497. [CrossRef]
51. Farghaly, H.S.; Metwalley, K.A.; Raafat, D.M.; Algowhary, M.; Said, G.M. Epicardial Fat Thickness in Children with Subclinical Hypothyroidism and Its Relationship to Subclinical Atherosclerosis: A Pilot Study. *Horm. Res. Paediatr.* **2019**, *92*, 99–105. [CrossRef]
52. Doğan, A.; Karabulut, A.; Kilinç, F.; Pekkolay, Z.; Tuzcu, A.K. Evaluation of epicardial fat thickness and carotid intima-media thickness in the patients with subclinical and overt hypothyroidism. *J. Contemp. Med.* **2019**, *9*, 145–150. [CrossRef]
53. Soto-García, A.J.; Elizondo-Riojas, G.; Rodriguez-Gutiérrez, R.; Mancillas-Adame, L.G.; González-González, J.G. Carotid Intima-Media Thickness in Patients with Subclinical Hypothyroidism: A Prospective Controlled Study. *Clin. Investig. Med.* **2021**, *44*, E39–E45. [CrossRef]
54. Asoğlu, E.; Akbulut, T.; Doğan, Z.; Asoğlu, R. Evaluation of the aortic velocity propagation, epicardial fat thickness, and carotid intima-media thickness in patients with subclinical hypothyroidism. *Rev. Cardiovasc. Med.* **2021**, *22*, 959–966. [CrossRef] [PubMed]
55. El Hini, S.H.; Mahmoud, Y.Z.; Saedii, A.A.; Mahmoud, S.S.; Amin, M.A.; Mahmoud, S.R.; Matta, R.A. Angiopoietin-like proteins 3, 4 and 8 are linked to cardiovascular function in naïve sub-clinical and overt hypothyroid patients receiving levothyroxine therapy. *Endocr. Connect.* **2021**, *10*, 1570–1583. [CrossRef] [PubMed]
56. Gönülalan, G.; Tanrikulu, Y. The New Anthropometric Measures in Patients with Hypothyroidism Hipotiro idi Hastalarında Yeni Antropometrik Ölçümler. *J. Harran Univ. Med. Fac.* **2021**, *18*, 149–154.
57. Sahu, M.; Mishra, I.; Baliarsinha, A.K.; Choudhury, A.K.; Routray, S.N. Utility of Epicardial Fat Thickness in Subclinical Hypothyroid Children to Determine Existence of Subclinical Atherosclerosis in Them. *Indian J Endocrinol. Metab.* **2022**, *26*, 483–489. [CrossRef] [PubMed]
58. Sharma, M.; Singh, R.; Kaur, H.; Jasdeep, K.G. Study of carotid intima media thickness (Cimt) in patients of subclinical hypothyroidism (SCH). *Eur. J. Mol. Clin. Med.* **2022**, *9*, 572–577.
59. DerSimonian, R.; Laird, N. Meta-analysis in clinical trials. *Control. Clin. Trials* **1986**, *7*, 177–188. [CrossRef] [PubMed]
60. Cochran, W.G. The combination of estimates from different experiments. *Biometrics* **1954**, *10*, 101–129. [CrossRef]
61. Gao, N.; Zhang, W.; Zhang, Y.-Z.; Yang, Q.; Chen, S.-H. Carotid intima-media thickness in patients with subclinical hypothyroidism: A meta-analysis. *Atherosclerosis* **2013**, *227*, 18–25. [CrossRef]
62. Yao, K.; Zhao, T.; Zeng, L.; Yang, J.; Liu, Y.; He, Q.; Zou, X. Non-invasive markers of cardiovascular risk in patients with subclinical hypothyroidism: A systematic review and meta-analysis of 27 case control studies. *Sci. Rep.* **2018**, *8*, 4579. [CrossRef]
63. Sahoo, R.; Krishna, V.; Subrahmaniyan, D.; Dutta, T.; Elangovan, S. Common carotid intima-media thickness in acute ischemic stroke: A case control study. *Neurol. India* **2009**, *57*, 627–630. [CrossRef]
64. Polak, J.F.; Pencina, M.J.; Pencina, K.M.; O'Donnell, C.J.; Wolf, P.A.; D'Agostino, R.B., Sr. Carotid-Wall Intima–Media Thickness and Cardiovascular Events. *N. Engl. J. Med.* **2011**, *365*, 213–221. [CrossRef]
65. Inoue, K.; Ritz, B.; Brent, G.A.; Ebrahimi, R.; Rhee, C.M.; Leung, A.M. Association of Subclinical Hypothyroidism and Cardiovascular Disease with Mortality. *JAMA Netw. Open* **2020**, *3*, e1920745. [CrossRef] [PubMed]
66. Vayá, A.; Giménez, C.; Sarnago, A.; Alba, A.; Rubio, O.; Hernández-Mijares, A.; Cámara, R. Subclinical hypothyroidism and cardiovascular risk. *Clin. Hemorheol. Microcirc.* **2014**, *58*, 1–7. [CrossRef] [PubMed]
67. Godinjak, A.; Velija-Ašimi, Z.; Bureković, A.; Kulić, M.; Gicić, S.; Serdarević, F. Subclinical inflammation: The link between increased cardiovascular riskand subclinical hypothyroidism in postmenopausal women. In CMBEBIH 2017: Proceedings of the International Conference on Medical and Biological Engineering 2017, Sarajevo, Bosnia and Herzegovina, 16–18 March 2017; Badnjevic, A., Ed.; Springer: Singapore, 2017; pp. 235–240.
68. Rizos, C.V.; Elisaf, M.S.; Liberopoulos, E.N. Effects of thyroid dysfunction on lipid profile. *Open Cardiovasc. Med. J.* **2011**, *5*, 76–84. [CrossRef] [PubMed]
69. Åsvold, B.O.; Vatten, L.J.; Nilsen, T.I.; Bjøro, T. The association between TSH within the reference range and serum lipid concentrations in a population-based study. The HUNT Study. *Eur. J. Endocrinol.* **2007**, *156*, 181–186. [CrossRef] [PubMed]
70. Kc, R.; Khatiwada, S.; Deo Mehta, K.; Pandey, P.; Lamsal, M.; Majhi, S. Cardiovascular Risk Factors in Subclinical Hypothyroidism: A Case Control Study in Nepalese Population. *J. Thyroid. Res.* **2015**, *2015*, 305241. [CrossRef]
71. Balagopal, P.; De Ferranti, S.D.; Cook, S.; Daniels, S.R.; Gidding, S.S.; Hayman, L.L.; McCrindle, B.W.; Mietus-Snyder, M.L.; Steinberger, J. Nontraditional Risk Factors and Biomarkers for Cardiovascular Disease: Mechanistic, Research, and Clinical Considerations for Youth. *Circulation* **2021**, *123*, 2749–2769. [CrossRef] [PubMed]
72. Wells, B.J.; Hueston, W.J. Are thyroid peroxidase antibodies associated with cardiovascular disease risk in patients with subclinical hypothyroidism? *Clin. Endocrinol.* **2005**, *62*, 580–584. [CrossRef]
73. Yoo, W.S.; Chung, H.K. Subclinical Hypothyroidism: Prevalence, Health Impact, and Treatment Landscape. *Endocrinol. Metab.* **2021**, *36*, 500–505. [CrossRef]
74. Urgatz, B.; Razvi, S. Subclinical hypothyroidism, outcomes and management guidelines: A narrative review and update of recent literature. *Curr. Med. Res. Opin.* **2023**, *39*, 351–365. [CrossRef]
75. Sato, Y.; Yoshihisa, A.; Kimishima, Y.; Kiko, T.; Watanabe, S.; Kanno, Y.; Abe, S.; Miyata, M.; Sato, T.; Suzuki, S.; et al. Subclinical Hypothyroidism Is Associated with Adverse Prognosis in Heart Failure Patients. *Can. J. Cardiol.* **2018**, *34*, 80–87. [CrossRef]
76. Kannan, L.; Shaw, P.A.; Morley, M.P.; Brandimarto, J.; Fang, J.C.; Sweitzer, N.K.; Cappola, T.P.; Cappola, A.R. Thyroid Dysfunction in Heart Failure and Cardiovascular Outcomes. *Circ. Heart Fail.* **2018**, *11*, e005266. [CrossRef]

77. Corona, G.; Croce, L.; Sparano, C.; Petrone, L.; Sforza, A.; Maggi, M.; Chiovato, L.; Rotondi, M. Thyroid and heart, a clinically relevant relationship. *J. Endocrinol. Investig.* **2021**, *44*, 2535–2544. [CrossRef]
78. Zhao, T.; Chen, B.; Zhou, Y.; Wang, X.; Zhang, Y.; Wang, H.; Shan, Z. Effect of levothyroxine on the progression of carotid intima-media thickness in subclinical hypothyroidism patients: A meta-analysis. *BMJ Open* **2017**, *7*, e016053. [CrossRef]
79. Aziz, M.; Kandimalla, Y.; Machavarapu, A.; Saxena, A.; Das, S.; Younus, A.; Nguyen, M.; Malik, R.; Anugula, D.; Latif, M.A.; et al. Effect of Thyroxin Treatment on Carotid Intima–Media Thickness (CIMT) Reduction in Patients with Subclinical Hypothyroidism (SCH): A Meta-Analysis of Clinical Trials. *J. Atheroscler. Thromb.* **2017**, *24*, 643–659. [CrossRef] [PubMed]
80. Willeit, P.; Tschiderer, L.; Allara, E.; Reuber, K.; Seekircher, L.; Gao, L.; Liao, X.; Lonn, E.; Gerstein, H.C.; Yusuf, S.; et al. Carotid Intima-Media Thickness Progression as Surrogate Marker for Cardiovascular Risk: Meta-Analysis of 119 Clinical Trials Involving 100 667 Patients. *Circulation* **2020**, *142*, 621–642. [CrossRef]
81. Blum, M.R.; Gencer, B.; Adam, L.; Feller, M.; Collet, T.-H.; da Costa, B.R.; Moutzouri, E.; Dopheide, J.; Depairon, M.; Sykiotis, G.P.; et al. Impact of Thyroid Hormone Therapy on Atherosclerosis in the Elderly With Subclinical Hypothyroidism: A Randomized Trial. *J. Clin. Endocrinol. Metab.* **2018**, *103*, 2988–2997. [CrossRef] [PubMed]
82. Pearce, S.H.; Brabant, G.; Duntas, L.H.; Monzani, F.; Peeters, R.P.; Razvi, S.; Wemeau, J.-L. 2013 ETA Guideline: Management of Subclinical Hypothyroidism. *Eur. Thyroid. J.* **2013**, *2*, 215–228. [CrossRef] [PubMed]
83. Razvi, S.; Weaver, J.U.; Butler, T.J.; Pearce, S.H.S. Levothyroxine treatment of subclinical hypothyroidism, fatal and nonfatal cardiovascular events, and mortality. *Arch. Intern. Med.* **2012**, *172*, 811–817. [CrossRef]
84. Surks, M.I.; Hollowell, J.G. Age-specific distribution of serum thyrotropin and antithyroid antibodies in the US population: Implications for the prevalence of subclinical hypothyroidism. *J. Clin. Endocrinol. Metab.* **2007**, *92*, 4575–4582. [CrossRef]

Journal of
Cardiovascular Development and Disease

MDPI

Article

Epidemiological Association of Current Smoking Status with Hypertension and Obesity among Adults Including the Elderly in Korea: Multivariate Analysis of a Nationwide Cross-Sectional Study Excluding Grades 2–3 Hypertension Cases

Sung-Eun Park [1,†], Seyong Jang [2,†], Wi-Young So [3,*,‡] and Junsu Kim [4,*,‡]

1 Sport Medicine Major, Korea National Sport University, Seoul 05541, Republic of Korea; qkrtjddms2@naver.com
2 Department of Taekwondo, College of Arts and Physical Education, Gachon University, Seongnam 13120, Republic of Korea; naganolala@gachon.ac.kr
3 Sport Medicine Major, College of Humanities and Arts, Korea National University of Transportation, Chungju-si 27469, Republic of Korea
4 Department of Sports and Outdoors, College of Bio Convergence, Eulji University, Seongnam 13135, Republic of Korea
* Correspondence: wowso@ut.ac.kr (W.-Y.S.); kim2019@eulji.ac.kr (J.K.); Tel.: +82-43-841-5991 (W.-Y.S.); +82-31-951-3878 (J.K.); Fax: +82-43-841-5990 (W.-Y.S.); +82-50-4177-7005 (J.K.)
† The first two authors (Sung-Eun Park and Seyong Jang) contributed equally to this work.
‡ The corresponding two authors (Wi-Young So and Junsu Kim) contributed equally to this work.

Abstract: Smoking is a major global health issue that contributes to various chronic diseases, while hypertension and obesity are considered significant health concerns due to their associated complications, such as cardiovascular diseases and metabolic disorders. In this study, we investigated the associations between current smoking status, hypertension, and obesity among the Korean population, excluding individuals with high blood pressure (systolic blood pressure $\geq$ 160 mmHg or diastolic blood pressure $\geq$ 100 mmHg) and those taking antihypertensive medications. Data from the 2015 Korea National Fitness Assessment, encompassing 3457 individuals, were analyzed. Logistic regression analysis was used to examine the effects of current smoking and other variables on hypertension and obesity. The results showed that, among the population that excludes specific hypertension criteria, current smoking status was not significantly associated with hypertension or obesity. However, sex and body mass index were significantly associated with hypertension, and age, sex, and blood pressure were significantly associated with obesity. Future research should utilize larger sample sizes and longitudinal designs to confirm these findings and include a broader range of hypertensive participants to better control for potential confounding variables.

Keywords: cross-sectional study; current smoking; epidemiology; hypertension; Korean population; multivariate analysis; obesity

1. Introduction

Smoking, as a worldwide habit, is considered a major risk factor for coronary artery disease, lung cancer, and stroke [1–3]. As a leading cause of death, it is also believed to be preventable through cessation [4]; however, smoking is difficult to quit because of its addictive nature. In fact, it has been reported that over 80% of smokers express a desire to quit, but only approximately 33% actually succeed, with approximately 80% returning to smoking within 6 months [5,6]. In 2015, the global prevalence of hypertension was estimated at approximately 1.13 billion, with a projected increase to 1.5 billion by 2025 and an expected annual death toll of 9.4 million due to complications such as heart disease, stroke, and kidney failure [7,8].

In 2017, smoking and increased systolic blood pressure were reported to be the highest risk factors for premature death in men worldwide [9]. Smoking, considered a major cause of cardiovascular disease, particularly for young adults, is associated with a significantly increased risk of cardiovascular disease later in life [10]. However, the association between smoking and hypertension has not been consistently reported. Some prospective cohort studies have reported smoking to be associated with an increased risk of developing hypertension [11,12], with older male smokers in the UK having higher systolic blood pressure than nonsmokers [13]. In a study in France, smoking was found to be a significant risk factor for hypertension in French men but not in French women [14]. However, other studies have shown that smokers have lower blood pressure than nonsmokers [15–17], indicating that smoking is not a risk factor for hypertension [18–20].

Besides smoking and hypertension, obesity is also a major public health concern worldwide. It is the fifth leading cause of global mortality, with approximately 800 million people classified as obese in 2016, and this is expected to reach approximately 1.12 billion by 2030 [21,22]. The life expectancy of smokers with obesity is approximately 13 years shorter than that of non-obese nonsmokers [23]. However, the relationship between smoking and obesity has also not been fully explored. The World Health Organization (WHO) has reported that regular smokers have a lower body mass index (BMI) than nonsmokers [24], and a cross-sectional study in the UK has reported a lower likelihood of obesity among smokers than among nonsmokers [25]. In contrast, other studies have reported no significant association between smoking and BMI [26,27]. Among Koreans, current smokers have a higher likelihood to have central obesity than nonsmokers, as evaluated by waist circumference [28].

Therefore, health issues, such as smoking, hypertension, and obesity, remain important global concerns, while the relationships among them remain unclear. Ongoing efforts to understand these relationships are crucial for addressing current public health issues. The prevalence of hypertension among Koreans has been steadily increasing, reflecting the aging population of Korea [29]. Additionally, among Korean adolescents, a consistent upward trend in the prevalence of hypertension has been observed, with an annual average change of 6.4%, particularly among those who are overweight or obese, indicating a higher risk of developing hypertension [30]. Similarly, obesity rates have been steadily increasing among Koreans, raising concerns about metabolic health issues, such as diabetes [31,32]. Both hypertension and obesity impose significant economic burdens on the country in terms of healthcare costs [33,34], and the increasing prevalence of these conditions suggests a growing economic burden. Furthermore, smoking remains an important public health issue in Korea. Despite ongoing anti-smoking campaigns, the smoking rate among Korean men remains high, with over 26.3% of males aged 15 and above reported as current smokers as of 2021 [35]. This high prevalence of smoking contributes to various health problems, including respiratory and cardiovascular diseases.

Therefore, in this study, we aimed to investigate the epidemiological associations between current smoking status, hypertension, and obesity in Korean men and women. By analyzing data from a representative national survey, we sought to understand how these factors are interrelated and identify the potential risk factors specific to the Korean population. It is crucial to explore these health issues by considering the unique characteristics and lifestyle factors of Korean men and women. The results of this study are expected to provide foundational data for developing public health strategies focused on the prevention and management of hypertension and obesity, complementing the existing research and guiding future health policies in Korea.

2. Materials and Methods

2.1. Participants

To analyze the relationships between current smoking status, hypertension, and obesity in Korea, the data from the 2015 Korea National Physical Fitness Survey were examined. The survey employed a multistage, stratified random sampling method based on sex, age, and region, using the Neyman allocation method to ensure representativeness. The appropriate sample size was determined, and samples were allocated by region, with the population including male and female adults aged ≥19 years nationwide, excluding Jeju Island. The measurements were conducted by local measurement agencies under the supervision of the main agency and collaborative research institutions [36].

The entire sample of the original survey included 3457 Korean individuals, with 1946 males and 1511 females. The age of all the participants in the survey ranged from 19 to 89 years, with the 89-year-old participants being present only in the male group. Their basic characteristics are presented in Table 1. The raw data did not include any identifiable information, such as name, phone number, home address, or resident registration number; thus, further ethical approval was not pursued. All research procedures were conducted under the control and approval of the Korea Institute of Sport Science and the Korea Ministry of Culture, Sports, and Tourism, adhering to the principles of the Helsinki Declaration.

Table 1. Physical characteristics of the participants.

Variables	Males (n = 1946)	Females (n = 1511)	p
Age (years)	42.77 ± 16.75	47.66 ± 18.79	<0.001 ***
Height (cm)	172.12 ± 6.51	158.53 ± 6.23	<0.001 ***
Weight (kg)	72.28 ± 9.77	56.91 ± 7.59	<0.001 ***
Systolic blood pressure (mmHg)	125.67 ± 11.54	122.17 ± 11.65	<0.001 ***
Diastolic blood pressure (mmHg)	77.05 ± 8.61	74.88 ± 9.15	<0.001 ***
Prevalence of hypertension (n, %)	303 (15.8%)	164 (11.0%)	<0.001 ***
Body mass index (kg/m^2)	24.37 ± 2.81	22.68 ± 3.02	<0.001 ***
Prevalence of obesity (n, %)	720 (37.6%)	310 (20.8%)	<0.001 ***
Smoker (yes/no)	512 (26.7%)	31 (2.1%)	<0.001 ***
Breakfast (yes/no)	977 (51.0%)	813 (54.7%)	0.034 *
Sleeping hours (hours/day)	6.58 ± 1.08	6.61 ± 1.14	0.604
Exercise (frequency per week)	2.66 ± 2.01	2.56 ± 2.01	0.215
High stress level (yes/no)	451 (23.6%)	306 (20.6%)	0.039 *

Results are expressed as mean ± standard deviation or n (%). * $p < 0.05$ and *** $p < 0.001$, tested by Mann–Whitney U test and χ^2 test.

2.2. Current Smoking Status

Participants were asked about their current smoking status through a questionnaire, where they selected one of three responses: currently smoking, smoked in the past but no longer smoking, or never smoked. Notably, the detailed information on smoking intensity and frequency was not provided. Therefore, participants were classified as smokers or nonsmokers based on their smoking status at the time of the survey, with former smokers included in the nonsmoking group.

2.3. Hypertension

Blood pressure was measured by nurses using a mercury sphygmomanometer (ALPK, Tokyo, Japan) and a stethoscope. Participants who visited the measurement agency for project participation wore the blood pressure cuff on their right upper arm after a 5 min rest in the seated position. Blood pressure was measured twice with a 2 min interval, and the average systolic blood pressure (SBP) and diastolic blood pressure (DBP) were recorded. The raw data used in this study excluded individuals who were taking antihypertensive medications and those with extremely high blood pressure (Grade 2–3 hypertension, SBP ≥ 160 mmHg or DBP ≥ 100 mmHg), as they had potential risks and limitations for participating in the various measurements [36]. The remaining participants were then classified as having Grade 1 hypertension (SBP ≥ 140 mmHg or DBP ≥ 90 mmHg) or normotensive based on the criteria defined by the American Heart Association [37] and the Korean Society of Hypertension [38]. The blood pressure measurement was conducted only once during the survey, which may not fully account for natural variations and potential measurement errors.

2.4. Obesity

BMI was used to assess obesity. It is calculated by dividing an individual's weight (kg) by the square of their height (m) and is highly correlated with body fat percentage. The WHO Regional Office for the Western Pacific and the Korean Society for the Study of Obesity [39] define obesity as a BMI ≥ 25 kg/m^2. This differs slightly from the criterion that classifies a BMI of $\geq$30 kg/m^2 as indicative of obesity.

2.5. Breakfast Habits, Sleeping Hours, Exercise Frequency, and Stress Level

To analyze the relationships between current smoking status and hypertension and obesity, factors that can influence smoking, such as breakfast habits, sleep duration, exercise frequency, and stress levels, were explored. Participants were asked whether they regularly had breakfast, with response options of "regular breakfast", "irregular breakfast", "skipping breakfast daily", and "replacing with snacks". Those who reported having regular breakfast were classified as having a breakfast habit. Participants were also asked about their average daily sleep duration and the number of times per week they exercised for at least 30 min and broke a sweat. Additionally, participants were asked to rate their daily stress levels on a 5-point scale, and those who responded "very high" or "high" were classified as the high stress group, and those who responded "moderate", "low", or "very low" as the moderate stress group.

2.6. Procedure and Statistical Analysis

All data are presented as mean $\pm$ standard deviation or frequency (%). Mann–Whitney U tests were used to compare continuous variables between groups, and chi-square tests were applied for categorical variables. To evaluate the impact of current smoking on hypertension and obesity, we performed multivariate logistic regression analysis, adjusting for potential confounding factors such as age, sex, blood pressure, BMI, dietary habits (regular breakfast consumption), exercise frequency, sleep duration, and stress levels. The significance level for all statistical tests was set at $p < 0.05$. Statistical analyses were conducted using IBM SPSS Statistics for Windows, Version 26.0 (IBM Corp., Armonk, NY, USA).

3. Results

3.1. Effects of Current Smoking on Hypertension

The logistic regression analysis aimed to examine the impact of smoking on hypertension, excluding individuals with hypertension (SBP $\geq$ 160 mmHg or DBP $\geq$ 100 mmHg) and those taking antihypertensive medications. The results showed that smoking was not a significant predictor of hypertension among the remaining participants. Specifically, the odds ratio for hypertension in smokers, compared with that of nonsmokers, was not statistically significant ($p = 0.731$). This indicates that smoking status did not have a major influence on hypertension, particularly when participants with extremely high blood pressure or those taking antihypertensive medications were excluded. Age was also not a significant predictor of hypertension ($p = 0.338$). Regarding sex, females had a significantly lower probability of hypertension than males, with an odds ratio of 0.721 ($p = 0.004$). Exercise frequency did not significantly predict hypertension ($p = 0.123$), and regular breakfast consumption was also not significant ($p = 0.555$). Similarly, sleep duration was not a significant predictor of hypertension ($p = 0.469$), and high stress levels were not significantly associated with hypertension, compared with moderate stress levels ($p = 0.236$). However, BMI was an important predictor, with a 7.3% increase in the probability of hypertension for every one-unit increase in BMI ($p < 0.001$) (see Table 2).

Table 2. Effect of current smoking on hypertension.

Adults	Beta	S.E.	Wald	df	*p*	Exp (B)	95% C.I. for Exp (B)
Smoker (vs. nonsmoker)	−0.048	0.140	0.118	1	0.731	0.953	(0.725–1.254)
Age (years)	0.003	0.003	0.918	1	0.338	1.003	(0.997–1.009)
Sex (female vs. male)	−0.327	0.115	8.136	1	0.004 **	0.721	(0.576–0.903)
Body mass index (kg/m^2)	0.070	0.017	16.745	1	<0.001 ***	1.073	(1.037–1.109)
Exercise (frequency per week)	−0.041	0.026	2.375	1	0.123	0.960	(0.912–1.011)
Breakfast (yes vs. no)	−0.064	0.108	0.349	1	0.555	0.938	(0.760–1.159)
Sleeping hours (hours/day)	0.033	0.046	0.525	1	0.469	1.034	(0.945–1.130)
Stress (high vs. moderate)	0.142	0.119	1.407	1	0.236	1.152	(0.912–1.456)
Constant	−3.626	0.538	45.365	1	<0.001 ***	0.027	

S.E.: standard error; df: degree of freedom; Exp (B): the odds ratio; C.I.: confidence interval. Note: the reference groups for the categorical variables are nonsmokers for current smoking status, males for sex, individuals who do not eat breakfast regularly for breakfast consumption, and those experiencing moderate stress for stress levels. ** $p < 0.01$ and *** $p < 0.001$, tested by logistic regression analysis.

3.2. Effects of Current Smoking on Obesity

The logistic regression analysis showed that, after excluding individuals with extremely high blood pressure and those taking antihypertensive medications, there was no significant association between current smoker (vs. nonsmoker) and obesity ($p = 0.112$, Exp (B) = 1.184). Age was a significant predictor, with each one-year increase in age associated with a 2.1% increase in the odds of obesity ($p < 0.001$, Exp (B) = 1.021). Women had significantly lower odds of obesity, compared with men, with an odds ratio of 0.428 ($p < 0.001$). Exercise frequency was not a significant predictor of obesity ($p = 0.679$, Exp (B) = 0.992) nor was regular breakfast consumption ($p = 0.233$, Exp (B) = 0.905). Sleep duration was also not a significant predictor ($p = 0.130$, Exp (B) = 0.948), and high stress levels were not significantly associated with obesity, compared with moderate stress ($p = 0.281$, Exp (B) = 1.107). However, both SBP and DBP were significant predictors of obesity. Each one-unit increase in SBP was associated with a 1.0% increase in the odds of obesity ($p = 0.009$, Exp (B) = 1.010), and each one-unit increase in DBP was associated with a 1.8% increase in the odds of obesity ($p < 0.001$, Exp (B) = 1.018) (see Table 3).

Table 3. Effect of current smoking on obesity.

Adults	Beta	S.E.	Wald	df	*p*	Exp (B)	95% C.I. for Exp (B)
Smoker (vs. nonsmoker)	0.169	0.106	2.522	1	0.112	1.184	(0.961–1.458)
Age (years)	0.020	0.002	72.163	1	<0.001 ***	1.021	(1.016–1.025)
Sex (female vs. male)	−0.849	0.087	94.967	1	<0.001 ***	0.428	(0.361–0.508)
Systolic blood pressure (mmHg)	0.010	0.004	6.874	1	0.009 **	1.010	(1.002–1.017)
Diastolic blood pressure (mmHg)	0.018	0.005	12.900	1	<0.001 ***	1.018	(1.008–1.028)
Exercise (frequency per week)	−0.008	0.020	0.171	1	0.679	0.992	(0.953–1.032)
Breakfast (yes vs. no)	−0.099	0.083	1.422	1	0.233	0.905	(0.769–1.066)
Sleeping hours (hours/day)	−0.054	0.036	2.290	1	0.130	0.948	(0.884–1.016)
Stress (high vs. moderate)	0.102	0.094	1.164	1	0.281	1.107	(0.920–1.332)
Constant	−3.656	0.537	46.417	1	<0.001 ***	0.026	

S.E.: standard error; df: degree of freedom; Exp (B): the odds ratio; C.I.: confidence interval. Note: The reference groups for the categorical variables are nonsmokers for current smoking status, males for sex, individuals who do not eat breakfast regularly for breakfast consumption, and those experiencing moderate stress for stress levels. ** $p < 0.01$ and *** $p < 0.001$, tested by logistic regression analysis.

4. Discussion

In this study, we aimed to examine the relationships between current smoking status, hypertension, and obesity among Korean adults and older individuals, excluding individuals with high blood pressure (SBP $\geq$ 160 mmHg or DBP $\geq$ 100 mmHg) and those taking antihypertensive medications. Our research findings showed no significant associations between current smoking status and hypertension or obesity, but it is important to note that the generalizability of the results may be limited by the exclusion of certain hypertensive patients. Additionally, the non-significant associations observed in our study may be attributable to the cross-sectional design, which limited the ability to establish causal relationships. Furthermore, potential confounding factors, such as age-related health interventions and socioeconomic status, may have influenced the results.

However, these findings contrast with several previous studies that have confirmed the important associations between smoking and these health outcomes. For instance, Bowman et al. [11] and Halperin et al. [12] reported that smoking was significantly associated with an increased risk of hypertension over time. The cross-sectional design of our study may have limited the ability to detect such long-term effects, and the discrepancy in results may be due to the differences in research design. Cross-sectional studies provide a snapshot of data at a single point in time, which means they cannot determine the direction of relationships between variables or explain changes over time.

Furthermore, the varying outcomes may be attributed to differences in population demographics and health-related behaviors. For example, our study focused on the Korean population, which may have distinct lifestyle factors and genetic predispositions, compared with the populations explored in previous studies. The influence of cultural and social norms on smoking and health-related behaviors in Korea may also have contributed to the observed differences.

Potential confounding factors, such as age, socioeconomic status, and healthcare accessibility, may have also influenced the results. For instance, as people age, they generally have more frequent blood pressure monitoring, and smoking cessation is often recommended as an intervention for hypertension management with increased attention. This increased attention and medical intervention could act as confounding factors, potentially obscuring the direct effects of smoking on hypertension. Another potential confounding factor is socioeconomic status, which can influence health behaviors, access to healthcare, and overall health outcomes. This behavior may impact the associations between smoking, hypertension, and obesity. Therefore, future research should include socioeconomic variables to more effectively control these confounding factors.

Additionally, while the sample size of our study is substantial, it may not be large enough to detect more subtle associations or interactions between smoking, hypertension, and obesity. These limitations can impact the accuracy and generalizability of our findings. Therefore, the results of this study should be interpreted with caution, and future research should consider a longitudinal design and larger sample sizes to provide more definitive conclusions about causal relationships.

Previous longitudinal studies have examined the relationships between smoking, hypertension, and obesity over time, providing more robust evidence of causal pathways. For instance, some studies have shown that smoking cessation can lead to weight gain, which might complicate the relationship between smoking and hypertension due to the confounding effect of obesity [40,41]. In comparison, our study did not find a significant association between current smoking status and hypertension or obesity. This contrasts with some longitudinal studies that observed a higher incidence of hypertension among smokers over time [11,12]. For example, Bowman et al. found that women who smoked had an increased risk of developing hypertension over a 10-year period, and Halperin et al. reported a significant association between smoking and hypertension in middle-aged and older men, which were not consistent with our findings.

In this study, BMI and blood pressure were identified as significant predictors of hypertension and obesity, while smoking was not a significant factor. This is consistent with some longitudinal studies that have also reported non-significant associations between smoking and hypertension after adjusting for BMI and other covariates [16,17]. Additionally, our study found that females had a significantly lower probability of hypertension than males ($p = 0.004$), and for each unit increase in BMI, the odds of developing hypertension increased by 7.3% ($p < 0.001$). This aligns with general findings that higher BMI is a risk factor for hypertension.

Nicotine increases energy expenditure, suppresses appetite, and can mimic satisfaction derived from food [42,43]. Smoking one cigarette has been shown to increase energy expenditure by 3% within 30 min [44], while smoking four cigarettes can increase it by 3.3% within 3 h [45]. Many people, especially women and adolescents, believe that smoking can prevent obesity [46,47], and the effects of nicotine serve as evidence. In fact, a higher BMI in young women has been associated with smoking, and higher body dissatisfaction has been reported to increase the risk of smoking in both males and females [48]. Smoking initiated by such motivations can prompt overweight individuals to continue or increase their smoking [49]. From a physiological perspective, a higher BMI is associated with increased total blood volume and adipose tissue, which can lead to changes in metabolism, resulting in lower nicotine levels in the bloodstream for the same amount of smoking, potentially leading to increased smoking [49–51]. Additionally, the addictive nature of smoking can make quitting difficult or raise concerns regarding weight gain after quitting [25,52]. More than 80% of smokers express a desire to quit smoking; however, the actual percentage of those who successfully quit smoking is only approximately 33% [5,53]. Among those who successfully quit smoking, more than 80% experience weight gain [40] and 75–80% of quitters return to smoking within 6 months [6].

Previous studies conducted over a long period support the concept that smokers tend to have lower body weight and BMI than nonsmokers [41,54]. Despite these trends, it is important to note that smoking and obesity have a complex relationship influenced by factors such as sex, age, geographical characteristics, physical activity, dietary habits, mental health, and genetic traits [49]. Although a few studies have reported on the chronic metabolic effects of smoking, one study reported that the resting metabolic rate in women decreased by 16% after smoking cessation and remained unchanged until day 60. However, women who resumed smoking on day 30 experienced a 12% decrease in their resting metabolic rate, which returned to baseline by day 60 [55]. This study reported that weight gain occurred due to a decrease in the resting metabolic rate and an increased calorie intake. However, considering that physical activity increases the metabolic rate and that smokers tend to be less physically active than nonsmokers [56], the level of physical activity should be analyzed along with the relationship between smoking and obesity.

Some studies have indicated that weight gain in Caucasians is similar between smokers and nonsmokers, while others have shown that weight gain among African American smokers is lower than that in nonsmokers, implying that smoking does not always reflect a positive impact on weight control [57]. It has also been reported that excessive smoking increases the risk of obesity, while ex-smokers have a higher likelihood of obesity than current smokers and nonsmokers [25]. However, despite many studies confirming weight gain after smoking cessation, there can be individual differences in the amount of weight gain [49]. Additionally, because there may be a U-shaped relationship between smoking and BMI, the complexity of this relationship needs to be considered [55].

In this study, current smokers were defined as those who were smoking at the time of the survey. This limits our understanding of the nuanced relationship between current smoking status, hypertension, and obesity. Additionally, the lack of detailed information on smoking intensity and frequency may affect the accuracy of the research findings on smoking exposure. Future studies should consider not only current smoking status but also the quantity and duration of smoking to address the diversity of smoking behaviors. This should include the impact of previous smoking history and secondhand smoke exposure. Furthermore, self-reported data on smoking status may be subject to bias; hence, the use of objective measurements and biomarkers could help address this limitation. For example, a previous cross-sectional study of Koreans before 2013 found that abdominal obesity was more likely to occur in smokers based on waist circumference but not BMI [28]. Given the evidence that smoking is associated with abdominal obesity, fat distribution, and insulin resistance [58,59], incorporating additional obesity indicators, such as waist circumference, could strengthen the analysis. Exploring the relationship between smoking and diabetes could also provide additional insights into the metabolic consequences of smoking. The blood pressure measurements were conducted only once during the survey, which may not fully account for natural variations and potential measurement errors. Future research should consider integrating multiple measurements over time to obtain more reliable average values.

Given these limitations, future studies should consider including larger and more diverse samples of smokers, as well as a broader range of hypertensive participants. Additionally, the use of longitudinal research designs to track changes over time and the integration of various obesity and metabolic health indicators should be explored in future studies. Particularly, the cultural and social norms around smoking and dietary habits in the context of Korean society may influence health outcomes. Understanding these contextual factors could provide a more comprehensive understanding of the relationships between smoking, hypertension, and obesity. Additionally, expanding the scope of the investigation could contribute to more nuanced discussions on the health impacts of smoking and inform public health strategies to mitigate the adverse effects of smoking. The data used in this study are from 2015; hence, there may be limitations in interpreting and applying the findings to the current situation. While the relationships examined are likely still relevant, future research using more recent data would be necessary to confirm our findings.

5. Conclusions

This study specifically investigated the relationships between current smoking status, hypertension, and obesity among the Korean population, excluding individuals with high blood pressure (SBP $\geq$ 160 mmHg or DBP $\geq$ 100 mmHg) and those taking antihypertensive medications. The results showed no significant associations between active smoking and hypertension or obesity in this limited population. Our findings indicated that current smoking status was not significantly associated with hypertension or obesity, which is consistent with previous reports [16,17] of non-significant associations even after adjusting for confounding factors. However, this contrasts with the findings of prospective studies [11,12], which have indicated important associations in diverse populations. These discrepancies may be attributable to differences in study populations, research designs, measurement methods, and confounding control.

This study adopted a cross-sectional design to collect and analyze large-scale data within limited resources and time. While this was suitable for exploring the initial associations between current smoking status, hypertension, and obesity among Korean adults, the limitations of cross-sectional studies in establishing causal relationships prevented the study from making an appropriate contribution to scientific discussion. To address this, future research efforts should aim to elucidate the causal relationships between smoking, hypertension, and obesity through longitudinal study designs. Furthermore, including larger sample sizes and a broader range of hypertensive participants in future research would enhance the generalizability of the findings, allowing for a more detailed investigation into the complex relationships between smoking, hypertension, and obesity, and their implications for public health.

Author Contributions: Conceptualization, S.-E.P. and S.J.; methodology, W.-Y.S. and J.K.; data collection, S.-E.P. and S.J.; formal analysis, W.-Y.S. and J.K.; investigation, S.-E.P. and S.J.; project administration, W.-Y.S. and J.K.; writing—original draft preparation, S.-E.P. and S.J.; writing—review, and editing, W.-Y.S. and J.K.; visualization, S.-E.P. and S.J.; validation, S.-E.P. and S.J.; supervision, W.-Y.S. and J.K. All authors have read and agreed to the published version of the manuscript.

Funding: This study received no external funding.

Institutional Review Board Statement: Since data sets of the raw data from the Korea National Sports Survey did not include private identifier information, such as name, telephone numbers, home addresses, and social security numbers, ethical approval was not required. Moreover, all study procedures were approved by the Korean Ministry of Culture, Sports and Tourism and conducted in accordance with the principles outlined in the Declaration of Helsinki (protocol code: 2015, approval date: 1 March 2015).

Informed Consent Statement: Informed consent was obtained from all the participants involved in the study.

Data Availability Statement: The data presented in this study are available upon request from the corresponding author. The data are not publicly available because of the protection of personal information.

Acknowledgments: The authors thank the study participants who willingly volunteered to participate in the present study.

Conflicts of Interest: The authors declare no conflicts of interest.

References

1. Tolstrup, J.S.; Hvidtfeldt, U.A.; Flachs, E.M.; Spiegelman, D.; Heitmann, B.L.; Bälter, K.; Goldbourt, U.; Hallmans, G.; Knekt, P.; Liu, S.; et al. Smoking and Risk of Coronary Heart Disease in Younger, Middle-Aged, and Older Adults. *Am. J. Public Health* **2014**, *104*, 96–102. [CrossRef]
2. Hong, S.; Mok, Y.; Jeon, C.; Jee, S.H.; Samet, J.M. Tuberculosis, Smoking and Risk for Lung Cancer Incidence and Mortality. *Int. J. Cancer* **2016**, *139*, 2447–2455. [CrossRef] [PubMed]
3. Peters, S.A.; Huxley, R.R.; Woodward, M. Smoking as a Risk Factor for Stroke in Women Compared with Men: A Systematic Review and Meta-analysis of 81 Cohorts, Including 3,980,359 Individuals and 42,401 Strokes. *Stroke* **2013**, *44*, 2821–2828. [CrossRef] [PubMed]
4. Doll, R.; Peto, R.; Boreham, J.; Sutherland, I. Mortality in Relation to Smoking: 50 Years' Observations on Male British Doctors. *BMJ* **2004**, *328*, 1519. [CrossRef] [PubMed]
5. Hughes, J.R. Motivating and Helping Smokers to Stop Smoking. *J. Gen. Intern. Med.* **2003**, *18*, 1053–1057. [CrossRef] [PubMed]
6. United States Public Health Service; Office of the Surgeon General; Center for Chronic Disease Prevention, & Health Promotion; Office on Smoking: US. *The Health Benefits of Smoking Cessation: A Report of the Surgeon General;* US Department of Health and Human Services, Public Health Service, Centers for Disease Control, Center for Chronic Disease Prevention and Health Promotion, Office on Smoking and Health: Washington, DC, USA, 1990.
7. Cham, B.; Scholes, S.; Ng Fat, L.; Badjie, O.; Mindell, J.S. Burden of Hypertension in the Gambia: Evidence from a National World Health Organization (WHO) STEP Survey. *Int. J. Epidemiol.* **2018**, *47*, 860–871. [CrossRef] [PubMed]
8. Mendis, S.; Puska, P.; Norrving, B.; World Health Organization. *Global Atlas on Cardiovascular Disease Prevention and Control;* World Health Organization: Geneva, Switzerland, 2011.
9. World Health Organization. *Findings from the Global Burden of Disease Study 2017;* Institute for Health Metrics and Evaluation: Seattle, WA, USA, 2018; pp. 23–24.
10. Navar, A.M.; Fine, L.J.; Ambrosius, W.T.; Brown, A.; Douglas, P.S.; Johnson, K.; Khera, A.V.; Lloyd-Jones, D.; Michos, E.D.; Mujahid, M.; et al. Earlier Treatment in Adults with High Lifetime Risk of Cardiovascular Diseases: What Prevention Trials Are Feasible and Could Change Clinical Practice? Report of a National Heart, Lung, and Blood Institute (NHLBI) Workshop. *Am. J. Prev. Cardiol.* **2022**, *12*, 100430. [CrossRef]
11. Bowman, T.S.; Gaziano, J.M.; Buring, J.E.; Sesso, H.D. A Prospective Study of Cigarette Smoking and Risk of Incident Hypertension in Women. *J. Am. Coll. Cardiol.* **2007**, *50*, 2085–2092. [CrossRef] [PubMed]
12. Halperin, R.O.; Gaziano, J.M.; Sesso, H.D. Smoking and the Risk of Incident Hypertension in Middle-Aged and Older Men. *Am. J. Hypertens.* **2008**, *21*, 148–152. [CrossRef]
13. Primatesta, P.; Falaschetti, E.; Gupta, S.; Marmot, M.G.; Poulter, N.R. Association Between Smoking and Blood Pressure: Evidence from the Health Survey for England. *Hypertension* **2001**, *37*, 187–193. [CrossRef]
14. Radi, S.; Lang, T.; Lauwers-Cancès, V.; Chatellier, G.; Fauvel, J.P.; Larabi, L.; De Gaudemaris, R.; IHPAF Group. One-Year Hypertension Incidence and Its Predictors in a Working Population: The IHPAF Study. *J. Hum. Hypertens.* **2004**, *18*, 487–494. [CrossRef] [PubMed]
15. Karvonen, M.; Orma, E.; Keys, A.; Fidanza, F.; Brozek, J. Cigarette Smoking, Serum-Cholesterol, Blood-Pressure, and Body Fatness; Observations in Finland. *Lancet* **1959**, *1*, 492–494. [CrossRef] [PubMed]
16. Green, M.S.; Jucha, E.; Luz, Y. Blood Pressure in Smokers and Nonsmokers: Epidemiologic Findings. *Am. Heart J.* **1986**, *111*, 932–940. [CrossRef]
17. Okubo, Y.; Miyamoto, T.; Suwazono, Y.; Kobayashi, E.; Nogawa, K. An Association Between Smoking Habits and Blood Pressure in Normotensive Japanese Men. *J. Hum. Hypertens.* **2002**, *16*, 91–96. [CrossRef] [PubMed]

18. Li, H.; Tong, W.; Wang, A.; Lin, Z.; Zhang, Y. Effects of Cigarette Smoking on Blood Pressure Stratified by BMI in Mongolian Population, China. *Blood Press.* **2010**, *19*, 92–97. [CrossRef] [PubMed]
19. Thuy, A.B.; Blizzard, L.; Schmidt, M.D.; Luc, P.H.; Granger, R.H.; Dwyer, T. The Association Between Smoking and Hypertension in a Population-Based Sample of Vietnamese Men. *J. Hypertens.* **2010**, *28*, 245–250. [CrossRef] [PubMed]
20. Lee, S.H.; Kim, Y.S.; Sunwoo, S.; Huh, B.Y. A Retrospective Cohort Study on Obesity and Hypertension Risk Among Korean Adults. *J. Korean Med. Sci.* **2005**, *20*, 188–195. [CrossRef] [PubMed]
21. World Health Organization. *Obesity Fact Sheet*; WHO: Geneva, Switzerland, 2016.
22. Kelly, T.; Yang, W.; Chen, C.S.; Reynolds, K.; He, J. Global Burden of Obesity in 2005 and Projections to 2030. *Int. J. Obes.* **2008**, *32*, 1431–1437. [CrossRef]
23. Peeters, A.; Barendregt, J.J.; Willekens, F.; Mackenbach, J.P.; Al Mamun, A.A.; Bonneux, L.; NEDCOM, the Netherlands Epidemiology and Demography Compression of Morbidity Research Group. Obesity in Adulthood and Its Consequences for Life Expectancy: A Life-Table Analysis. *Ann. Intern. Med.* **2003**, *138*, 24–32. [CrossRef]
24. Molarius, A.; Seidell, J.C.; Kuulasmaa, K.; Dobson, A.J.; Sans, S. Smoking and Relative Body Weight: An International Perspective from the WHO MONICA Project. *J. Epidemiol. Community Health* **1997**, *51*, 252–260. [CrossRef]
25. Dare, S.; Mackay, D.F.; Pell, J.P. Relationship Between Smoking and Obesity: A Cross-Sectional Study of 499,504 Middle-Aged Adults in the UK General Population. *PLoS ONE* **2015**, *10*, e0123579. [CrossRef] [PubMed]
26. Zbikowski, S.M.; Jack, L.M.; McClure, J.B.; Deprey, M.; Javitz, H.S.; McAfee, T.A.; Catz, S.L.; Richards, J.; Bush, T.; Swan, G.E. Utilization of Services in a Randomized Trial Testing Phone- and Web-Based Interventions for Smoking Cessation. *Nicotine Tob. Res.* **2011**, *13*, 319–327. [CrossRef]
27. de Oliveira Fontes Gasperin, L.; Neuberger, M.; Tichy, A.; Moshammer, H. Cross-Sectional Association Between Cigarette Smoking and Abdominal Obesity Among Austrian Bank Employees. *BMJ Open* **2014**, *4*, e004899. [CrossRef] [PubMed]
28. Kim, Y.; Jeong, S.M.; Yoo, B.; Oh, B.; Kang, H.C. Associations of Smoking with Overall Obesity, and Central Obesity: A Cross-Sectional Study from the Korea National Health and Nutrition Examination Survey (2010–2013). *Epidemiol. Health* **2016**, *38*, e2016020. [CrossRef]
29. Kim, H.C.; Cho, S.M.J.; Lee, H.; Lee, H.H.; Baek, J.; Heo, J.E.; Korean Society of Hypertension (KSH)—Hypertension Epidemiology Research Working Group. Korea Hypertension Fact Sheet 2020: Analysis of Nationwide Population-Based Data. *Clin. Hypertens.* **2021**, *27*, 8. [CrossRef] [PubMed]
30. Park, P.G.; Park, E.; Kang, H.G. Increasing Trend in Hypertension Prevalence Among Korean Adolescents from 2007 to 2020. *BMC Public Health* **2024**, *24*, 617. [CrossRef]
31. Rhee, E.J. Prevalence and Current Management of Cardiovascular Risk Factors in Korean Adults Based on Fact Sheets. *Endocrinol. Metab.* **2020**, *35*, 85–94. [CrossRef] [PubMed]
32. Choi, H.H.; Choi, G.; Yoon, H.; Ha, K.H.; Kim, D.J. Rising Incidence of Diabetes in Young Adults in South Korea: A National Cohort Study. *Diabetes Metab. J.* **2022**, *46*, 803–807. [CrossRef]
33. World Health Organization. First WHO Report Details Devastating Impact of Hypertension and Ways to Stop It. Available online: https://www.who.int/thailand/news/detail/19-09-2023-first-who-report-details-devastating-impact-of-hypertension-and-ways-to-stop-it (accessed on 12 April 2024).
34. Tremmel, M.; Gerdtham, U.G.; Nilsson, P.M.; Saha, S. Economic Burden of Obesity: A Systematic Literature Review. *Int. J. Environ. Res. Public Health* **2017**, *14*, 435. [CrossRef]
35. Organization for Economic Cooperation and Development. *OECD Data Explorer*; Organization for Economic Cooperation and Development: Republic of Korea, 2023. Available online: https://data-viewer.oecd.org?chartId=4ee5d407-e8da-4ab8-8821-8fc4d81035fa (accessed on 2 June 2024).
36. Korea Institute of Sport Science. *2015 National Physical Fitness Survey Final Results Report*; Korea Ministry of Culture, Sports, and Tourism: Sejong, Republic of Korea, 2016.
37. American Heart Association. High Blood Pressure. Available online: http://www.heart.org/en/health-topics/high-blood-pressure (accessed on 12 April 2024).
38. Korean Society of Hypertension. Hypertension Treatment Guidelines. Available online: http://www.koreanhypertension.org/ (accessed on 12 April 2024).
39. Korean Society for the Study of Obesity (KSSO). Diagnosis and Evaluation of Obesity. Available online: http://www.kosso.or.kr/ (accessed on 12 April 2024).
40. Aubin, H.J.; Farley, A.; Lycett, D.; Lahmek, P.; Aveyard, P. Weight Gain in Smokers After Quitting Cigarettes: Meta-analysis. *BMJ* **2012**, *345*, e4439. [CrossRef]
41. Pednekar, M.S.; Gupta, P.C.; Shukla, H.C.; Hebert, J.R. Association Between Tobacco Use and Body Mass Index in Urban Indian Population: Implications for Public Health in India. *BMC Public Health* **2006**, *6*, 70. [CrossRef] [PubMed]
42. Hofstetter, A.; Schutz, Y.; Jéquier, E.; Wahren, J. Increased 24-Hour Energy Expenditure in Cigarette Smokers. *N. Engl. J. Med.* **1986**, *314*, 79–82. [CrossRef] [PubMed]
43. Audrain-McGovern, J.; Benowitz, N.L. Cigarette Smoking, Nicotine, and Body Weight. *Clin. Pharmacol. Ther.* **2011**, *90*, 164–168. [CrossRef] [PubMed]
44. Dallosso, H.M.; James, W.P.T. The Role of Smoking in the Regulation of Energy Balance. *Int. J. Obes.* **1984**, *8*, 365–375. [PubMed]

45. Collins, L.C.; Cornelius, M.F.; Vogel, R.L.; Walker, J.F.; Stamford, B.A. Effect of Caffeine and/or Cigarette Smoking on Resting Energy Expenditure. *Int. J. Obes. Relat. Metab. Disord.* **1994**, *18*, 551–556. [PubMed]
46. Potter, B.K.; Pederson, L.L.; Chan, S.S.; Aubut, J.A.L.; Koval, J.J. Does a Relationship Exist Between Body Weight, Concerns About Weight, and Smoking Among Adolescents? An Integration of the Literature with an Emphasis on Gender. *Nicotine Tob. Res.* **2004**, *6*, 397–425. [CrossRef] [PubMed]
47. White, M.A. Smoking for Weight Control and Its Associations with Eating Disorder Symptomatology. *Compr. Psychiatry* **2012**, *53*, 403–407. [CrossRef] [PubMed]
48. Howe, L.J.; Trela-Larsen, L.; Taylor, M.; Heron, J.; Munafò, M.R.; Taylor, A.E. Body Mass Index, Body Dissatisfaction and Adolescent Smoking Initiation. *Drug Alcohol Depend.* **2017**, *178*, 143–149. [CrossRef] [PubMed]
49. Taylor, A.E.; Richmond, R.C.; Palviainen, T.; Loukola, A.; Wootton, R.E.; Kaprio, J.; Relton, C.L.; Davey Smith, G.; Munafò, M.R. The Effect of Body Mass Index on Smoking Behaviour and Nicotine Metabolism: A Mendelian Randomization Study. *Hum. Mol. Genet.* **2019**, *28*, 1322–1330. [CrossRef]
50. Prather, R.D.; Tu, T.G.; Rolf, C.N.; Gorsline, J. Nicotine Pharmacokinetics of NicoDerm (Nicotine Transdermal System) in Women and Obese Men Compared with Normal-Sized Men. *J. Clin. Pharmacol.* **1993**, *33*, 644–649. [CrossRef]
51. Jain, R.B.; Bernert, J.T. Effect of Body Mass Index and Total Blood Volume on Serum Cotinine Levels Among Cigarette Smokers: NHANES 1999–2008. *Clin. Chim. Acta* **2010**, *411*, 1063–1068. [CrossRef] [PubMed]
52. Beebe, L.A.; Bush, T. Post-cessation Weight Concerns Among Women Calling a State Tobacco Quitline. *Am. J. Prev. Med.* **2015**, *48* (Suppl. S1), S61–S64. [CrossRef] [PubMed]
53. Rigotti, N.A. Clinical Practice. Treatment of Tobacco Use and Dependence. *N. Engl. J. Med.* **2002**, *346*, 506–512. [CrossRef] [PubMed]
54. Sneve, M.; Jorde, R. Cross-Sectional Study on the Relationship Between Body Mass Index and Smoking, and Longitudinal Changes in Body Mass Index in Relation to Change in Smoking Status: The Tromsø Study. *Scand. J. Public Health* **2008**, *36*, 397–407. [CrossRef] [PubMed]
55. Moffatt, R.J.; Owens, S.G. Cessation from Cigarette Smoking: Changes in Body Weight, Body Composition, Resting Metabolism, and Energy Consumption. *Metabolism* **1991**, *40*, 465–470. [CrossRef] [PubMed]
56. Klesges, R.C.; Eck, L.H.; Isbell, T.R.; Fulliton, W.; Hanson, C.L. Smoking Status: Effects on the Dietary Intake, Physical Activity, and Body Fat of Adult Men. *Am. J. Clin. Nutr.* **1990**, *51*, 784–789. [CrossRef] [PubMed]
57. Klesges, R.C.; Ward, K.D.; Ray, J.W.; Cutter, G.; Jacobs, D.R., Jr.; Wagenknecht, L.E. The Prospective Relationships Between Smoking and Weight in a Young, Biracial Cohort: The Coronary Artery Risk Development in Young Adults Study. *J. Consult. Clin. Psychol.* **1998**, *66*, 987–993. [CrossRef] [PubMed]
58. Eliasson, B. Cigarette Smoking and Diabetes. *Prog. Cardiovasc. Dis.* **2003**, *45*, 405–413. [CrossRef]
59. Houston, T.K.; Person, S.D.; Pletcher, M.J.; Liu, K.; Iribarren, C.; Kiefe, C.I. Active and Passive Smoking and Development of Glucose Intolerance Among Young Adults in a Prospective Cohort: CARDIA Study. *BMJ* **2006**, *332*, 1064–1069. [CrossRef]

Journal of
Cardiovascular Development and Disease

MDPI

Article

Cutoff Values of Aldosterone and the Aldosterone–Renin Ratio for Predicting Primary Aldosteronism in Patients with Resistant Hypertension: A Real-Life Study

João Vicente da Silveira [1,2], Carine Sangaleti [3], Cleber Camacho [1], Ana Alice Wolf Maciel [4], Maria Claudia Irigoyen [2], Thiago Macedo [2], José Jayme G. De Lima [2], Luciano F. Drager [2,4], Luiz Aparecido Bortolotto [2], Heno Ferreira Lopes [2,*], Madson Q. Almeida [5], Brent M. Egan [6,7] and Fernanda Marciano Consolim-Colombo [1,2]

1 Medical School, Universidade Nove de Julho—Uninove, São Paulo 04101-200, Brazil; joao.silveira@uol.com.br (J.V.d.S.); camacho@uninove.br (C.C.); hipfernada@incor.usp.br (F.M.C.-C.)
2 Cardiology Department, Unidade de Hipertensão, Instituto do Coração—Universidade de São Paulo—HC-FMUSP, São Paulo 05403-000, Brazil; hipirigoyen@gmail.com (M.C.I.); thiago.cardio@gmail.com (T.M.); jose.lima@incor.usp.br (J.J.G.D.L.); luciano.drager@incor.usp.br (L.F.D.); hipbortolotto@gmail.com (L.A.B.)
3 Nurse Department, Universidade Estadual do Centro-Oeste—Unicentro, Guarapuava 85040-167, Brazil; carineteles@unicentro.br
4 Unidade de Hipertensão, Disciplina de Nefrologia—Universidade de São Paulo—HC-FMUSP, São Paulo 05403-010, Brazil; anaalice.wolf@gmail.com
5 Laboratório de Endocrinologia Molecular e Celular LIM/25, Disciplina de Endocrinologia e Metabologia, Hospital das Clínicas, Faculdade de Medicina da Universidade de São Paulo (FMUSP), São Paulo 05403-010, Brazil; madsonalmeida@gmail.com
6 Cardiovascular Health, American Medical Association, Medical University of South Carolina, Greenville, SC 29425, USA; brent.egan@ama-assn.org
7 Medicine and Nursing, Medical University of South Carolina, Charleston, SC 29425, USA
* Correspondence: hipheno@gmail.com

Abstract: Primary aldosteronism (PA) is commonly associated with resistant hypertension. Biochemical tests can be clinically useful in the screening and diagnosis of primary aldosteronism. This study aimed to identify the cutoff values of aldosterone levels (A) and the aldosterone–renin ratio (ARR) for an accurate prediction of PA in patients with apparent resistant hypertension in a real-life scenario. This database-based study included a historical cohort of male and female patients with apparent resistant hypertension, aged 18 years or older and surveyed for PA in a specialized center from 2008 to 2018. Aldosterone and plasma renin activity (PRA) or the plasma renin concentration (PRC) were measured in the treated hypertensive patients. The patients with positive screening results were subsequently referred to the endocrinology department for confirmatory tests. The patients with confirmed PA were included in the case group, and the others remained as controls. Receiver-operating characteristic (ROC) curves were used to identify the cutoff points for aldosterone and the ARR, thereby analyzing their sensitivity and specificity for confirmed PA. Among the 3464 patients (59 $\pm$ 13 years old, 41% male) who had apparent resistance hypertension screened, PA was confirmed in 276 individuals (8%). A $\geq$ 16.95 ng/dL (95% CI: 0.908–0.933) had an odds ratio of 6.24 for PA, while A/PRA $\geq$ 29.88 (95% CI: 0.942–0.984) or an A/PRC $\geq$ 2.44 (95% CI: 0.978–0.990) had an odds ratio of 216.17 for PA diagnoses. Our findings suggest that a positive PA screening with aldosterone $\geq$ 17 ng/dL associated with A/PRA $\geq$ 29.88 or an A/PRC ratio of $\geq$2.44 should be sufficient to confirm the diagnosis of PA without confirmatory testing.

Keywords: primary aldosteronism; secondary hypertension; aldosterone–renin ratio; aldosterone; apparently resistant hypertension; reference value

1. Introduction

Recent guidelines define primary aldosteronism (PA) as a group of disorders in which aldosterone production is inappropriately high and relatively autonomous from the physiological control of the renin–angiotensin system [1–6]. Such inappropriate aldosterone production causes sodium retention and potassium excretion, hypertension, cardiovascular damage, and the suppression of plasma renin [7,8].

Initially, PA was considered a rare form of secondary hypertension. However, cross-sectional and prospective studies report PA in 3 to 10% of hypertensive patients in general, reaching a higher prevalence in particular settings such as resistant hypertension (patients with a blood pressure greater than 140/90 mmHg using three antihypertensive drugs, including diuretics) [9–12]. There are two main etiologies of PA: aldosterone-producing adenoma, as described by Cohn in 1955, which accounts for approximately 30–40% of cases, and idiopathic aldosteronism or bilateral adrenal hyperplasia, which is detected in approximately 60–70% of cases [13,14]. Germline mutations affecting genes in aldosterone synthesis may generate a small fraction of rare cases of PA [15]. The early detection of PA enables targeted treatment, enhances blood pressure control rates, and reduces associated cardiovascular morbidity and mortality. Unfortunately, recent studies indicate insufficient rates of PA screening among hypertensive patients, including those with apparent treatment-resistant hypertension (only 2%) [16–18]. Screening for PA aims to distinguish between this secondary cause of hypertension and essential (primary) hypertension [18].

A high plasma aldosterone concentration is a hallmark of PA, while the most reliable tool for PA screening is a high aldosterone–renin ratio (ARR) [19]. Current guidelines suggest that aldosterone levels surpassing 12–15 ng/dL are a reliable indicator of PA [1,6]. Plasma renin activity (PRA) [20,21] or the direct plasma renin concentration (PRC) [22,23] are considered the main methods for conducting screening tests in patients with PA. Nevertheless, the consensus on the definitive cutoff values for the ARR must be improved, as they may vary depending on several factors, including the use of medications [22–25]. The actual advised cutoff for the A/PRA ratio is 20 to 30 (ng/d)/(ng/mL/h). Regarding the A/PRC ratio, the guidelines suggest a cutoff of 2.0 to 2.5 ng/dl, but several publications consider a more extensive range of values from 1.0 to 5.7 (ng/dL)/(μU/mL) [26–28].

After a positive screening, subsequent evaluations are mandatory to confirm PA and its etiology. These assessments include protocols to evaluate the adrenal gland at functional, structural, and even molecular levels and require specialized centers and economic resources [7,8,14,15]. In this scenario, the delayed detection of PA negatively impacts the prognosis of the patients [18,19].

In the present study, we aimed to investigate the cutoff values of the aldosterone level, the A/PRA ratio, and the A/PRC ratio that best predict PA in a large cohort of patients who were referred to a tertiary hospital for the evaluation of treatment-resistant hypertension. This information would reinforce the importance of PA screening and reduce delays in the diagnosis and appropriate treatment of PA in this high-risk population.

2. Material and Methods

2.1. Study Population

This study analyzed medical records from hypertensive individuals treated at the University of São Paulo's Heart Institute/Clinical Hospital between 2008 and 2018, with ethical approval by the Institution's Human Research Committee of Hospital das Clinicas—Sao Paulo University (Protocol SDC-COP 105.19.011, approved on 30 March 2019). Adult patients with treatment-resistant severe hypertension underwent aldosterone and renin testing while on antihypertensive medication. However, the patients were instructed to discontinue mineralocorticoid receptor antagonists four weeks prior to the test, in accordance with guidelines [1–6]. We removed duplicates and incomplete records, and excluded patients with chronic kidney disease, dialysis, or severe systemic diseases. The data collected included demographics, blood pressure measures, and laboratory test results, such as creatinine, electrolytes, glucose, and HbA1C. The estimated glomerular filtration rate (eGFR) was determined using appropriate formulas, and 24 h urine sodium was measured.

Morning venous blood samples were collected after the patients had been out of bed for at least 2 h and typically after they had been seated for 5–15 min for aldosterone and renin assays. In 2012, the assay method transitioned from radioimmunoassay to chemiluminescence-based methods [7,25].

We set the aldosterone thresholds at 10 ng/dL for proceeding with the PA investigation, adjusting the PRA and PRC values to reduce false positives. An A/PRA ratio $\geq$ 30 ng/mL/h and an A/PRC ratio $\geq$ 2.5 ng/dL indicated positive screening.

Positive screening led to referral for further PA confirmation and etiology assessment at the Endocrine Division, which included functional tests and adrenal imaging [7,25]. Only the patients who completed the diagnostic process and received PA treatment were included in the case group, and the rest served as controls (Figure 1).

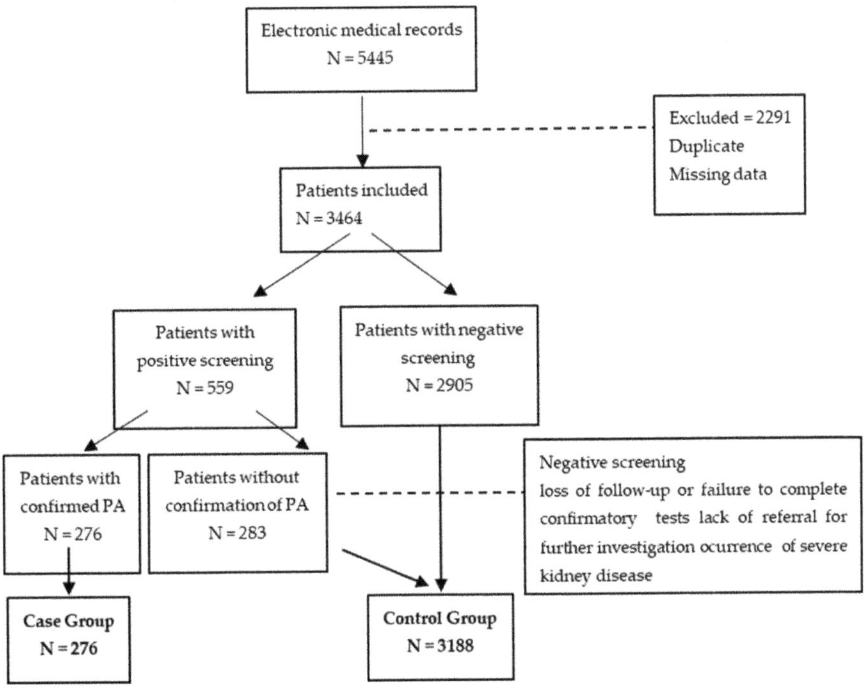

Figure 1. Flow chart of the protocol.

2.2. Statistical Analysis

The descriptive statistics included frequencies and summary statistics, and the data are expressed as the mean $\pm$ SD. Chi-square tests were used to analyze the categorical variables, while nonparametric tests (Mann–Whitney or Fisher's Exact tests) were used for the data that were not normally distributed. ROC curves determined the cutoffs for aldosterone and the ARR, while logistic regressions evaluated the predictors of PA. The Hosmer and Lemeshow test assessed the model fit, with the CHAID (Chi-Square Interaction Detector) algorithm aiding in the multivariate analysis. The Bonferroni correction was applied, and a 5% significance level was used for all the tests. The analyses were conducted using IBM SPSS Software, version 25.0 (Armonk, NY, USA).

3. Results

The database initially held 5445 records; after exclusions, 3464 the patients remained for the analysis. Of these, 559 (16.1%) had a positive PA screen with aldosterone >10 ng/dL and a high ARR; 276 were diagnosed with PA and constituted the case group, while the others were considered as controls.

Table 1 describes the study cohort, showing an average age of 59 years, an overweight status, and a high systolic blood pressure, despite treatment. Serum potassium was normal on average, while creatinine and HbA1c were slightly elevated. Most the patients (70%) had the PRA measured, with an average A/APR ratio of 17.4 ± 3.7 and a median of 8.0. The PRC was available for 30%, yielding an average A/PRC ratio of 1.9 ± 0.4). The study population was predominantly female (60%). Compared to the men, the women had higher blood pressure and HbA1C values, while the men had higher creatinine levels, a lower eGFR, and higher urinary sodium excretion.

Table 1. Characteristics of all included patients and stratified by sex-based groups.

	Total	Mean ± SD	Female	Mean ± SD	Male	Mean ± SD	p
	Number		Number		Number		
Age (years old)	(3464)	58.90 ± 13.1	2060	59.60 ± 12.90	1404	57.80 ± 13.2	<0.001
BMI (kg/m^2)	(3302)	29.01 ± 5.60	1965	29.89 ± 6.02	1337	29.33 ± 4.90	0.109
SBP (mmHg)	(3328)	159.58 ± 30.84	1978	160.71 ± 31.14	1350	157.92 ± 30.32	0.007
DBP (mmHg)	(3328)	95.75 ± 17.94	1978	95.59 ± 17.70	1350	95.98 ± 18.30	0.857
Creatinine (mg/dL)	(3432)	1.28 ± 1.14	2036	1.10 ± 0.87	1396	1.54 ± 1.41	<0.001
GFR (mL/min/1.73 m^2)	(3305)	86.30 ± 38.72	1969	91.45 ± 39.86	1336	78.71 ± 35.64	<0.001
K$^+$ (mEq/L)	(3259)	4.25 ± 0.57	2040	4.28 ± 0.52	1390	4.24 ± 0.58	0.857
Urinary Na$^+$ (mEq/L)	(2205)	173.84 ± 82.04	1329	157.37 ± 71.97	876	198.88 ± 89.71	<0.001
HbA1c (%)	(2979)	6.51 ± 2.21	1787	6.57 ± 2.48	1192	6.42 ± 1.72	0.021
Aldosterone (ng/dL)	(3464)	13.45 ± 16.70	2060	13.13 ± 18.69	1404	13.92 ± 13.24	<0.001
PRA (ng/mL/h)	(2414)	3.88 ± 8.83	1366	2.13 ± 4.48	1048	6.15 ± 12.01	<0.001
A/PRA	(2414)	17.44 ± 36.97	1366	18.57 ± 44.29	1048	15.96 ± 24.28	<0.001
PRC (μUI/mL)	(1050)	57.74 ± 108.44	694	48.41 ± 93.07	356	75.92 ± 131.68	0.157
A/PRC	(1050)	1.87 ± 3.83	694	1.74 ± 3.75	356	2.12 ± 3.97	0.459

Data are expressed as the mean ± SD. BMI: body mass index; SBP: systolic blood pressure, DBP: diastolic blood pressure; GFR: glomerular filtration rate; K$^+$: concentration of serum potassium; HbA1c: glycated hemoglobin; A/PRA: aldosterone to plasma renin activity ratio; A/PRC: aldosterone to plasma renin concentration ratio.

Table 2 indicates that using an A/PRA ratio ≥ 30, 14.7% of the patients screened positively, while with an A/PRC ratio ≥ 2.0, the value was 19.5%. The men had a higher positive screening prevalence. Of the patients with positive screens, 347 were further investigated at the Endocrine Service, 276 had confirmed PA, and 71 did not. The case group (n = 276) was used for the statistical analysis, with the remainder serving as controls (n = 3188).

The ROC curve analysis (Table 3) showed that an aldosterone level of ≥16.95 ng/dL had a sensitivity of 84.8% and a specificity of 83.4%, but the accuracy was 8.5%. An A/PRA ratio ≥ 29.88 and an A/PRC ratio ≥ 2.44 demonstrated high accuracy (90.4% and 93.8%, respectively), sensitivity, and specificity, with high positive and negative predictive values.

The cases (Table 4) were younger and had lower blood pressures and potassium levels compared to the controls. As expected, the mean aldosterone level was higher in the case group. Additionally, the median A/PRA and A/PRC levels were notably higher in the case group than in the controls.

Table 2. Prevalence of positive screening for primary aldosteronism according to sex, considering both aldosterone and aldosterone–renin ratios.

	Total		Sex				p
			Female		Male		
	Cases/Total	% (95% CI)	Cases/Total	% (95% CI)	Cases/Total	% (95% CI)	
Aldosterone > 10 and A/PRA ≥ 30 or A/PRC ≥ 2.5	559/3464	16.1 (14.9–17.4)	297/2060	14.4 (1.9–15.9)	262/1404	18.7 (16.6–20.7)	<0.001
Aldosterone > 10 and A/PRA ≥ 30	354/2414	14.7 (13.3–16.1)	174/1366	12.7 (11.0–14.5)	180/1048	17.2 (14.9–19.5)	<0.001
Aldosterone > 10 and A/PRC ≥ 2.5	205/1050	19.5 (17.1–21.9)	123/694	17.7 (14.9–20.6)	82/356	23.0 (18.6–27.4)	0.120

Data are expressed as the mean ± SD and median; p = descriptive level of the Chi-square test. A/PRA: aldosterone to plasma renin activity ratio; A/PRC: aldosterone to plasma renin concentration ratio.

Table 3. Cutoff, sensitivity, specificity, and positive and negative predictive values (% and 95% confidence intervals) of clinical variables for confirmed primary aldosteronism.

	Cutoff Value	Sensitivity % (95% CI)	Specificity % (95% CI)	Predictive Value Positive % (95% CI)	Predictive Value Negative % (95% CI)	Overall Accuracy [1] (%)	ROC (95% CI)	N
Aldosterone (ng/dL)	≥16.95	84.8 (80.0–88.8)	83.4 (82.1–84.7)	30.7 (27.4–34.1)	98.4 (97.9–98.9)	8.5	0.920 (0.908–0.933)	3464
A/PRA	≥29.88	96.2 (91.4–98.8)	90.1 (88.8–91.3)	35.9 (30.9–41.1)	99.8 (99.4–99.9)	90.4	0.963 (0.942–0.984)	2414
A/PRC	≥2.44	99.3 (96.2–100.0)	92.9 (91.1–94.5)	69.2 (62.5–75.4)	99.9 (9.3–100.0)	93.8	0.984 (0.978–0.990)	1050

[1] Overall accuracy = percentage of correct classification.

Table 4. Comparison of clinical and laboratory parameters between confirmed cases (primary aldosteronism) and control groups.

	Groups		p
	Control	Case	
Male, number/total (%)	40.5%	40.9%	0.885[a]
Age (years old) N, Mean ± SD	59.2 ± 13.1	54.8 ± 12	<0.001
BMI (kg/m^2) N, Mean ± SD	29.68 ± 5.65	29.31 ± 4.83	0.426
SBP (mmHg) N, Mean ± SD	160.43 ± 30.6	147.7 ± 31.73	<0.001
DBP (mmHg) N, Mean ± SD	96.12 ± 17.94	90.52 ± 17.19	<0.001
Creatinine (mg/dL) N, Mean ± SD	1.29 ± 1.18	1.10 ± 0.54	0.021
K^+ (mEq/L) N, Mean ± SD	4.29 ± 0.52	3.72 ± 0.84	<0.001
Urinary Na^+ (mEq/L) N, Mean ± SD	174.2 ± 82.25	160.05 ± 73.11	0.301
HbA1c (%) N, Mean ± SD	6.51 ± 1.53	6.55 ± 6.37	0.803
Aldosterone (ng/dL) N, Mean ± SD	11.19 ± 10.48	39.57 ± 38.67	<0.001
A/PRA N, Mean ± SD	12.64 ± 18.04	100.13 ± 101.58	<0.001
A/PRC N, Mean ± SD	0.81 ± 1.29	8.46 ± 6.75	<0.001

BMI: body mass index; SBP: systolic blood pressure, DBP: diastolic blood pressure; K^+: concentration of serum potassium; HbA1c: glycated hemoglobin; A/PRA: aldosterone to plasma renin activity ratio; A/PRC: aldosterone to plasma renin concentration ratio.

Multivariate logistic regression (Table 5) showed that for every 1 mEq/L increase in potassium, the odds of PA decreased by 45%. The patients with aldosterone ≥ 16.95 ng/dL or an A/APR ≥ 29.88 or an A/PRC ≥ 2.44 were substantially more likely to have confirmed PA, highlighting the need for precise evaluation in these patients.

Table 5. Adjusted odds ratio of potassium, aldosterone, and aldosterone–renin ratios in predicting primary aldosteronism.

	Final Model	
	Adjusted Odds Ratio (95% CI)	***p***
K^+ (mEq/L)	0.55 (0.39–0.77)	<0.001
Aldosterone ≥ 16.95 ng/dL (ROC)	6.24 (3.97–9.81)	<0.001
A/PRA ≥ 29.88 or A/PRC ≥ 2.44	216.17 (86.34–541.22)	<0.001

A/PRA: aldosterone to plasma renin activity ratio; A/PRC: aldosterone to plasma renin concentration ratio.

4. Discussion

Primary aldosteronism, marked by high aldosterone and suppressed renin levels, is often under-recognized, despite its prevalence of up to 20% in resistant hypertension. Our retrospective, single-center study confirmed a significantly higher likelihood of diagnosing PA with higher aldosterone levels and a higher ARR. We focused on the patients with uncontrolled hypertension who were on multiple medications, finding a mean blood pressure of almost 160/96 mmHg across the cohort. The average age was 58.9 years, with the females being slightly older, and the males showing lower glomerular filtration rates, indicating a high cardiovascular risk profile requiring diligent evaluation for secondary hypertension. Medication adjustments were avoided due to the risks involved in our severely hypertensive cohort. Our aldosterone threshold (>10 ng/dL) was lower than the guidelines suggest, minimizing the potential false negatives. Over a decade, we screened 2414 the patients with PRA and 1050 with PRC, identifying a significant PA prevalence.

Among the patients completing the diagnostic algorithm, 80% confirmed PA, with a higher-than-average incidence of adenoma (68%). Those with bilateral hyperplasia received targeted medication. The 20% false-positive rate for PA screening was lower than previously reported, suggesting our tests effectively minimized unnecessary confirmatory testing. Although in a recent review the authors suggested repeating aldosterone and renin measurements to increase the sensitivity of the ARR in diagnosing PA, in our study, only one sample proved to be sensitive for diagnosing PA [29].

The ROC curve analysis helped refine the diagnostic criteria, though a potential verification bias exists due to the absence of confirmatory tests for "negative" screening results. Our control group definition aligned with those of recent studies, which vary considerably in similar research. The aldosterone cutoff of ≥16.95 ng/dL exceeded guideline recommendations, yielding high sensitivity and specificity, but a modest positive predictive value. The A/PRA ratio threshold closely matched the upper guideline limit, with high accuracy and an excellent negative predictive value. The A/PRC ratio cutoff demonstrated high accuracy and excellent predictive values, outperforming those in the patients who ceased antihypertensives in previous studies. The multivariate analysis indicated that an aldosterone level ≥ 16.95 ng/dL and ARR values above our cutoffs substantially increased the PA risk. The cases of confirmed PA were generally younger, with lower blood pressures and potassium levels, but no single clinical or laboratory feature stood out as a definitive PA indicator. Plasma renin and aldosterone levels usually decrease with age, but renin decreases more, raising the A/R ratio in older individuals. Optimal A/PRC ratio cutoffs vary by age group: >3.7 for those ≥60 years, 2.0 for 40–59 years, and 1.0 for <40 years. Our study, with an average participant age of 60 years and a chosen A/PRC cutoff of ≥2.44, suggests that age-related adjustments may be necessary. Although the mean serum potassium was within the normal range, the lower levels identified in the case group support that normokalaemia does not rule out PA, as most of the patients would be missed. Our analysis also indicated that every 1 mEq/L increase in potassium decreased the PA odds by

45%. Hypokalemia is indeed a common feature of primary aldosteronism (PA), although it is not always present [1–6]. Studies have shown that only approximately 30–40% of patients with PA exhibit significant hypokalemia [1–6]. This study's result demonstrated that a 1 mEq/L increase in serum potassium was associated with a 45% decrease in the odds of PA. Conversely, higher serum potassium levels may suggest a lower likelihood of PA, as the excess aldosterone would typically drive potassium levels down. The multivariate logistic regression analysis, which likely accounted for potential confounders, strengthened the validity of this association between serum potassium and the odds of PA. The aldosterone/potassium (A/K) ratio, also known as the aldosterone–potassium ratio (APR), has been proposed as a simple screening tool for PA [30]. An elevated APR suggests an increased likelihood of PA, and some studies have demonstrated its usefulness in identifying the patients who should undergo further testing for PA.

Moreover, a recent publication by Puar et al. (2020) [30] described that the aldosterone-to-lowest-potassium ratio is a convenient score to guide the clinicians of patients of various ethnicities on the probability of the primary aldosteronism subtype. The authors concluded that using the APR to identify the patients more likely to benefit from adrenal vein sampling (AVS) may be a cost-effective strategy to manage this common condition. We intend to calculate the aldosterone–potassium ratio and compare the results with the aldosterone–renin ratio (ARR) in a future publication, as it was not the main objective of the present study.

Some final considerations need to be addressed. Renin synthesis is influenced by prostaglandins and cyclooxygenase (COX) activity, with NSAIDs impacting these factors and consequently affecting renin levels [31]. Prostaglandins such as prostacyclin (PGI2) and prostaglandin E2 (PGE2) stimulate renin secretion and are synthesized by COX-1 and COX-2. NSAIDs inhibit COX activity, reducing prostaglandin synthesis and, thus, renin secretion [31]. Research indicates that COX-2 inhibitors can significantly decrease plasma renin levels and renal renin activity [32,33]. Randomized crossover studies in healthy individuals have shown that COX-2 inhibitors, like rofecoxib and meloxicam, inhibit renin release when administered with furosemide or a low-sodium diet [33]. Consequently, NSAID use can affect the interpretation of the aldosterone–renin ratio (ARR), and it is advisable to discontinue these medications before testing. In our study, we did not differentiate the data based on NSAID use, nor did we specifically screen for chronic NSAID use. Although the patients were instructed to avoid NSAIDs before the confirmatory tests, we cannot rule out short-term use at the time of screening. This represents a limitation of our study and may have influenced the results. Future research should collect detailed information on NSAID use and account for this factor in the data analysis.

Limitations of the Study

While our study provides valuable insights into PA screening, several limitations merit consideration. The single-center, retrospective design may limit the generalizability across diverse populations. Although justified by our high-risk cohort, the absence of an antihypertensive medication washout period could have influenced the screening outcomes. Future research should stratify the results by ethnicity, age group, and medication use, including NSAIDs, to offer more nuanced insights. The potential verification bias due to the absence of confirmatory tests for negative screenings necessitates a prospective study design with universal confirmatory testing. Lastly, our study did not explore the aldosterone–potassium ratio (APR) as a screening tool, which recent studies suggest may be valuable, particularly in diverse ethnic populations.

5. Conclusions

In conclusion, our data suggest that aldosterone $\geq$ 17 ng/dL with an A/PRA $\geq$ 29.88 or an A/PRC $\geq$ 2.44 could reliably diagnose PA without additional testing.

Author Contributions: Project development, J.V.d.S., A.A.W.M., T.M., J.J.G.D.L. and L.F.D.; research design, F.M.C.-C., J.V.d.S., M.Q.A. and M.C.I.; the responsibility for the data analysis, J.V.d.S., C.S. and C.C.; the interpretation of the results, F.M.C.-C., L.F.D., L.A.B., M.Q.A., B.M.E. and H.F.L.; manuscript writing, F.M.C.-C., L.F.D., L.A.B., M.Q.A. and H.F.L.; manuscript editing, H.F.L., F.M.C.-C. and M.Q.A. All authors have read and agreed to the published version of the manuscript.

Funding: L.F.D., L.A.B., M.C.I., M.Q.A. and F.M.C.-C. received financial support from governmental agencies, the CNPQ (Conselho Nacional de Desenvolvimento Científico e Tecnológico) and the FAPESP (Fundacao de Amparo a Pesquisa do Estado de São Paulo).

Institutional Review Board Statement: This study was conducted in accordance with the Declaration of Helsinki and approved by the Institution's Human Research Committee of Hospital das Clinicas—Sao Paulo University (Protocol SDC-COP 105.19.011, approved on 30 March 2019).

Informed Consent Statement: Informed consent was obtained from all the subjects involved in the study.

Data Availability Statement: The data that support the findings of this study are available from the corresponding author (H.F.L.) upon reasonable request.

Acknowledgments: The authors would like to thank the Endocrinology Department at HC-FMUSP for their valuable collaboration in carrying out confirmatory tests for primary aldosteronism.

Conflicts of Interest: The authors declare no conflict of interest.

References

1. Funder, J.W.; Carey, R.M.; Mantero, F.; Murad, M.H.; Reincke, M.; Shibata, H.; Stowasser, M.; Young, W.F. The Management of primary aldosteronism: Case detection, diagnosis, and treatment: An endocrine society clinical practice guideline. *J. Clin. Endocrinol. Metab.* **2016**, *101*, 1889–1916. [CrossRef] [PubMed]
2. Williams, T.A.; Reincke, M. Diagnosis and management of primary aldosteronism: The Endocrine Society guideline 2016 revisited. *Eur. J. Endocrinol.* **2016**, *179*, R19–R29. [CrossRef]
3. Williams, B.; Mancia, G.; Spiering, W.; Agabiti Rosei, E.; Azizi, M.; Burnier, M.; Clement, D.L.; Coca, A.; De Simone, G.; Dominiczak, A.; et al. 2018 ESC/ESH Guidelines for the management of arterial hypertension. *Eur. Heart J.* **2018**, *39*, 3021–3104. [CrossRef] [PubMed]
4. Barroso, W.S.; Rodrigues, S.; Bortolotto, A.; Mota-Gomes, A.; Brandão, A.; de Feitosa, M.; Machado, A.; Poli-de-Figueiredo, E.; Amodeo, C.; Júnior, D.M.; et al. Diretriz Brasileira de Hipertensão Arterial—2020. *Arq. Bras. Cardiol.* **2021**, *116*, 516–518. [CrossRef]
5. Naruse, M.; Katabami, T.; Shibata, H.; Sone, M.; Takahashi, K.; Tanabe, A.; Izawa, S.; Ichijo, T.; Otsuki, M.; Omura, M.; et al. Japan Endocrine Society clinical practice guideline for the diagnosis and management of primary aldosteronism 2021. *Endocr. J.* **2022**, *69*, 327–359. [CrossRef] [PubMed]
6. Rossi, G.P. Primary Aldosteronism. JACC State-of-the-Art Review. *J. Am. Coll. Cardiol.* **2019**, *74*, 2799–2811. [CrossRef] [PubMed]
7. Vilela, L.A.P.; Almeida, M.Q. Diagnosis and management of primary aldosteronism. *Arch. Endocrinol. Metab.* **2017**, *61*, 305–312. [CrossRef]
8. Gordon, R.D.; Ziesak, M.D.; Tunny, T.J.; Stowasser, M.; Klemm, S.A. Evidence that primary aldosteronism may not be uncommon: 12% incidence among antihypertensive drug trial volunteers. *Clin. Exp. Pharmacol. Physiol.* **1993**, *20*, 296–298. [CrossRef]
9. Rossi, G.P.; Bernini, G.; Caliumi, C.; Desideri, G.; Fabris, B.; Ferri, C.; Ganzaroli, C.; Giacchetti, G.; Letizia, C.; Maccario, M.; et al. A prospective study of the prevalence of primary aldosteronism in 1125 hypertensive patients. *J. Am. Coll. Cardiol.* **2006**, *48*, 2293–2300. [CrossRef]
10. Calhoun, D.A. Is there an unrecognized epidemic of primary aldosteronism? *Hypertension* **2007**, *50*, 447–453. [CrossRef]
11. Kline, G.A.; Ally, P.H.P.; Alexander, A.L.; Ernesto, L.S. Primary aldosteronism: A common cause of resistant hypertension. *Cmaj* **2017**, *189*, E773–E778. [CrossRef] [PubMed]
12. Douma, S.; Petidis, K.; Doumas, M.; Papaefthimiou, P.; Triantafyllou, A.; Kartali, N.; Papadopoulos, N.; Vogiatzis, K.; Zamboulis, C. Prevalence of primary hyperaldosteronism in resistant hypertension: A retrospective observational study. *Lancet* **2008**, *371*, 1921–1926. [CrossRef] [PubMed]
13. Mulatero, P.; Sechi, L.A.; Williams, T.A.; Lenders, J.W.M.; Reincke, M.; Satoh, F.; Januszewicz, A.; Naruse, M.; Doumas, M.; Veglio, F.; et al. Subtype diagnosis, treatment, complications and outcomes of primary aldosteronism and future direction of research: A position statement and consensus of the Working Group on Endocrine Hypertension of the European Society of Hypertension. *J. Hypertens.* **2020**, *38*, 1929–1936. [CrossRef]
14. Mulatero, P.; Monticone, S.; Deinum, J.; Amar, L.; Prejbisz, A.; Zennaro, M.C.; Beuschlein, F.; Rossi, G.P.; Nishikawa, T.; Morganti, A.; et al. Genetics, prevalence, screening and confirmation of primary aldosteronism: A position statement and consensus of the Working Group on Endocrine Hypertension of the European Society of Hypertension. *J. Hypertens.* **2020**, *38*, 1919–1928. [CrossRef]

15. Hannemann, A.; Bidlingmaier, M.; Friedrich, N.; Manolopoulou, J.; Spyroglou, A.; Völzke, H.; Beuschlein, F.; Seissler, J.; Rettig, R.; Felix, S.B.; et al. Screening for primary aldosteronism in hypertensive subjects: Results from two German epidemiological studies. *Eur. J. Endocrinol.* **2012**, *167*, 7–15. [CrossRef]
16. Xu, Z.; Yang, J.; Hu, J.; Song, Y.; He, W.; Luo, T.; Cheng, Q.; Ma, L.; Luo, R.; Fuller, P.J.; et al. Primary aldosteronism in patients in China with recently detected hypertension. *J. Am. Coll. Cardiol.* **2020**, *75*, 1913–1922. [CrossRef]
17. Jaffe, G.; Gray, Z.; Krishnan, G.; Stedman, M.; Zheng, Y.; Han, J.; Chertow, G.M.; Leppert, J.T.; Bhalla, V. Screening rates for primary aldosteronism in resistant hypertension. *Hypertension* **2020**, *75*, 650–659. [CrossRef]
18. Ohno, Y.; Sone, M.; Inagaki, N.; Yamasaki, T.; Ogawa, O.; Takeda, Y.; Kurihara, I.; Itoh, H.; Umakoshi, H.; Tsuiki, M.; et al. Prevalence of Cardiovascular Disease and Its Risk Factors in Primary Aldosteronism: A Multicenter Study in Japan. *Hypertension* **2018**, *71*, 530–537. [CrossRef]
19. Hiramatsu, K.; Yamada, T.; Yukimura, Y.; Komiya, I.; Ichikawa, K.; Ishihara, M.; Nagata, H.; Izumiyama, T. A screening test to identify aldosterone-producing adenoma by measuring plasma renin activity. Results in hypertensive patients. *Arch. Intern. Med.* **1981**, *141*, 1589–11593. [CrossRef]
20. Maiolino, G.; Rossitto, G.; Bisogni, V.; Cesari, M.; Seccia, T.M.; Plebani, M.; Rossi, G.P.; Semplicini, A.; Ganzaroli, C.; Pessina, A.C.; et al. Quantitative value of aldosterone-renin ratio for detection of aldosterone-producing adenoma: The Aldosterone-Renin Ratio for Primary Aldosteronism (AQUARR) study. *J. Am. Heart Assoc.* **2017**, *6*, e005574. [CrossRef] [PubMed]
21. Rossi, G.P.; Ceolotto, G.; Rossitto, G.; Seccia, T.M.; Maiolino, G.; Berton, C.; Basso, D.; Plebani, M. Prospective validation of an automated chemiluminescence-based assay of renin and aldosterone for the work-up of arterial hypertension. *Clin. Chem. Lab. Med.* **2016**, *54*, 1441–1450. [CrossRef] [PubMed]
22. Hung, A.; Ahmed, S.; Gupta, A.; Davis, A.; A Kline, G.; A Leung, A.; Ruzicka, M.; Hiremath, S.; Hundemer, G.L. Performance of the aldosterone to renin ratio as a screening test for primary aldosteronism. *J. Clin. Endocrinol. Metab.* **2021**, *106*, 2423–2435. [CrossRef] [PubMed]
23. Li, X.; Goswami, R.; Yang, S.; Li, Q. Aldosterone/direct renin concentration ratio as a screening test for primary aldosteronism: A meta-analysis. *J. Renin-Angiotensin-Aldosterone Syst.* **2016**, *17*. [CrossRef] [PubMed]
24. Stowasser, M.; Ahmed, A.H.; Pimenta, E.; Taylor, P.J.; Gordon, R.D. Factors affecting the aldosterone/renin ratio. *Horm. Metab. Res.* **2012**, *44*, 170–176. [CrossRef]
25. Maciel, A.A.W.; Freitas, T.C.; Fagundes, G.F.C.; Petenuci, J.; Vilela, L.A.P.; Brito, L.P.; Goldbaum, T.S.; Zerbini, M.C.N.; Ledesma, F.L.; Tanno, F.Y.; et al. Intra-individual Variability of Serum Aldosterone and Implications for Primary Aldosteronism Screening. *J. Clin. Endocrinol. Metab.* **2023**, *108*, 1143–1153. [CrossRef] [PubMed]
26. Seiler, L.; Rump, L.C.; Schulte-Mönting, J.; Slawik, M.; Borm, K.; Pavenstädt, H.; Beuschlein, F.; Reincke, M. Diagnosis of primary aldosteronism: Value of different screening parameters and influence of antihypertensive medication. *Eur. J. Endocrinol.* **2004**, *150*, 329–337. [CrossRef] [PubMed]
27. Burrello, J.; Monticone, S.; Buffolo, F.; Lucchiari, M.; Tetti, M.; Rabbia, F.; Mengozzi, G.; Williams, T.A.; Veglio, F.; Mulatero, P. Diagnostic accuracy of aldosterone and renin measurement by chemiluminescent immunoassay and radioimmunoassay in primary aldosteronism. *J. Hypertens.* **2016**, *34*, 920–927. [CrossRef]
28. Lijmer, J.G.; Mol, B.W.; Heisterkamp, S.; Bonsel, G.J.; Prins, M.H.; van der Meulen, J.H.; Bossuyt, P.M. Empirical evidence of design-related bias in studies of diagnostic tests. *JAMA* **1999**, *282*, 1061–1066. [CrossRef]
29. Lin, C.-H.; Lin, C.-H.; Chung, M.-C.; Hung, C.-S.; Tseng, F.-Y.; Er, L.K.; Hou, C.J.-Y.; Lin, Y.-H.; Wu, V.-C.; Cheng, H.-M.; et al. Aldosterone-to-renin ratio (ARR) as a screening tool for primary aldosteronism (PA). *J. Formos. Med. Assoc.* **2024**, *123*, S98–S103. [CrossRef]
30. Puar, T.H.; Loh, W.J.; Lim, D.S.; Loh, L.M.; Zhang, M.; Foo, R.S.; Lee, L.; Swee, D.S.; Khoo, J.; Tay, D.; et al. Aldosterone-potassium ratio predicts primary aldosteronism subtype. *J. Hypertens.* **2020**, *38*, 1375–1383. [CrossRef]
31. Kim, G.H. Renal effects of prostaglandins and cyclooxygenase-2 inhibitors. *Electrolyte Blood Press.* **2008**, *6*, 35–41. [CrossRef]
32. Castrop, H.; Schweda, F.; Schumacher, K.; Wolf, K.; Kurtz, A. Role of renocortical cyclooxygenase-2 for renal vascular resistance and macula densa control of renin secretion. *J. Am. Soc. Nephrol.* **2001**, *12*, 867–874. [CrossRef]
33. Stichtenoth, D.O.; Marhauer, V.; Tsikas, D.; Gutzki, F.M.; Frölich, J.C. Effects of specific COX-2-inhibition on renin release and renal and systemic prostanoid synthesis in healthy volunteers. *Kidney Int.* **2005**, *68*, 2197–2207. [CrossRef]

Journal of
Cardiovascular Development and Disease

MDPI

Article

Effect of Prior Moderate Aerobic Exercise to Prolonged Sitting on Peripheral and Central Cardiovascular Measures in Young Women

Abdullah Bandar Alansare [1,*], Rawan Tuayes Alotaibi [1], Ali Mufrih Albarrati [2], Lee Stoner [3] and Bethany Barone Gibbs [4]

1 Department of Exercise Physiology, College of Sport Sciences and Physical Activity, King Saud University, King Khalid Rd., Riyadh 80200, Saudi Arabia; ronzaotb3@gmail.com
2 Rehabilitation Sciences Department, College of Applied Medical Sciences, King Saud University, King Khalid Rd., Riyadh 80200, Saudi Arabia; albarrati@ksu.edu.sa
3 Department of Sport and Exercise, University of North Carolina, Chapel Hill, NC 27599, USA; stonerl@email.unc.edu
4 Department of Epidemiology and Biostatistics, West Virginia University School of Public Health, Morgantown, WV 26506, USA; bethany.gibbs@hsc.wvu.edu
* Correspondence: aalansare@ksu.edu.sa; Tel.: +966-555-061381

Abstract: Background: Prolonged sitting is a risk factor for cardiovascular disease (CVD). We examined whether moderate aerobic exercise prior to prolonged sitting (EX + SIT) has protective effects on peripheral and central cardiovascular and autonomic measures. Methods: Young women ($n = 26$; 23.4 ± 4.3 years old; BMI = 23.1 ± 4.3) completed two sessions in random order: (1) EX + SIT, which consisted of 25 min of moderate aerobic exercise followed by a 3 h prolonged sitting bout, and (2) a 3 h prolonged sitting bout only (SIT-only). Seated peripheral and central blood pressure (BP), pulse wave velocity (PWV), and heart rate variability (HRV) were measured at baseline and after 1 h, 2 h, and 3 h of sitting. Generalized linear mixed models with random effects examined the effects of conditions (i.e., EX + SIT vs. SIT) on BP, PWV, and HRV while adjusting for baseline values. Results: Only peripheral and central diastolic BP ($\beta = 2.18$; $p = 0.016$ and $\beta = 1.99$; $p = 0.034$, respectively) were significantly lower in the EX + SIT condition compared to the SIT-only condition. No differences were detected in other BP, PWV, or HRV variables between the two conditions ($p > 0.05$ for all). Conclusions: Performing moderate aerobic exercise in the morning before engaging in prolonged sitting bouts may reduce some of the prolonged-sitting-induced cardiovascular impairments in young women. Further research is needed to confirm these findings in males and middle-aged/older adults.

Keywords: blood pressure; pulse wave velocity; heart rate variability; sedentary lifestyle; physical activity

1. Introduction

Sedentary behavior (SB) such as prolonged, uninterrupted sitting is increasing at an alarming rate worldwide [1,2]. SB is now recognized as a significant risk factor for cardiovascular diseases (CVDs) and mortality [3]. Strong evidence suggests that the associations of SB with CVDs and mortality may be explained by several unfavorable cardiovascular and autonomic responses to prolonged sitting [3–5]. For instance, acute bouts of prolonged, uninterrupted sitting increase CVD risk factors such as blood pressure (BP) and pulse wave velocity (PWV), a non-invasive measure of vascular stiffness [6–9]. Over time, persistent elevations of BP and PWV may lead to CVD and mortality. As such, public health efforts to mitigate the adverse effects of too much SB have emerged, including the construction of local and global recommendations to reduce SB and prolonged SB patterns [10–12].

In general, adults are recommended to limit overall SB and take frequent breaks during prolonged sitting bouts [10–12]. Strategies to break up prolonged sitting include intermittent standing [13], short bouts of walking or other aerobic exercise [13,14], or bouts of resistance exercise [15]. However, in some work scenarios (e.g., official meetings) and often while traveling or commuting, these strategies are not feasible, and individuals may be required to engage in prolonged sitting and the associated health hazards. As such, exploring alternative approaches to combat the negative impacts of prolonged sitting is necessary to improve health and prevent cardiovascular hazards.

Some research has explored whether exercise prior to prolonged sitting is an effective strategy to prevent the unfavorable cardiovascular alterations that are induced by prolonged sitting. However, the effects of exercise prior to prolonged sitting on CVD risk factors are inconsistent. For example, recent investigations revealed that prolonged-sitting-induced endothelial dysfunctions were prevented by performing aerobic exercise prior to prolonged sitting in young adults [16,17]. Nonetheless, implementing aerobic exercise prior to prolonged sitting did not attenuate BP or PWV increases in young males or mixed-sex samples [18–20]. Yet, importantly, previous research has indicated that aerobic exercise breaks (i.e., those performed during prolonged sitting bouts) attenuate BP responses to prolonged sitting to a greater extent in women than in men [14]. Accordingly, the inclusion of only males or mixed samples could have masked the beneficial cardiovascular effects of aerobic exercise prior to prolonged sitting on BP and PWV in previous studies [18,19]. As such, further research that examines the effects of exercise prior to prolonged sitting based on various cardiovascular and autonomic measurements taken from female samples is needed to achieve a more comprehensive understanding of its cardiovascular and autonomic benefits. Furthermore, including only young females is of particular importance, as recent data suggest that young-to-middle-aged females have experienced no improvements in rates of CVD, while similarly aged males and older females have experienced decreasing CVD rates [21,22].

Therefore, this study aims to examine whether moderate aerobic exercise prior to prolonged sitting (EX + SIT) attenuates the effects of prolonged sitting (SIT) on peripheral and central BP, PWV, and HRV in young women. It was hypothesized that performing moderate aerobic exercise prior to prolonged sitting would have a protective effect on cardiovascular and autonomic measures compared to prolonged sitting that did not occur after aerobic exercise.

2. Materials and Methods

This study was reported following CONSORT (Consolidated Standards of Reporting Trials) guidelines [23]. The ethical approval was obtained from the Institutional Review Board at King Saudi University (No. 23/0074/IRB-A). All participants provided written informed consent before participating in the study.

2.1. Participants

Potential participants were recruited via advertisements posted in King Saud University buildings, sent via emails, and posted on social media platforms. Participants responding to advertisements were enrolled in the study if they met the following inclusion criteria: women aged from 18 to 40 years old, with resting systolic BP (SBP) $\leq$ 139 mmHg and resting diastolic BP (DBP) $\leq$ 89 mmHg [24], with a body mass index (BMI) < 30 kg/m^2, who self-reported being able to perform prolonged sitting and moderate aerobic exercise, were free of any disease that may affect the study's outcomes, and were not using antihypertensive or glucose-lowering drugs. Participants were excluded during screening if they were currently pregnant or breastfeeding. The entire study took place in the Exercise Physiology Laboratory at King Saud University.

2.2. Experimental Design

This randomized cross-over study consisted of two experimental conditions that were performed on two different days and separated by a one-week interval [19,25] (Figure 1). Before each visit, the participants were instructed to refrain from consuming food for 12 h and to abstain from caffeine and self-perceived heavy exercise for 24 h. These abstentions were verbally confirmed upon arrival (between 6:00 am and 10:00 am). After informed consent was provided, baseline measurements, including BP eligibility measurements, were performed. Participants who met the study's criteria were randomly assigned to perform a moderate aerobic exercise followed by 3 h of uninterrupted sitting (EX + SIT) or 3 h of uninterrupted sitting only (SIT). Cardiovascular measurements, including BP, PWV, and HRV, were obtained at four timepoints (i.e., baseline and after 1, 2, and 3 h of sitting). The same measurement procedures were followed during the two experimental visits for all participants.

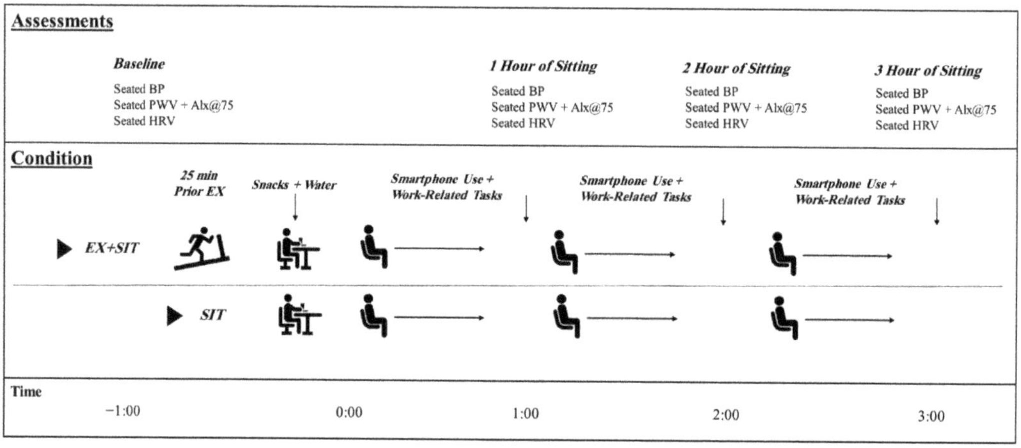

The participants arrived at the laboratory between 6:00 and 10:00 a.m. Seated BP, PWV, AIX@75, and HRV were assessed, respectively, at four timepoints (baseline, 1 h, 2 h, and 3 h of sitting). For the EX + SIT condition, baseline assessments were completed, the participants performed moderate aerobic exercise for 25 min, snacks and water were consumed, and then the prolonged uninterrupted sitting bout started. For the SIT condition, baseline assessments were completed, snacks and water were consumed, and then the prolonged uninterrupted siting bout started. AIx@75 — the normalized augmentation index to 75 beat/minute, BP — blood pressure, EX + SIT — the exercise prior to sitting condition, HRV — heart rate variability, PWV — pulse wave velocity, SIT — the sit-only condition, ▶ — indicates the start of condition.

Figure 1. Experimental conditions.

2.3. Randomization

A simple randomization technique was performed to assign the order of experimental conditions for each participant. Research personnel wrote EX + SIT or SIT on two pieces of paper that were folded to hide the writing. The participant picked up one piece of paper and completed the selected condition.

2.4. Sample Size

The required sample size for the current study was calculated using the G Power software (G* Power Version 3.1.9.4), as follows. Assuming a within-subject correlation of 0.7, a type I error rate of 0.05, and 80% power, 21 participants were required to detect a standardized effect size of 0.25 within participants across the two experimental conditions (i.e., EX + SIT and SIT). To account for potential missing data or withdrawal, 28 participants were recruited.

2.5. Prolonged Sitting

During the study, each participant performed two separate bouts of prolonged, uninterrupted sitting. One bout was performed during the EX + SIT condition and the other was completed during the SIT condition. Each sitting bout lasted for three consecutive hours. Before starting, the participants were instructed to empty their bladders, if needed. Furthermore, during both sitting bouts, participants sat on a chair with the soles of both feet flat on the floor while maintaining a 90-degree angle at the knee and pelvic joints. Throughout the sitting period, the participants were allowed to use their smartphones and were provided with a computer to complete work-related tasks.

2.6. Exercise Session

During the EX + SIT condition, each participant performed aerobic exercise on a treadmill (h/p/cosmos, Inc., Nußdorf, Germany®) prior to the prolonged sitting bout. The exercise intensity was selected based on two factors: the participant's safety and previous evidence suggesting that the chosen intensity can improve cardiovascular outcomes. To achieve this, the relative moderate intensity of 60% heart rate max (HR_{max}) was selected [26–28]. The targeted heart rate was determined by using the following formula: $60\%HR_{max} = (220 - age) * 0.6$ [27]. According to the American College of Sports Medicine, this intensity is classified as light-intensity aerobic exercise [27]. Each participant performed moderate aerobic exercise for 25 min while following the Balke protocol [29]. In addition to its beneficial effects on health [30], this duration was selected because it is a manageable starting point for many young females, which promotes achieving the current physical activity recommendation (i.e., 150 min/week of moderate aerobic exercise throughout the week) [31].

To elaborate, the participants began with a 5 min walking warm-up. Next, the participants jogged or ran at a constant speed (5.3 km/h) for 25 min. The incline of the treadmill began at 0% and increased by 1% every minute, when needed, to ensure that each participant was exercising at their targeted intensity (i.e., $60\%HR_{max}$) during the entire exercise period, and the participant's heart rate was monitored with a chest heart rate strap (T31; Polar Electro, Inc., Helsinki, Finland®). Afterward, the participants performed a 5 min walk to cool down.

2.7. Snacks and Water

During the two experimental conditions, the participants were provided with a standardized snack and water (i.e., 16 ounces) to minimize potential distractions such as hunger, hypoglycemia, or physiological effects on the cardiovascular system while fasting. The snacks provided were Nature Valley® (Minneapolis, MN, USA) oats and honey granola bars, which consisted of 190 calories per bar. Each participant received an individualized amount of the bars which fulfilled 30% of their total daily energy needs, which was determined by the Harris–Benedict equation [32]. The snack and water were provided to the participants during both experimental conditions, just before the start of the prolonged uninterrupted sitting bouts (Figure 1).

2.8. Measurements

2.8.1. Participants' Characteristics and Physical Activity Level

The participants self-reported their age and education level. Body height was measured in duplicate by a wall-mounted stadiometer (Perspective Enterprises, Portage, MI, USA), whereas body weight was measured in duplicate by a digital scale (WB-110A, Tanita, Tokyo, Japan). These duplicated measures were averaged to calculate the body mass index (BMI) (BMI = body weight in kg/body height in m^2). The short version of the International Physical Activity Questionnaire was utilized to estimate the number of minutes participants spent performing MVPA.

2.8.2. Peripheral Blood Pressure

Seated BP measurements were completed using a validated oscillometric device (MobilOGraph 24 h PWA Monitor®, Aachen, Germany) with an appropriately sized cuff based on the arm circumcenter [33,34]. The monitor was programmed to operate automatically. To begin the BP measurements, the participants sat in a chair for 10 min with their back supported, both feet on the floor, and both arms supported at their heart level. The cuff was placed on the left arm and two consecutive BP measurements were performed with a one-minute rest interval in between [34]. The average of the two measurements during the first assessment was used to determine eligibility. The same procedures were utilized to complete the BP measurements at baseline and each hour during the sitting protocol during both experimental conditions (Figure 1). After completing these measurements, the oscillometric device (MobilOGraph 24 h PWA Monitor®, Aachen, Germany) was connected to the IEM on Life's Side software through Bluetooth to process and calculate the peripheral BP values, which included SBP, DBP, and mean arterial pressure (MAP).

2.8.3. Central Blood Pressure, Pulse Wave Velocity, and Augmentation Index

The MobilOGraph 24 h PWA Monitor is also a valid oscillometric device that is commonly used to estimate the central BP, PWV, and augmentation index by using the cuff-based method [35]. After acquiring the seated peripheral BP measurements, the device inflates the cuff to the DBP value and records pulse waves for 10 consecutive seconds [36,37]. Then, an algorithm called ARCSolver (Austrian Institute of Technology, Vienna, Austria) estimates several variables, including seated central SBP (cSPB), DBP (cDBP), pulse pressure (cPP), PWV, augmentation pressure (AP), and the normalized augmentation index to 75 beat/min (Alx@75) [34,38]. In parallel with the peripheral BP measurements, these central cardiovascular estimations were performed at baseline and each hour during the sitting protocol during both experimental conditions (Figure 1). To be included in the current analysis, each participant was required to have at least one successful pulse wave analysis for each timepoint.

2.8.4. Heart Rate Variability

The time intervals between consecutive heartbeats were measured to calculate seated HRV indices by using a validated instrument (Polar V800 monitor with Polar H10 heart rate strap; Polar Electro, Inc., Helsinki, Finland®) [39]. The heart rate strap was placed on the participants' chest under their chest muscles while they were resting and prior to the BP measurements. During the measurement, participants were instructed to remain quiet, breathe normally, and not to move or to talk. A 5 min record of time intervals was collected at each timepoint (i.e., at baseline and every hour into sitting) during both experimental conditions (Figure 1).

To process and derive HRV indices, the time interval data were downloaded using PolarFlow. These data were imported into Kubios Premium analysis software (version 3.3.1, MATLAB, The MathWorks, Inc. Portola Valley, CA, United States of America). To clean the data, the current guidelines [40] were utilized as follows: (1) the automatic correction was used to ensure data had ≤5% artifacts, and (2) further visual inspection of the existence of any distortion in the data was performed. Then, two HRV indices were calculated, including the standard deviation of normal R-R intervals (SDNN) (i.e., a measure of overall variability) and the root mean square of successive differences (RMSSDs) (i.e., a measure of cardiac parasympathetic activity). Natural log transformation was performed for SDNN and RMSSD due to skewness. These HRV indices were chosen in the current study due to their ability to predict CVD, as well as its well-understood statistical and physiological basis [40].

2.9. Statistical Analysis

The characteristics of the participants were summarized as means and standard deviations (SDs) or frequencies and percentages (%), as appropriate. To assess the study's hypotheses, generalized linear mixed (GLM) models with random effects examined the effects of conditions (i.e., EX + SIT vs. SIT) on BP, PWV, and HRV variables while adjusting for baseline values [41]. The estimated β coefficients in these models represented whether the average of the outcome was lower during the EX + SIT condition than the SIT condition. In addition, the strength of the effects was evaluated by calculating Cohen's d as follows: $d = \beta$/the standard deviation of baseline values of the cardiovascular and autonomic variables. The magnitude of effects was considered large ($d = 0.8$), medium ($d = 0.5$), or small ($d = 0.2$) using conventional thresholds [42]. The statistical significance level was set as $\alpha < 0.05$. Stata version 14 (StataCorp, LLC, College Station, TX, USA) was utilized for the data analyses.

3. Results

Out of the 28 women who were enrolled, 2 participants did not complete both experimental conditions (i.e., EX + SIT and SIT). Thus, a sample of 26 participants was analyzed and included in the presented results. These participants had complete data for HRV variables ($n = 26$), though only $n = 25$ participants were included in the BP and PWV analyses because one participant had no peripheral and central BP and PWV data for a condition (i.e., EX + SIT) due to a technical error. Participant characteristics are reported in Table 1. Overall, the participants tended to be young with healthy BMIs, BPs, and PWVs.

Table 1. Participant characteristics ($n = 26$).

Variable	Mean (SD) or *n* (%)
Age, years	23.4 (4.3)
Education	
High School Degree or less	18 (69.2)
Bachelor's Degree or higher	8 (30.8)
MVPA, min/week	82.5 (79.3)
Height, cm	158.7 (6.5)
Weight, kg	58.3 (11.9)
BMI, kg/m^2	23.1 (4.3)
SBP, mmHg *	113.6 (9.7)
DBP, mmHg *	72.1 (7.5)
MAP, mmHg *	91.0 (8.0)
cSPB, mmHg *	103.7 (9.1)
cDBP, mmHg *	72.7 (7.8)
cPP, mmHg *	31.0 (6.2)
PWV, m/s *	4.8 (0.4)
AIX@75, % *	26.7 (8.8)
SDNN, ln	3.6 (0.3)
RMSSD, ln	3.3 (0.5)

Abbreviations: AIX@75—normalized augmentation index to 75 beat/minute, DBP—diastolic blood pressure, cDBP—central diastolic blood pressure, cPP—central pulse pressure, cSBP—central systolic blood pressure, cm—centimeter, kg—kilogram, ln—natural log transformation, m^2—meter squared, m/s—meters per second, mmHg—millimeter of mercury, MVPA—moderate-to-vigorous physical activity, *n*—number, PWV—pulse wave velocity, RMSSD—root of mean successive differences, SBP—systolic blood pressure, SD—standard deviation, SDNN—standard deviation of normal R-R, * indicates $n = 25$.

Cardiovascular Responses to Prolonged Sitting with and without Prior Exercise

Figure 2 and Supplemental Table S1 display peripheral BP differences between the EX + SIT vs. SIT condition. Both SBP ($\beta = 0.77$; $p = 0.512$) and MAP ($\beta = 1.53$; $p = 0.054$) were not significantly different between the two conditions. However, DBP ($\beta = 2.18$; $p = 0.016$) was significantly lower in the EX + SIT condition compared to the SIT condition. The size of this difference was small ($d = 0.29$). Furthermore, Figure 3 and Supplemental Table S1 show central BP differences between the two conditions. Neither cSBP ($\beta = 1.39$; $p = 0.255$) nor cPP ($\beta = -0.48$; $p = 0.635$) significantly differed when comparing the EX + SIT vs. SIT condition. Yet, cDBP ($\beta = 1.99$; $p = 0.034$) was significantly lower in the EX + SIT condition compared to the SIT condition. The size of this difference was mild ($d = 0.26$).

Figures 4 and 5 and Supplemental Table S1 also reveal the vascular stiffness and HRV differences between the two conditions. No significant differences were observed in PWV ($\beta = 0.02$; $p = 0.616$), AIX@75 ($\beta = -0.99$; $p = 0.253$), lnSDNN ($\beta = 0.04$; $p = 0.323$), or lnRMSSD ($\beta = 0.01$; $p = 0.926$) between the EX + SIT vs. SIT condition.

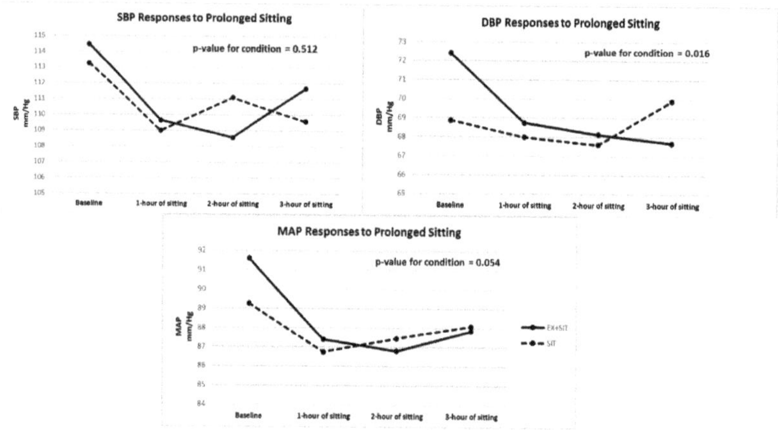

Abbreviations: DBP — diastolic blood pressure, EX + SIT — exercise prior to sit condition, mmHg — millimeter of mercury, SBP — systolic blood pressure, SIT — sit-only condition.

Figure 2. Peripheral BP responses to prolonged sitting with and without prior exercise (n = 25).

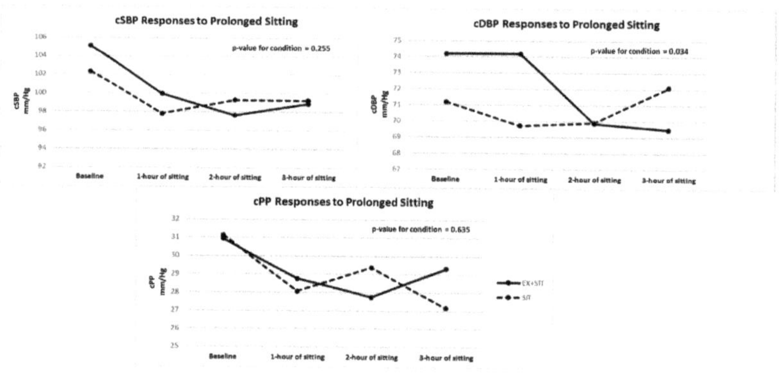

Abbreviations: cDBP — central diastolic blood pressure, cPP — central pulse pressure, cSBP — central systolic blood pressure; EX + SIT — prior exercise to sit condition, mmHg — millimeter of mercury, SIT — sit-only condition.

Figure 3. Central BP responses to prolonged sitting with and without prior exercise (n = 25).

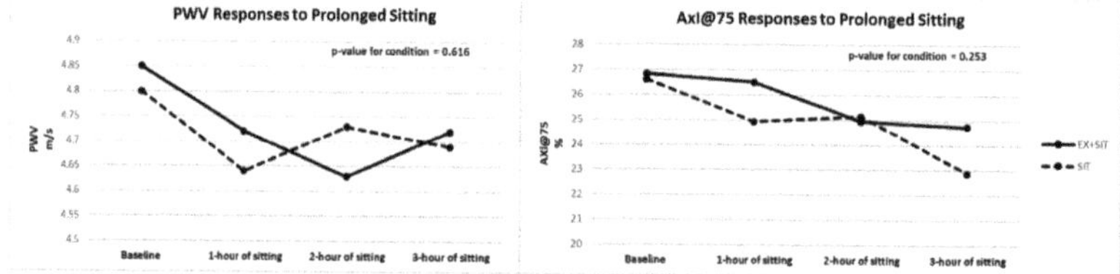

Abbreviations: AIX@75 — normalized augmentation index to 75 beat/minute, EX + SIT — prior exercise to sit condition, m/s — meter per second, PWV — pulse wave velocity, SIT — sit only condition.

Figure 4. Vascular stiffness responses to prolonged sitting with and without prior exercise (n = 25).

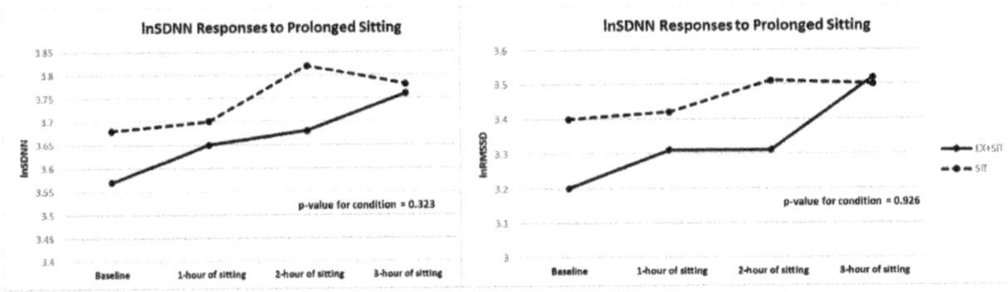

Abbreviations: EX + SIT—prior exercise to sit condition, ln—natural log transformation, RMSSD—root of mean successive differences, SDNN—standard deviation of normal R-R, SIT—sit only condition.

Figure 5. HRV responses to prolonged sitting with and without prior exercise (n = 26).

4. Discussion

This study uniquely assessed seated peripheral and central cardiovascular and autonomic responses to EX + SIT vs. SIT-only conditions in young women. We revealed favorable effects of EX + SIT on peripheral and central DBP in young women; the sizes of these effects were small ($d < 0.3$ for both measures). Yet, other cardiovascular and autonomic measures were comparable when comparing the EX + SIT with the SIT-only condition. These findings suggest that while prolonged sitting may detrimentally affect cardiovascular and autonomic health, performing EX + SIT may be an effective strategy to prevent prolonged-sitting-induced DBP increases in young women.

4.1. Strengths and Limitations of the Study

This study has notable strengths. First, previous evidence suggested that there are sex differences in cardiovascular responses to aerobic exercise during prolonged sitting, with women having greater cardiovascular benefits [14]. Accordingly, this study included female participants only to clarify sex-specific effects. Moreover, the randomized crossover (within-subject) design is another strength of the study, which allowed us to control for potential inter-participant variability [43]. In contrast to previous prolonged sitting studies [6,7,14], we simultaneously assessed peripheral and central cardiovascular and autonomic variables. Thus, our study provides a more comprehensive understanding of the cardiovascular and autonomic responses to prolonged sitting.

Nevertheless, a few drawbacks should be considered when interpreting the study's findings. First, we did not measure or control for the menstrual cycle of the included participants. Although it is suggested not to control for the menstrual cycle in cardiovascular research to improve the external validity of the results [44], the counterpoint view suggests controlling for it to avoid the direct and indirect influence of ovarian hormones on cardiovascular regulations [45]. As such, future studies could account for such a debatable viewpoint. Moreover, our study enrolled healthy young women only. Thus, the effects of EX + SIT on peripheral and central cardiovascular and autonomic health may be different in older women, individuals with cardiovascular or other chronic diseases, or in their male counterparts [14,46]. Therefore, further investigations that enroll participants with these different characteristics are warranted.

4.2. Peripheral Cardiovascular Responses

To the best of our knowledge, only two existing studies have examined the effect of prior aerobic exercise on peripheral BP responses to prolonged sitting. The first study included a mixed-sex sample of young adults (n = 10; female n = 4) and reported that 30 min of moderate aerobic exercise significantly increased seated peripheral MAP during a 5 h prolonged, uninterrupted sitting bout compared to no prior exercise condition [20]. The other study enrolled young men only (n = 15) and found that 30 min of moderate aerobic exercise did not influence seated peripheral SBP, DBP, or MAP during prolonged sitting [18]. In contrast to these findings, we observed significantly lower seated peripheral

DBP when 25 min of moderate aerobic exercise was performed prior to a 3 h prolonged sitting bout compared to no prior exercise condition in young women ($n = 25$).

The discrepancies observed between these studies may be most likely explained by sex and exercise modality differences. For example, the previous two studies enrolled a mixed-sex sample [20] or men only [18], whereas our study included women only. As mentioned earlier, data suggest the existence of sex differences in response to prolonged sitting [47] and aerobic exercise during prolonged sitting, with females likely acquiring greater cardiovascular benefits [14]. Moreover, while we observed significantly lower seated peripheral BP (i.e., DBP) when young women performed moderate aerobic exercise on a treadmill (i.e., jogging or running at 60% HRmax), the study that included a mixed-sex sample of young adults (i.e., men and women) found significantly higher seated peripheral BP (i.e., MPA) when moderate aerobic exercise was performed on a cycling ergometer (i.e., cycling at 90% power-evoking gas exchange threshold) [20]. Robust evidence indicates that the favorable effects of aerobic exercise on peripheral BP are much clearer and stronger when exercise is performed on a treadmill vs. a cycling ergometer [48–50]. Together, these findings suggest that the evidence about the effects of prior exercise to prolonged sitting on peripheral cardiovascular health remains mixed and warrants further investigation.

4.3. Central Cardiovascular and Autonomic Responses

Comparable to the prolonged sitting and peripheral cardiovascular health literature, no existing study examined the influence of aerobic exercise prior to prolonged sitting on central autonomic health and only two recent studies assessed the effects on central cardiovascular measures [18,19]. The first study examined the influence of 30 min of moderate aerobic exercise prior to a 3 h prolonged sitting bout on central seated SBP, DBP, MAP, and supine carotid–femoral PWV (cfPWV) in young men [18]. It was revealed that moderate aerobic exercise prevented prolonged-sitting-induced increases in central SBP, DBP, and MAP but failed to mitigate cfPWV increase [18]. Conversely, the other study found that 30 min of moderate aerobic exercise prior to a 2.5 h prolonged sitting bout prevented an increase in supine brachial–femoral PWV (bfPWV) in a sample of mixed young adults ($n = 22$; 50% males); yet it failed to prevent the supine femoral–ankle PWV (faPWV) increase [19]. In our current study, performing 25 min of moderate aerobic exercise prior to a 3 h prolonged sitting bout decreased central seated DBP in young women ($n = 25$). However, neither of the other central seated BP values, nor seated PWV or HRV, were significantly different from the SIT-only condition. In summary, the current evidence suggests that performing aerobic exercise prior to prolonged sitting may prevent prolonged-sitting-induced central DBP increases in male and female adults. However, the responses of SBP, central vascular stiffness, and autonomic measures to moderate aerobic exercise prior to prolonged sitting remain variable. Possible reasons for disparate results require further research and may include sex and measurement posture [6,51].

4.4. Potential Mechanisms

Previous studies showed that a single bout of prolonged sitting can reduce venous return, stroke volume, cardiac output, and vasoactive substances and increase sympathetic activation, leading to increased BP [7,51]. In contrast, a single bout of moderate aerobic exercise can potentially reverse these adverse cardiovascular changes, leading to reduced BP—a phenomenon known as post-exercise hypotension [52]. In our current study, all cardiovascular risk factors seem to oppose findings from previous studies [7,51] and showed improvements from baseline across the prolonged sitting bout, regardless of the prior exercise. Even though explanations for these discrepancies appear to be complex and need further investigation, a previous systematic review and meta-analysis suggest that the contradicting cardiovascular responses to movement behaviors, such as exercise in adults, may be explained by ethnicity and genes [53]. Nevertheless, peripheral and central DBPs were significantly lower in the EX + SIT vs. SIT-only condition. Although these effects do not appear to be the result of improved autonomic regulation (i.e., unchanged HRV), they may be due to reduced vascular resistance during the moderate aerobic exercise which persisted into the prolonged sitting bout. However, further research is needed to confirm this hypothesis.

4.5. Clinical Significance

The current SB recommendations suggest limiting SB but do not specify the best approaches to confront the adverse impacts of excessive, unavoidable SB on cardiovascular health [10–12]. Individuals are suggested to take frequent breaks during prolonged sitting bouts. While this recommendation may work in circumstances such as during leisure time, it may be challenging in other times such as during formal meetings and while driving. Our study provides preliminary evidence that performing moderate aerobic exercise in the morning before engaging in prolonged sitting bouts may be an alternative strategy to partially avert prolonged-sitting-induced BP increases, particularly for DBP in young women. These findings add further evidence and strategy to the current SB recommendations that aim at improving cardiovascular health.

5. Conclusions

In summary, this study uniquely assessed the effects of EX + SIT vs. SIT-only on peripheral and central cardiovascular and autonomic measures in young women. As hypothesized, EX + SIT appeared to have favorable effects on peripheral and central DBP. However, no effects on other measures of peripheral or central BP, PWV, or HRV were observed. As such, performing moderate aerobic exercise in the morning before engaging in prolonged sitting bouts may confront some but not all of the prolonged-sitting-induced cardiovascular impairments. Further research is needed to confirm these findings in different population groups, such as older women, and explore the potential mechanisms.

Supplementary Materials: The following supporting information can be downloaded at https://www.mdpi.com/article/10.3390/jcdd11100307/s1, Table S1: Cardiovascular and autonomic responses to prolonged sitting with and without prior exercise (n = 25).

Author Contributions: A.B.A. and R.T.A. designed the study and performed the experiments. A.B.A. and B.B.G. analyzed the data. A.B.A., R.T.A., A.M.A., L.S. and B.B.G. interpreted the data and wrote the first manuscript. All authors have read and agreed to the published version of the manuscript.

Funding: This research received no external funding.

Institutional Review Board Statement: The study was conducted in accordance with the Declaration of Helsinki and approved by the Institutional Review Board of King Saudi University (No. 23/0074/IRB-A).

Informed Consent Statement: Informed consent was obtained from all participants involved in the study.

Data Availability Statement: The datasets used and/or analyzed during the current study are available from the corresponding author on reasonable request.

Acknowledgments: The authors would like to thank the Researchers Supporting Project Number (RSPD2024R587), King Saud University, Riyadh, Saudi Arabia.

Conflicts of Interest: The authors declare no conflicts of interest.

References

1. Alansare, A.B. Post-COVID-19 Total and Domain-specific Sedentary Behaviors in Saudi Adults. *Am. J. Health Behav.* **2023**, *47*, 765–776. [CrossRef]
2. Mclaughlin, M.; Atkin, A.; Starr, L.; Hall, A.; Wolfenden, L.; Sutherland, R.; Wiggers, J.; Ramirez, A.; Hallal, P.; Pratt, M. Worldwide surveillance of self-reported sitting time: A scoping review. *Int. J. Behav. Nutr. Phys. Act.* **2020**, *17*, 111. [CrossRef] [PubMed]
3. Li, S.; Lear, S.A.; Rangarajan, S.; Hu, B.; Yin, L.; Bangdiwala, S.I.; Alhabib, K.F.; Rosengren, A.; Gupta, R.; Mony, P.K. Association of sitting time with mortality and cardiovascular events in high-income, middle-income, and low-income countries. *JAMA Cardiol.* **2022**, *7*, 796–807. [CrossRef] [PubMed]

4. Dempsey, P.C.; Matthews, C.E.; Dashti, S.G.; Doherty, A.R.; Bergouignan, A.; Van Roekel, E.H.; Dunstan, D.W.; Wareham, N.J.; Yates, T.E.; Wijndaele, K.; et al. Sedentary behavior and chronic disease: Mechanisms and future directions. *J. Phys. Act. Health* **2020**, *17*, 52–61. [CrossRef]
5. Dempsey, P.C.; Larsen, R.N.; Dunstan, D.W.; Owen, N.; Kingwell, B.A. Sitting less and moving more: Implications for hypertension. *Hypertension* **2018**, *72*, 1037–1046. [CrossRef] [PubMed]
6. Credeur, D.P.; Miller, S.M.; Jones, R.; Stoner, L.; Dolbow, D.R.; Fryer, S.M.; Stone, K.; McCoy, S.M. Impact of prolonged sitting on peripheral and central vascular health. *Am. J. Cardiol.* **2019**, *123*, 260–266. [CrossRef]
7. Alansare, A.B.; Kowalsky, R.J.; Jones, M.A.; Perdomo, S.J.; Stoner, L.; Gibbs, B.B. The Effects of a Simulated Workday of Prolonged Sitting on Seated versus Supine Blood Pressure and Pulse Wave Velocity in Adults with Overweight/Obesity and Elevated Blood Pressure. *J. Vasc. Res.* **2020**, *57*, 355–366. [CrossRef]
8. Fuchs, F.D.; Whelton, P.K. High blood pressure and cardiovascular disease. *Hypertension* **2020**, *75*, 285–292. [CrossRef]
9. Valencia-Hernández, C.A.; Lindbohm, J.V.; Shipley, M.J.; Wilkinson, I.B.; McEniery, C.M.; Ahmadi-Abhari, S.; Singh-Manoux, A.; Kivimäki, M.; Brunner, E.J. Aortic pulse wave velocity as adjunct risk marker for assessing cardiovascular disease risk: Prospective study. *Hypertension* **2022**, *79*, 836–843. [CrossRef]
10. DiPietro, L.; Al-Ansari, S.S.; Biddle, S.J.; Borodulin, K.; Bull, F.C.; Buman, M.P.; Cardon, G.; Carty, C.; Chaput, J.-P.; Chastin, S. Advancing the global physical activity agenda: Recommendations for future research by the 2020 WHO physical activity and sedentary behavior guidelines development group. *Int. J. Behav. Nutr. Phys. Act.* **2020**, *17*, 143. [CrossRef]
11. Alfawaz, R.A.; Aljuraiban, G.S.; AlMarzooqi, M.A.; Alghannam, A.F.; BaHammam, A.S.; Dobia, A.M.; Alothman, S.A.; Aljuhani, O.; Aljaloud, K.S. The recommended amount of physical activity, sedentary behavior, and sleep duration for healthy Saudis: A joint consensus statement of the Saudi Public Health Authority. *Ann. Thorac. Med.* **2021**, *16*, 239. [CrossRef] [PubMed]
12. Katzmarzyk, P.T.; Powell, K.E.; Jakicic, J.M.; Troiano, R.P.; Piercy, K.; Tennant, B.; Committee, P.A.G.A. Sedentary behavior and health: Update from the 2018 physical activity guidelines advisory committee. *Med. Sci. Sports Exerc.* **2019**, *51*, 1227. [CrossRef] [PubMed]
13. Buffey, A.J.; Herring, M.P.; Langley, C.K.; Donnelly, A.E.; Carson, B.P. The acute effects of interrupting prolonged sitting time in adults with standing and light-intensity walking on biomarkers of cardiometabolic health in adults: A systematic review and meta-analysis. *Sports Med.* **2022**, *52*, 1765–1787. [CrossRef] [PubMed]
14. Wheeler, M.J.; Dunstan, D.W.; Ellis, K.A.; Cerin, E.; Phillips, S.; Lambert, G.; Naylor, L.H.; Dempsey, P.C.; Kingwell, B.A.; Green, D.J. Effect of morning exercise with or without breaks in prolonged sitting on blood pressure in older overweight/obese adults: Evidence for sex differences. *Hypertension* **2019**, *73*, 859–867. [CrossRef] [PubMed]
15. Kowalsky, R.J.; Jakicic, J.M.; Hergenroeder, A.; Rogers, R.J.; Gibbs, B.B. Acute cardiometabolic effects of interrupting sitting with resistance exercise breaks. *Appl. Physiol. Nutr. Metab.* **2019**, *44*, 1025–1032. [CrossRef]
16. Morishima, T.; Restaino, R.M.; Walsh, L.K.; Kanaley, J.A.; Padilla, J. Prior exercise and standing as strategies to circumvent sitting-induced leg endothelial dysfunction. *Clin. Sci.* **2017**, *131*, 1045–1053. [CrossRef]
17. Garten, R.S.; Scott, M.C.; Zúñiga, T.M.; Hogwood, A.C.; Fralin, R.C.; Weggen, J. A prior high-intensity exercise bout attenuates the vascular dysfunction resulting from a prolonged sedentary bout. *J. Phys. Act. Health* **2019**, *16*, 916–924. [CrossRef]
18. Wright, A.; Stavres, J.; Galloway, R.; Donahue, P.; Sha, Z.; McCoy, S. Aortic stiffness increases during prolonged sitting independent of intermittent standing or prior exercise. *Eur. J. Appl. Physiol.* **2023**, *123*, 533–546. [CrossRef]
19. Riley, S.; Paterson, C.; Bates-Fraser, L.C.; Ondrak, K.S.; Stoner, L.; Hanson, E.D. Uninterrupted prolonged sitting and arterial stiffness: Moderating effect of prior aerobic exercise in physically active adults. *Eur. J. Appl. Physiol.* **2024**, *124*, 1959–1967. [CrossRef]
20. Younger, A.M.; Pettitt, R.W.; Sexton, P.J.; Maass, W.J.; Pettitt, C.D. Acute moderate exercise does not attenuate cardiometabolic function associated with a bout of prolonged sitting. *J. Sports Sci.* **2016**, *34*, 658–663. [CrossRef]
21. Wilmot, K.A.; O'Flaherty, M.; Capewell, S.; Ford, E.S.; Vaccarino, V. Coronary heart disease mortality declines in the United States from 1979 through 2011: Evidence for stagnation in young adults, especially women. *Circulation* **2015**, *132*, 997–1002. [CrossRef] [PubMed]
22. Maas, A.H.; van der Schouw, Y.T.; Regitz-Zagrosek, V.; Swahn, E.; Appelman, Y.E.; Pasterkamp, G.; Ten Cate, H.; Nilsson, P.M.; Huisman, M.V.; Stam, H.C. Red alert for women's heart: The urgent need for more research and knowledge on cardiovascular disease in women: Proceedings of the workshop held in Brussels on gender differences in cardiovascular disease, 29 September 2010. *Eur. Heart J.* **2011**, *32*, 1362–1368. [CrossRef] [PubMed]
23. Moher, D. CONSORT Group (Consolidated Standards of Reporting Trials). The CONSORT statement: Revised recommendations for improving the quality of reports of parallel-group randomized trials. *Ann. Intern. Med.* **2001**, *134*, 657–662. [CrossRef] [PubMed]
24. McCormack, T.; Boffa, R.J.; Jones, N.R.; Carville, S.; McManus, R.J. The 2018 ESC/ESH hypertension guideline and the 2019 NICE hypertension guideline, how and why they differ. *Eur. Heart J.* **2019**, *40*, 3456–3458. [CrossRef]
25. Ballard, K.D.; Duguid, R.M.; Berry, C.W.; Dey, P.; Bruno, R.S.; Ward, R.M.; Timmerman, K.L. Effects of prior aerobic exercise on sitting-induced vascular dysfunction in healthy men. *Eur. J. Appl. Physiol.* **2017**, *117*, 2509–2518. [CrossRef]
26. Kang, S.-J.; Kim, E.-h.; Ko, K.-J. Effects of aerobic exercise on the resting heart rate, physical fitness, and arterial stiffness of female patients with metabolic syndrome. *J. Phys. Ther. Sci.* **2016**, *28*, 1764–1768. [CrossRef]

27. American College of Sports Medicine (ACSM). *ACSM's Guidelines for Exercise Testing and Prescription*; Lippincott Williams & Wilkins: Philadelphia, PA, USA, 2013.
28. Hespanhol Junior, L.C.; Pillay, J.D.; van Mechelen, W.; Verhagen, E. Meta-analyses of the effects of habitual running on indices of health in physically inactive adults. *Sports Med.* **2015**, *45*, 1455–1468. [CrossRef]
29. Balke, B.; Ware, R.W. An experimental study of physical fitness of Air Force personnel. *United States Armed Forces Med. J.* **1959**, *10*, 675–688.
30. Naugle, K.M.; Naugle, K.E.; Fillingim, R.B.; Samuels, B.; Riley, J.L., III. Intensity thresholds for aerobic exercise–induced hypoalgesia. *Med. Sci. Sports Exerc.* **2014**, *46*, 817. [CrossRef]
31. Piercy, K.L.; Troiano, R.P.; Ballard, R.M.; Carlson, S.A.; Fulton, J.E.; Galuska, D.A.; George, S.M.; Olson, R.D. The physical activity guidelines for Americans. *Jama* **2018**, *320*, 2020–2028. [CrossRef]
32. Harris, J.A.; Benedict, F.G. A biometric study of human basal metabolism. *Proc. Natl. Acad. Sci. USA* **1918**, *4*, 370–373. [CrossRef] [PubMed]
33. Wei, W.; Tölle, M.; Zidek, W.; van der Giet, M. Validation of the mobil-O-Graph: 24 h-blood pressure measurement device. *Blood Press. Monit.* **2010**, *15*, 225–228. [CrossRef] [PubMed]
34. Whelton, P.K.; Carey, R.M.; Aronow, W.S.; Casey, D.E.; Collins, K.J.; Dennison Himmelfarb, C.; DePalma, S.M.; Gidding, S.; Jamerson, K.A.; Jones, D.W. 2017 ACC/AHA/AAPA/ABC/ACPM/AGS/APhA/ASH/ASPC/NMA/PCNA guideline for the prevention, detection, evaluation, and management of high blood pressure in adults: A report of the American College of Cardiology/American Heart Association Task Force on Clinical Practice Guidelines. *J. Am. Coll. Cardiol.* **2018**, *71*, e127–e248. [PubMed]
35. Milan, A.; Zocaro, G.; Leone, D.; Tosello, F.; Buraioli, I.; Schiavone, D.; Veglio, F. Current assessment of pulse wave velocity: Comprehensive review of validation studies. *J. Hypertens.* **2019**, *37*, 1547–1557. [CrossRef]
36. Weber, T.; Wassertheurer, S.; Hametner, B.; Parragh, S.; Eber, B. Noninvasive methods to assess pulse wave velocity: Comparison with the invasive gold standard and relationship with organ damage. *J. Hypertens.* **2015**, *33*, 1023–1031. [CrossRef]
37. Papaioannou, T.G.; Argyris, A.; Protogerou, A.D.; Vrachatis, D.; Nasothimiou, E.G.; Sfikakis, P.P.; Stergiou, G.S.; Stefanadis, C.I. Non-invasive 24 hour ambulatory monitoring of aortic wave reflection and arterial stiffness by a novel oscillometric device: The first feasibility and reproducibility study. *Int. J. Cardiol.* **2013**, *169*, 57–61. [CrossRef]
38. Hametner, B.; Wassertheurer, S.; Kropf, J.; Mayer, C.; Eber, B.; Weber, T. Oscillometric estimation of aortic pulse wave velocity: Comparison with intra-aortic catheter measurements. *Blood Press. Monit.* **2013**, *18*, 173–176. [CrossRef]
39. Giles, D.; Draper, N.; Neil, W. Validity of the Polar V800 heart rate monitor to measure RR intervals at rest. *Eur. J. Appl. Physiol.* **2016**, *116*, 563–571. [CrossRef]
40. Laborde, S.; Mosley, E.; Thayer, J.F. Heart rate variability and cardiac vagal tone in psychophysiological research–recommendations for experiment planning, data analysis, and data reporting. *Front. Psychol.* **2017**, *8*, 213. [CrossRef]
41. Kenward, M.G.; Roger, J.H. The use of baseline covariates in crossover studies. *Biostatistics* **2010**, *11*, 1–17. [CrossRef]
42. Cohen, J. *Statistical Power Analysis for the Behavioral Sciences*; Academic Press: Cambridge, MA, USA, 2013.
43. Lim, C.-Y.; In, J. Considerations for crossover design in clinical study. *Korean J. Anesthesiol.* **2021**, *74*, 293. [CrossRef] [PubMed]
44. Stanhewicz, A.E.; Wong, B.J. Counterpoint: Investigators should not control for menstrual cycle phase when performing studies of vascular control that include women. *J. Appl. Physiol.* **2020**, *129*, 1117–1119. [CrossRef] [PubMed]
45. Wenner, M.M.; Stachenfeld, N.S. Point: Investigators should control for menstrual cycle phase when performing studies of vascular control that include women. *J. Appl. Physiol.* **2020**, *129*, 1114–1116. [CrossRef] [PubMed]
46. Parker, B.A.; Kalasky, M.J.; Proctor, D.N. Evidence for sex differences in cardiovascular aging and adaptive responses to physical activity. *Eur. J. Appl. Physiol.* **2010**, *110*, 235–246. [CrossRef]
47. Vranish, J.R.; Young, B.E.; Kaur, J.; Patik, J.C.; Padilla, J.; Fadel, P.J. Influence of sex on microvascular and macrovascular responses to prolonged sitting. *Am. J. Physiol. -Heart Circ. Physiol.* **2017**, *312*, H800–H805. [CrossRef]
48. Lakin, R.; Notarius, C.; Thomas, S.; Goodman, J. Effects of moderate-intensity aerobic cycling and swim exercise on post-exertional blood pressure in healthy young untrained and triathlon-trained men and women. *Clin. Sci.* **2013**, *125*, 543–553. [CrossRef]
49. de Fúcio Lizardo, J.H.; Modesto, L.K.; Campbell, C.S.G.; Simões, H.G. Post-exercise hypotension: Comparison between different intensities of exercise on a treadmill and a cycle ergometer. *Rev. Bras. Cineantropometria Desempenho Hum.* **2007**, *9*, 115–120.
50. Reed, J. Blood pressure responses of sedentary African American women during cycle and treadmill exercise. *Ethn. Dis.* **2007**, *17*, 59–64.
51. Stoner, L.; Barone Gibbs, B.; Meyer, M.L.; Fryer, S.; Credeur, D.; Paterson, C.; Stone, K.; Hanson, E.D.; Kowalsky, R.J.; Horiuchi, M. A primer on repeated sitting exposure and the cardiovascular system: Considerations for study design, analysis, interpretation, and translation. *Front. Cardiovasc. Med.* **2021**, *8*, 716938. [CrossRef]
52. Brasil, I.A.; Silva, J.C.P.; Pescatello, L.S.; Farinatti, P. Central and peripheral mechanisms underlying postexercise hypotension: A scoping review. *J. Hypertens.* **2024**, *42*, 751–763. [CrossRef]
53. Bruneau, M.L., Jr.; Johnson, B.T.; Huedo-Medina, T.B.; Larson, K.A.; Ash, G.I.; Pescatello, L.S. The blood pressure response to acute and chronic aerobic exercise: A meta-analysis of candidate gene association studies. *J. Sci. Med. Sport* **2016**, *19*, 424–431. [CrossRef] [PubMed]

Journal of
Cardiovascular Development and Disease

MDPI

Review

Diagnostic Methods of Atherosclerotic Plaque and the Assessment of Its Prognostic Significance—A Narrative Review

Paweł Gać [1,2,*], Anna Jakubowska-Martyniuk [1], Aleksandra Żórawik [1], Wojciech Hajdusianek [1], Dawid Żytkowski [1], Tomasz Matys [3] and Rafał Poręba [2]

1 Department of Environmental Health, Occupational Medicine and Epidemiology, Wroclaw Medical University, Mikulicza-Radeckiego 7, 50-368 Wroclaw, Poland
2 Centre of Diagnostic Imaging, 4th Military Hospital, Rudolfa Weigla 5, 50-981 Wrocław, Poland
3 Department of Angiology and Internal Diseases, Wroclaw Medical University, Borowska 213, 50-556 Wroclaw, Poland
* Correspondence: pawelgac@interia.pl or pawel.gac@umw.edu.pl

Abstract: Cardiovascular diseases (CVD) are a leading cause of death. The most notable cause of CVD is an atherosclerotic plaque. The aim of this review is to provide an overview of different diagnostic methods for atherosclerotic plaque relevant to the assessment of cardiovascular risk. The methods can be divided into invasive and non-invasive. This review focuses on non-invasive with attention paid to ultrasonography, contrast-enhanced ultrasonography, intravascular ultrasonography, and assessment of intima-media complex, coronary computed tomography angiography, and magnetic resonance. In the review, we discuss a number of Artificial Intelligence technologies that support plaque imaging.

Keywords: cardiovascular; atherosclerosis; diagnostics; plaque; prognosis

1. Introduction

Cardiovascular diseases are one of the leading causes of death in the European Union with ischemic heart disease and stroke responsible for the majority of deaths from cardiovascular disease. However, it should be emphasized that age-standardized death rates of cardiovascular diseases have decreased recently by approximately 10%. [1,2]. Given the seriousness of this problem, a great deal of scientific effort has been devoted to addressing this issue, resulting in the development of many guidelines, such as the European Society of Cardiology Guidelines. Of these, particular attention to the problem of atherosclerotic plaque was given in the 2021 ESC Guidelines on cardiovascular disease prevention in clinical practice [3]. The guidelines emphasize the importance of atherosclerotic cardiovascular disease and its risk factors such as, inter alia, low-density lipoprotein cholesterol, blood pressure, cigarette smoking, or diabetes mellitus leading to atherosclerotic plaque formation that leads to vascular occlusion. Atherosclerosis begins with the disruption of the most inner layer of the vascular wall, which is an endothelium, which is mainly caused by the exposition to cardiovascular risk factors. The plaque may be initially asymptomatic, and, in some patients, it may even remain so throughout their life; however, especially in patients with additional risk factors, it may lead to further complications [3,4].

Diagnostic imaging, however, participates not only in evaluation of risk in the area of cardiological prevention, but assists in diagnosing patients suspected of acute coronary syndromes. In particular, coronary computed tomography angiography (CCTA) can help to assess patients with no ECG changes and uncertain high-sensitivity cardiac troponin [5]. Similarly, for patients with suspected chronic coronary syndrome with an appropriate pre-test likelihood assessment of disease, CCTA is a recommended diagnostic procedure [6].

There are studies reporting that plaque can excessively enlarge in the months before clinical incident. In a study conducted by Hackett et al. it was based on the records of all their patients who happened to have had coronary arteriography performed during a clinically stable phase of their disease before and after AMI [7]. Therefore, appropriate imaging is particularly important [8,9].

The plaques have been histologically classified by Stary et al. based on their components [9,10]. Such components include, for instance, atherogenic lipoprotein, macrophage foam cells, lipid-laden smooth muscle cells, extracellular lipid droplets or calcium. It should be emphasized that some plaque poses a greater threat than others—particularly type IV and V. There is also a noticeable variation in the pattern of plaque growth. Plaque of types I–IV grow mainly due to lipid accumulation, whereas type V is caused by smooth muscle and collagen increase and type VI is caused by thrombosis or hematoma [10]. The main methodological concepts of current review are presented in Figure 1.

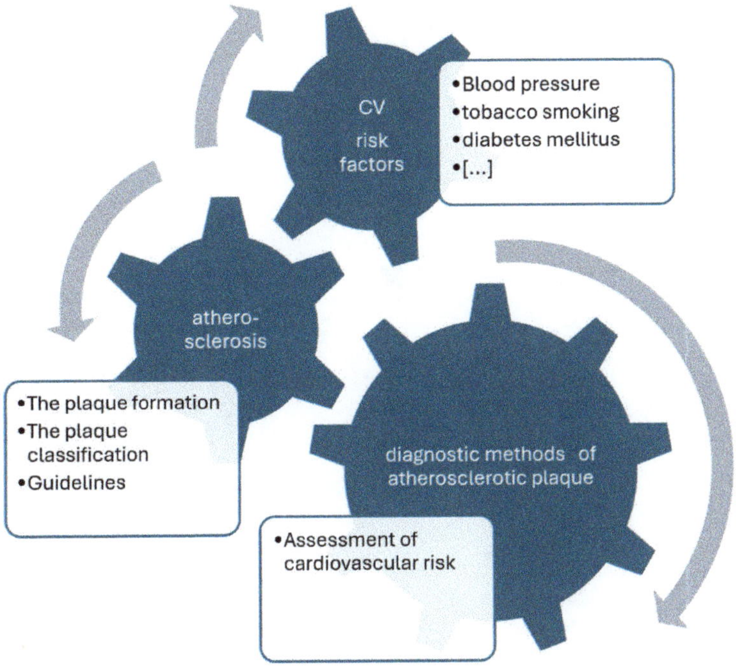

Figure 1. Methodological approach of the current review. CV—cardiovascular.

The aim of this review is to provide an overview of different radiological diagnostic methods: ultrasonography, computed tomography, magnetic resonance imaging, positron emission tomography of atherosclerotic plaque which are relevant to the assessment of cardiovascular risk.

2. Imaging of Atherosclerotic Plaque Morphology

Currently, many invasive and non-invasive imaging methods are used to study atherosclerosis; most specify lumen diameter or stenosis, wall thickness, and plaque volume [11]. A wide variety of techniques are used in clinical practice. They include ultrasound, computer tomography (CT), magnetic resonance tomography (MRI), positron emission tomography (PET), single-photon emission computed tomography (SPECT), and photon-counting detector CT (PCD-CT) [12,13]. The imaging of plaque is also the subject of guidelines of American Society of Neuroradiology, which emphasizes that not only the measurements of luminal stenosis, but also advanced wall imaging is important in identifying plaque that poses a greater risk. The main research concepts are presented in Figure 2.

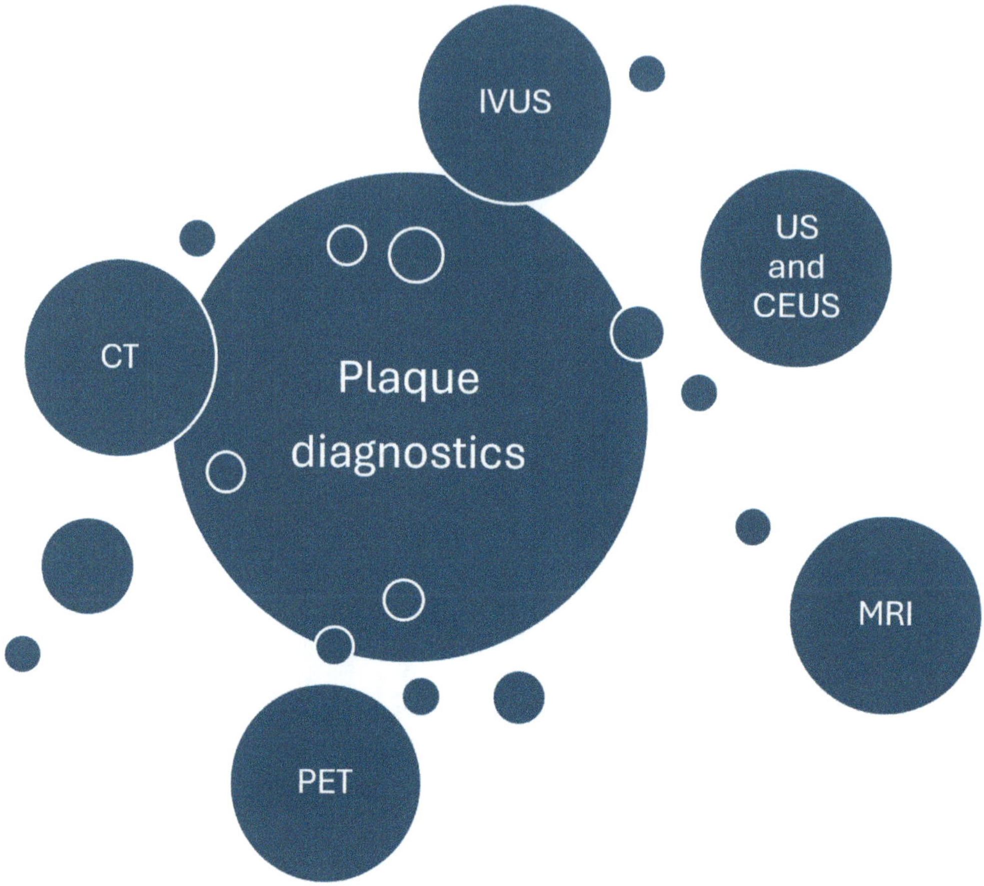

Figure 2. Main research concepts. CT—computed tomography, IVUS—intravascular ultrasound, CEUS—contrast—enhanced ultrasound, MRI—magnetic resonance imaging, PET—positron emission tomography, US—ultrasound.

2.1. *Ultrasound Imaging Techniques*

Ultrasound imaging techniques (USG) help to find vulnerable atherosclerotic plaques [12]. This method is based on transmitting and receiving high-frequency sound waves [11]. This provides the high spatial resolution required for measuring intima-media thickness (IMT). However, higher frequency is also limited by the depth of body penetration [14]. The time between transmission and reception of a wave is related to the distance between the source and the reflector [11]. Due to signal attenuation problems, non-invasive ultrasound for imaging blood vessel wall is generally limited to shallow vascular beds such as carotid, femoral, and other peripheral arteries. Atherosclerotic plaque can be directly visualized on B-mode ultrasound, intravascular ultrasound (IVUS), and three-dimensional (3D) ultrasound [15]. The thickness of the artery wall and the structure and composition of atherosclerotic plaque can be measured [14]. The echogenicity of the plaque reflects its characteristics. Hypoechoic heterogeneous plaque is associated with both intraplaque hemorrhage and lipids, whereas hyperechoic homogeneous plaque is mainly fibrous [11], Figure 3.

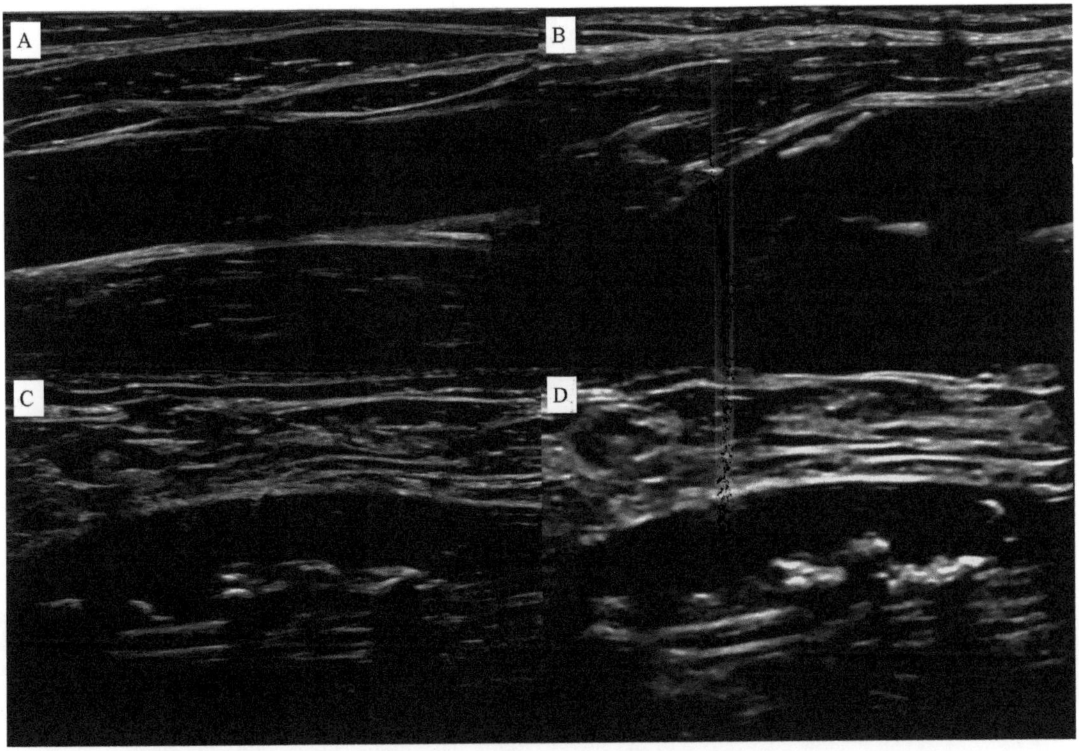

Figure 3. Atherosclerotic plaques on ultrasound examination: (**A**) heterogeneous plaque in the common carotid artery, (**B**) homogeneous hyperechoic plaques in the carotid bulb, (**C**) heterogeneous plaque in the superficial femoral artery, (**D**) hyperechoic plaque in the superficial femoral artery.

B-mode ultrasound of the carotid arteries can identify plaques and measure intima-media thickness (IMT) [16]. Abnormal thickening of the carotid IMT is thought to be a marker of generalized atherosclerotic disease. However, different sources provide nonidentical limit values for IMT. Ibanez et al. say that normal IMT has been determined to be approximately 0.5 to 1.1 mm, values > 1.1 mm may indicate the presence of atherosclerotic plaque [14]. However, the Mannheim consensus suggests at least 0.5 mm or 50% of the surrounding IMT value and thickness of at least 1.5 mm [17]. On the other hand, Chuan-Wei Yang et al. assume presence of the intima–media's focal thickening > 1 mm that bulges out into the carotid artery's lumen with at least twice the thickness of the IMT on either side [18]. And, finally, the American Society of Echocardiography defines plaque as any thickening of atherosclerotic origin that intrudes into the lumen of carotid artery, or an IMT of at least 1.5 mm [19]. Abnormal thickening of the carotid IMT is thought to be a marker of generalized atherosclerotic disease. Normal IMT has been determined to be approximately 0.5 to 1.1 mm, with values > 1.1 mm indicating the presence of atherosclerotic plaque. The use of this index as a vascular marker is based partly on the assumption that carotid IMT > 75th percentile for age indicates generalized atherosclerosis [14]. Although ultrasonography has the advantage of being non-invasive and enabling qualitative assessment of carotid plaques, image quality is limited by echo windows and calcification [16]. IMT measurement has proved to be a useful research technique when quality can be rigorously controlled and many patients are involved; however, it is less useful in a clinical setting for monitoring an individual patient [14]. An example IMT measurement is shown in Figure 4.

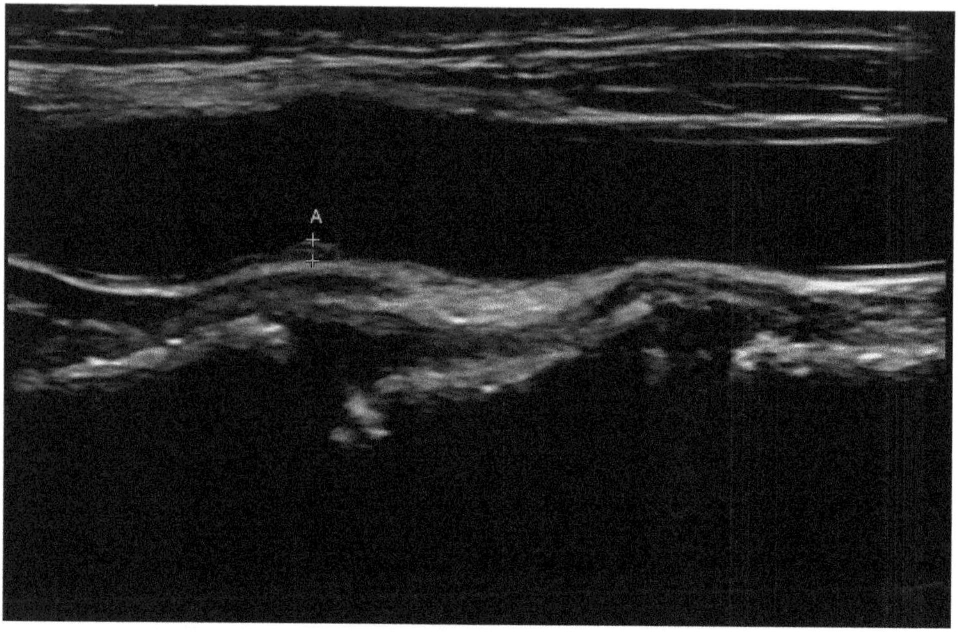

Figure 4. Example of measurement of intima media thickness (IMT) in ultrasound examination of the carotid arteries. A—IMT measurement, + measurement markers.

Due to limitations caused by the physics of ultrasound examinations, the examination is dependable only at the far arterial wall and does not indicate whether the thickening is because of intima or media infiltration or hypertrophy. As with other USG methods, this technique is operator-dependent and has lower reproducibility [11].

To indirectly find out if a patient has blood flow problems (for example due to stenosis caused by atherosclerotic plaque), other tests might be chosen, like a stress echocardiography. This test uses intravenous vasodilators such as adenosine or dobutamine. There are different stresses of similar diagnostic and prognostic accuracy. Among them dobutamine is the best for viability. The choice of one test over the other depends on patient characteristics, local drug costs, and the physician's preference. Stress echocardiography is a good choice due to it lower cost, wider availability and for the radiation-free nature [20,21].

2.2. The Use of Contrast in USG Imaging of Atherosclerosis

Another method is to inject a contrast agent into liposomes [12]. Contrast-enhanced ultrasound (CEUS) can provide information about plaque composition, and structural information [22]. The quantitative assessment of microbubble retention in the carotid plaque on CEUS is a technique that has promise as a tissue-specific marker of inflammation and a potential role in risk stratification of atherosclerotic carotid stenosis [23]. CEUS enables an assessment of myocardial perfusion, a function of left ventricle and intracardiac thrombus and endocardial borders [24]. Microbubbles are retained in inflamed tissue, it is possible that CEUS could be translated into clinical practice, where it may have a role in monitoring therapy or selecting patients for surgical procedures [22]. There are available USG devices that have preprogrammed settings for CEUS. To avoid destruction of the microbubbles, you select a low mechanical index, which allows continuous image acquisition (0.1–0.3) or middle-high (0.3–0.5) mechanical index, which requires intermittent imaging allowing the replenishment of destructed microbubbles [24]. UCAs (Ultrasound Contrast Agents) are administered safely in various applications [25] with a very low rate of adverse reactions (about 0.014%) [26,27]. Conducting a laboratory assessment of the liver, thyroid, or kidney function before administration is not required [28]. Contraindications for the contrast agent administration are allergy to the agent, large right to left shunt, and an unstable condition [24]. The overall reported rate of fatalities attributed to one UCA, SonoVue™ (Bracco, Milan), is low (14/2,447,083 exposed patients; 0.0006%) and compares favorably with the risk of fatal events reported for iodinated contrast agents (approximately 0.001%) [25]. The limitations of this method is that CEUS is significantly dependent on operator skill, the cost of contrast media is not negligible, and the image lacks a wide scope and therefore has difficulty exploring some deep regions [27].

The novel imaging technique is a 3-dimensional vascular ultrasound (3DVUS) [29]. There are reports that say that 3DVUS is a more comprehensive evaluation of overall atherosclerosis burden, which avoids the drawbacks of 2DVUS, and offers reproducibility of plaque measurements. The volumetric-linear probe uses the "mechanical-sweep" method and enables accurate measurements of atherosclerosis from early to more advanced disease stages regardless of plaque size [30].

Although 3DVUS allows for the detection and assessment of atherosclerotic plaques in arteries, such as the femoral or carotid artery, it is not accurate in measuring them in deeper vessels such as the aorta [30]. It is inexpensive and radiation-free and has the potential to become an important screening device for identifying patients in high-risk groups [29].

2.3. Intravascular Ultrasonography Assessment

Intravascular ultrasound (IVUS) is an innovative approach to arterial wall imaging, enabling direct real-time imaging of atherosclerosis and providing a cross-sectional, tomographic perspective of the vessel and atherosclerotic disease [11]. It is a catheter-based test, which, in addition to determining the size of the coronary lumen, allows for obtaining an image of the thickness and acoustic density of the entire vessel wall [14]. It is regulated by accurate and deeply penetrating imaging capabilities with a distributed signal converted in real time into a two-dimensional (2D) video image. Grayscale IVUS enabled the in vivo assessment of vessel wall dimensions, phenotypic features, distribution, and severity of atherosclerotic lesions [31]. The advantage of IVUS over regular US techniques is that it can provide data on the structure of atherosclerotic plaque. The liposome has a layered structure, which allows it to capture gas bubbles that can effectively reflect sound waves and produce acoustically reflective liposomes [12]. Liposomes can be conjugated to antibodies such as anti-fibrinogen or anti-ICAM-1 to enhance platelet recognition and targeting [12]. The current generation of catheters (incorporating a transducer) have a diameter of 0.96 to 1.17 mm and provide high image quality. Based on echogenicity, atherosclerotic plaque can be divided into three categories: (1) highly echogenic areas with acoustic shadows, often corresponding to calcified tissue; (2) hyperechoic areas indicating fibrosis or microcalcifications; or (3) hypoechoic areas consistent with thrombotic or lipid-rich tissue or a mixture of these [11].

Subsequent advances in IVUS processing, and, in particular, the analysis of the radiofrequency ultrasonic backscatter signal (IVUS-RF), also known as virtual histology intravascular ultrasound (VH-IVUS), allowed a real-time cross-sectional and longitudinal three-dimensional (3D) visualization of a vessel that broadened the knowledge on the composition and mechanical properties of the vulnerable plaque [31]. VH-IVUS can precisely detect the presence of fibrous, fibro-lipid, calcified, and necrotic areas in plaques [22]. The predictive accuracy of in vivo IVUS-VH can be degraded by the presence of intramural thrombus [15].

IVUS may be useful in selecting the most appropriate option of transcatheter therapy (rotational atherectomy, stents, etc.)—lesions with calcification would be expected to be more rigid and, therefore, prone to rupture in response to the mechanical stress of balloon dilation, whereas softer, lipid-rich, noncalcified plaque may stretch but not fracture [11].

Studies that have compared ultrasound measurements with histological findings have shown that the IMT of posterior (far) wall IMT of the carotid artery as measured with the use of US reflects the true thickness of the wall, although measurements recorded with US may be slightly different than estimates attained by histology. Values obtained by measuring the anterior (proximal) wall of the carotid artery are less accurate [14]. Based on research conducted by Gernot Schulte-Altedorneburg et al., it was noticed that values obtained by ultrasound always turned out to be smaller than those obtained histologically, indicating a systematic discrepancy [32]. One of USG's advantages is its great spatial resolution, due to its high frequency (up to 50 MHz). On the other hand, IVUS is an invasive procedure [33].

2.4. Computed Tomography Assessment

Computed tomography (CT) is fast and relatively inexpensive. With a bolus injection of a contrast agent, CT is suitable for detecting calcifications in atherosclerotic plaque and fibrous tissue [12]. However, the lipid-rich necrotic core could only be adequately quantified in certain subsets of plaque, and hemorrhage and thrombus could not reliably be distinguished from lipids. Plaque density measured in Hounsfield units showed significant overlap between densities associated with lipid-rich necrotic core, connective tissue, and hemorrhage [15]. This method is not effective in detecting other components of high-risk plaque: thin-capped fibroma and the presence of inflammatory cells [16]. Examples of hyperdense (calcified), mixed-dense, and hypodense (noncalcified) atherosclerotic plaques on CTA of coronary arteries are presented in Figure 5.

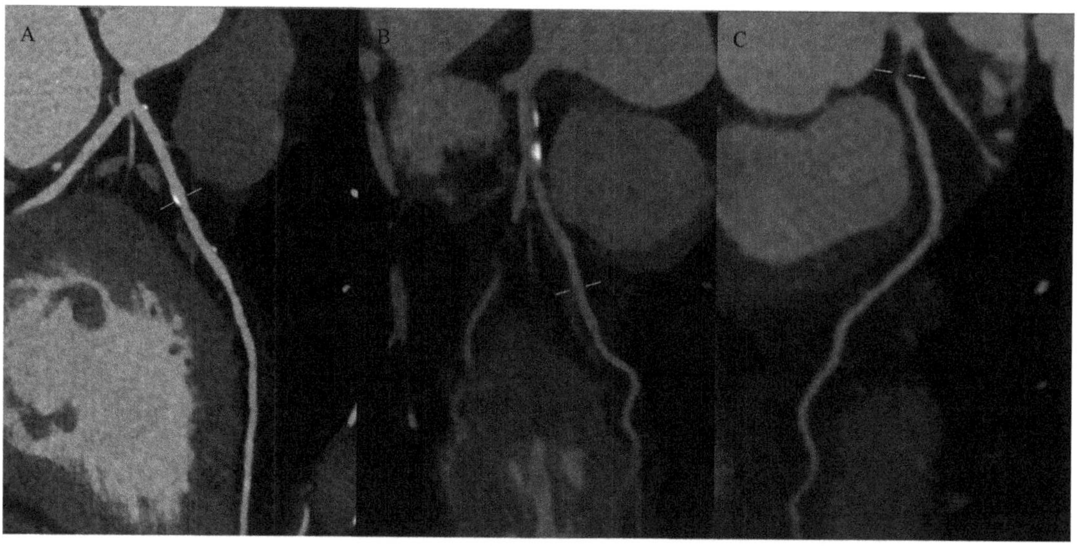

Figure 5. Atherosclerotic plaques on coronary computed tomography angiography: (**A**) calcified plaques in the left anterior descending artery (LAD), (**B**) mixed plaques in the LAD, (**C**) non-calcified concentric plaque in the LAD.

Computed tomography uses two techniques to image atherosclerosis: one is the more traditional angiographic technique (CTA), which allows the assessment of narrowing of the lumen of the artery but requires the use of a contrast agent. Another technique is direct calcium visualization and related calcium quantification methods such as calcium scoring [15]. An example of coronary artery calcium score measurement using CT is shown in Figure 6.

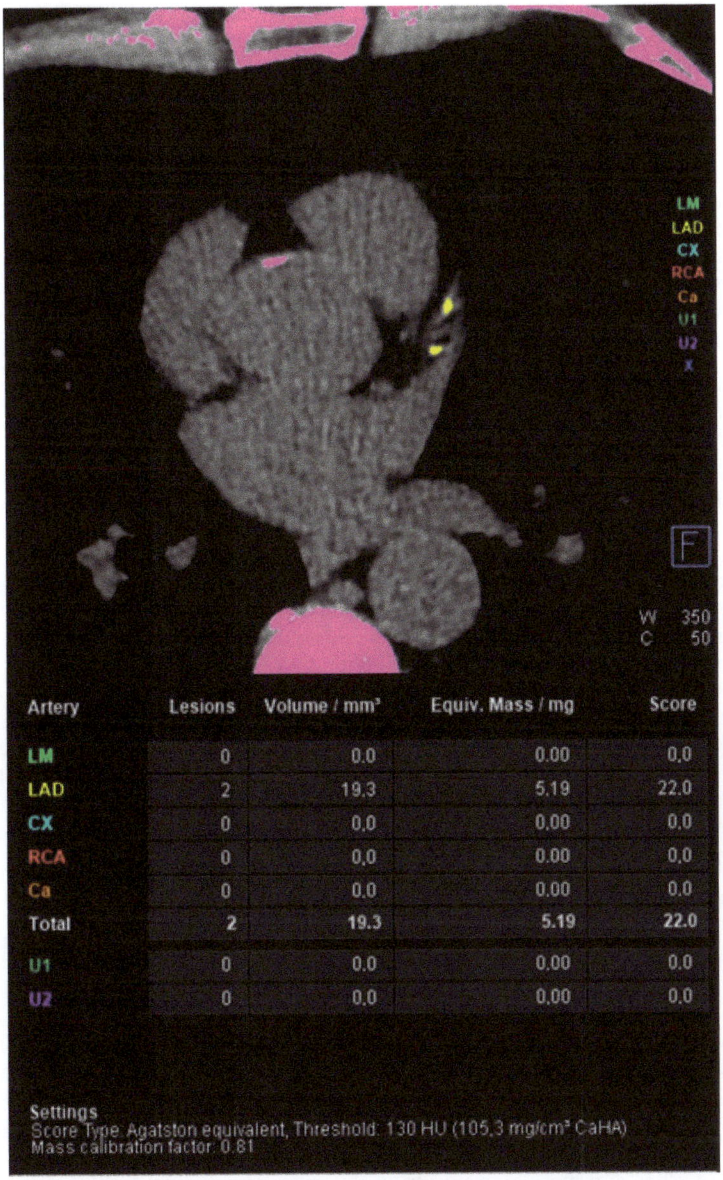

Figure 6. Coronary artery calcium score measurement using non-contrast computed tomography. Light green indicates calcifications in the left main (LM), yellow in the left anterior descending (LAD), blue in the left circumflex (CX), red in the right coronary artery (RCA), orange in other coronary branches (Ca), dark green and purple in extracoronary structures (U1 and U2). The application indicates voxels proposed as meeting the calcification criterion in pink.

It has been shown that the amount of calcium detected in coronary vessels correlates with the extent of coronary atherosclerosis detected histologically [22,34]. This allows more accurate assessment of coronary plaque burden. Assesses presence of both obstructive and non-obstructive disease and analysis of plaque composition [35]. The second category includes: electron-beam CT (EBCT), multiple-row detector CT (MDCT/MSCT) and dual-source tomography (DSCT). EBCT uses stationary tungsten rings to generate X-ray images at 3 mm slice thickness from which a coronary artery calcium score is calculated to assess cardiovascular risk. In contrast, the latter uses a continuously rotating X-ray source to obtain 0.5–0.75 mm slices during a single patient breath hold [22]. Dual source computed tomography (DSCT) is used in the assessment of atherosclerotic plaque by simultaneously capturing images from two X-ray systems, which can achieve increased temporal resolution and acquisition speed combined with significantly reduced radiation dose [16]. Nevertheless, this technique cannot be used to differentiate thin-cap fibroatheroma, only to assess the features of calcifications and fibro-fatty tissue in the coronary plaque [36]. Novel photon-counting detector CT (PCD-CT) has the potential to address the limitations of previous CT systems, such as insufficient spatial resolution, limited accuracy in detecting small low-contrast structures, or missing routine availability of spectral information [13]. The photon-counting computed tomography (PCCT) has a significant advantage in the imaging of coronary arteries and enables a wider examination of the plaque structure [37].

2.5. Optical Coherence Tomography

Recent studies have shown that optical coherence tomography (OCT) is an accurate method for assessing the thickness of the fibrous cap in atherosclerotic plaques [12], enabling the identification of thin caps and plaque ruptures and erosion [35]. OCT uses near-infrared light emitted through a fiberoptic wire with a rotating lens to achieve an exceptionally high spatial resolution (10–15 μm), providing accurate measurement of fibrous cap thickness with strong correlation to histology, and good sensitivity and specificity to distinguish plaque type [38]. OCT has proven useful in assessing intraplaque neovascularization, which is a key factor contributing to atherosclerotic plaque growth and instability [31]. Unfortunately, the distinction between calcium and lipids in plaques can be difficult with OCT due to limited tissue penetration (up to 3 mm), which makes it difficult to estimate the entire plaque volume [12]. Moreover, for image acquisition, a blood-free field is needed, which can be achieved through the supply of saline or contrast flushing during pullback [38]. OCT has been found to be useful for assessing developmental processes, including thrombus formation and calcifications important for atherosclerotic plaque progression [31,39].

2.6. Magnetic Resonance Imaging

Other commonly used methods include magnetic resonance imaging (MRI) and magnetic resonance angiography (MRA), which use gadolinium and iron oxide derivatives as contrast enhancement with a resolution of 10–100 microns to visualize the structure of atherosclerotic lesions [12]. In addition to the traditional contrast, MRI offers the ability to probe atherosclerotic plaque for diffusion, contrast uptake, dynamic contrast permeability, magnetization transfer, and others [15]. MR provides imaging without ionizing radiation and can be repeated sequentially over time [11]. Early studies have shown that the surface area of atherosclerotic plaque tissue components with a lipid-rich core assessed by MRI correlates with a histopathological assessment [16]. In clinical practice, MRI mainly visualizes signals from protons in free water, triglycerides, and free fatty acids [22], differentiates plaque components based on biophysical and biochemical parameters, such as chemical composition and concentration, water content, physical state, and molecular movement [11]. Macromolecules, for example proteins or cholesterol crystals, are not involved in conventional MR signals due to a noticeably short T2 signal [16,40]. MRI enables not only the quantitative assessment of the size of the atherosclerotic plaque, but also the assessment of intra-plaque hemorrhage and the integrity of the fibrous sheath [14], and it provides the ability to distinguish the vessel lumen from the vessel wall [41]. Non-contrast T1-weighted magnetic resonance imaging can identify the presence of high-risk plaques and thrombi [31], which uses a high T1 signal associated with methemoglobin, a key component of fresh thrombus [35]. Additionally, it can detect positive arterial remodeling in asymptomatic patients with subclinical atherosclerosis [31].

Coronary magnetic resonance imaging (MRI) is a rapidly developing method that, thanks to recent technological improvements, can provide reliable imaging of the proximal and middle vessels [38]. However, this technique is not optimal for quantifying lumen area/volume because it is prone to unwanted signal loss due to complex flow patterns [15]. When using "bright blood" contrast-free techniques for coronary MRA, which relies on a high T2/T1 ratio of blood to function as an internal contrast agent, there is a need to potentially avoid nephrotoxic contrast agents [38].

2.7. Positron Emission Tomography

Methods such as positron emission tomography (PET) and single photon emission computed tomography (SPECT) are gaining popularity because they use imaging elements such as 18F, 64Cu, 11C/99mTc, 123/124/125/131I, 111In tracers [14]. Radioisotope decay is detected in order to produce the signal, measured as standardized uptake values or tissue-to-background ratios [22]. The efficiency of PET is much greater, and the technique provides higher resolution, less noise, and less radiation exposure than SPECT [14]. Additionally, a prevalence of PET over other techniques, including SPECT and MRI, is its greater sensitivity in detecting molecular signals, but limited spatial resolution means that images must be co-registered (like SPECT) with CT or MR to accurately localize the anatomical signal PET [38]. The development of hybrid PET/CT scanners with improved imaging allowed the assessment of the activity of atherosclerotic disease [35]. PET is used to detect cellular activity and assess biological processes relevant to atherosclerosis, such as arterial inflammation, hypoxia, neo-angiogenesis, and microcalcification [31].

The PET study uses 18F-fluorodeoxyglucose (FDG), a commonly used radiolabeled glucose analog for various diagnostic purposes [38], which accumulates in proportion to metabolic activity [14] and is captured by macrophages [31]. It has been shown that numerous macrophages reside in ruptured plaques [12]. 18F-FDG accumulates in the arterial wall in direct proportion to the degree of cellular glycolysis, respectively, reflecting the density of atherosclerotic plaque macrophages and the degree of inflammation [31], as a non-specific marker [38]; therefore, it is worth noting that FDG uptake may have added value in detecting the condition inflammation (e.g., in psoriasis, RA or HIV) [22] or diabetes [35]. High uptake of 18F-FDG by myocardial cells often prevents the interpretation of coronary signals [38], but uptake can be reduced by preparation before the test with a low-carbohydrate, high-fat diet [23]. Importantly, FDG/PET-CT has been shown to be highly reproducible in assessing the degree of FDG uptake by the vessel wall [14]. FDG uptake can be decreased by medication. This may lead to adapting it as an endpoint in various trials which target the anti-inflammatory effects of different therapies [35].

Another PET tracer used for the dynamic assessment of microcalcifications in coronary vessels is 18F-sodium fluoride (18F-NaF), which is commonly used as a marker of bone mineralization in skeletal imaging [12]. In this case, uptake by the myocardium has no effect on the signal [31]. In aortic stenosis, areas of increased 18F fluoride activity predict where new macroscopic calcium deposits will be deposited, providing excellent prediction of progression in the valve calcification score [35].

The use of other tracers is also being studied, such as 68Ga-DOTATATE [31], 18F-fluorocholine (18F-FCH) or 11C-PK11195 [35]. There was decreased background heart cell uptake with tracers when compared with 18F-FDG. Therefore, they are preferable for coronary artery imaging [31].

Radioactive isotopes used to produce SPECT tracers typically have longer half-lives and are more widely available than those used in PET [16]. Additionally, SPECT is widely available (and cheaper) than PET, but is susceptible to artifacts, especially those caused by motion and soft tissue, and requires significant radiation exposure [42].

The table for comparison of the different imaging modalities is presented below as Table 1.

Table 1. The table presents comparison of the different imaging modalities.

Imaging Modality	Advantages	Limitations
USG	• Non invasive • Enables qualitative assessment of carotid plaques. • High spatial resolution required for measuring intima-media thickness.	• Limited to shallow vascular beds. • Quality is limited by echo windows and calcification. • Not indicating whether the thickening is because of intima or media infiltration or hypertrophy. • Operator-dependent and has lower reproducibility.
CEUS	• Gives information about plaque composition, and structure. • Low rate of adverse reactions.	• Strongly operator dependent. • Cost of contrast media.
IVUS	• High image quality • direct real-time imaging of atherosclerosis and the vessel. • Can assess the structure of atherosclerotic plaque.	• Invasive procedure.
CT	• Fast. • Relatively inexpensive. • Suitable for detecting calcifications in atherosclerotic plaque.	• Hemorrhage and thrombus could not reliably be distinguished from lipid. • Not effective in detecting other components of high-risk plaques: thin-capped fibroma and the presence of inflammatory cells. • X-rays patient exposition.
MRI	• Not exposing to ionizing radiation. • Enables the assessment of intra-plaque hemorrhage and the integrity of the fibrous sheath. • Detects positive arterial remodeling in asymptomatic patients with subclinical atherosclerosis.	• Prone to unwanted signal loss due to complex flow patterns.

USG—ultrasonography CEUS—contrast-enhanced ultra sonography, CT—computed tomography, MRI—magnetic resonance imaging.

2.8. Multimodality Imaging

Multimodality consists of combining two or more techniques [43]. One of the techniques consists of near-infrared spectroscopy (NIRS) and intravascular ultrasound (IVUS), in which NIRS is responsible for the assessment of plaque with high lipid content and IVUS is responsible for the dimension of plaque measurements [44]. This technique and other similar techniques are interesting aspects of multimodality, which is a development of dual-probe catheters for an invasive plaque assessment. Another available example is the combination of IVUS and optical coherence tomography [45]. Another example of multimodality is the combination of magnetic resonance imaging and positron emission tomography to enrich the examination with inflammation analysis due to the accumulation of radionuclide in macrophages [46].

3. Artificial Intelligence and Atherosclerotic Plaque Imaging

3.1. Artificial Intelligence in Atherosclerosis Assessment

Nowadays, there are attempts to increase the share of artificial intelligence (AI) in everyday diagnostics, including the detection of asymptomatic atherosclerosis. AI is playing an increasingly significant role in supporting image processing and interpretation, offering greater efficiency, fewer human errors, and better diagnostic accuracy, without increasing costs and workload [41], enabling accurate measurement of atherosclerotic plaque volume and stenosis severity based on CCTA scans [47]. Combining human knowledge with artificial intelligence can facilitate the reliable and accurate interpretation of images obtained using CT, MR, PET, intravascular ultrasound, and OCT [48]. One of the many applications of artificial intelligence is the creation of predictive models by exposure to substantial amounts of data in order to match or exceed the capabilities of simple visual assessment or manual measurement [47]. The use of AI, which is not guided by any generally accepted assumptions, allows the exploration of all available data for non-linear patterns that can predict the risk of a specific person, i.e., precise risk stratification [49]. At the same time, rapid improvements in artificial intelligence algorithms will facilitate full automation of software-based plaque quantification [50], an evolving field with the potential to have a profound impact on clinical practice [47].

3.2. Legal Aspects of Using Artificial Intelligence in Radiology

Artificial Intelligence (AI) in radiology represents one of the most innovative applications of technology in medicine. It enables the automatic analysis of medical images, assisting doctors in diagnosing diseases, monitoring treatment progress, and planning therapy. Despite numerous benefits, the implementation of AI in this field involves significant legal challenges.

Ensuring patient safety is a fundamental aspect of introducing AI into radiology. Legal regulations concerning medical devices, such as the European Parliament and Council Regulation (EU) 2017/745 on medical devices (MDR), require these devices to undergo rigorous conformity assessments before being placed on the market [51]. AI algorithms must be thoroughly evaluated for efficacy and safety, and their results must be transparent and accessible to regulatory bodies.

Processing medical data using AI in radiology imposes high requirements for data protection. According to the General Data Protection Regulation (GDPR), medical data are classified as a special category of data that requires additional protection [52]. Therefore, the use of AI for analyzing medical images must comply with principles of data minimization, purpose limitation, and data integrity and confidentiality. It is also necessary to obtain patient consent for processing their data unless there is another legal basis.

One of the biggest legal challenges related to AI in radiology is the issue of liability for diagnostic errors. Traditionally, the responsibility for diagnostic errors lies with the physician, but the use of AI complicates the situation. Three main scenarios of liability can be distinguished: the liability of the software manufacturer, the liability of the user (physician), and shared liability. In practice, resolving liability issues may require analyzing the specific circumstances of a given case, including whether the algorithm operated as intended and whether the user properly interpreted its results [53].

The dynamic development of AI in radiology requires flexible and adaptive legal regulations. Current legal frameworks may not keep pace with the rate of innovation, necessitating continuous updates. In particular, there is a need to develop specific regulations concerning the certification of AI algorithms, real-time monitoring of their performance, and ensuring transparency in AI decision-making processes. It is also important for these regulations to be harmonized at the international level to ensure consistency and facilitate data exchange and cross-border cooperation [54].

The application of artificial intelligence in radiology holds immense potential but also involves significant legal challenges. Key issues include ensuring patient safety, protecting personal data, and determining legal liability. Future legal regulations must be flexible and adapted to the dynamically evolving technology to effectively support its safe and efficient use in medical practice.

4. Discussion

Despite great progress and effort in reducing atherosclerotic plaque formation as part of the treatment of patients after acute coronary syndromes and in secondary prevention, the incidence of atherosclerosis is exceedingly high. The assessment of plaque stability remains an important prognostic factor, so the development of diagnostic methods remains an important therapeutic issue. Atherosclerosis appears to be an irreversible process, although studies to date report possible plaque regression with intensive drug therapy [55–59]. Atherosclerosis is a major contributor to cardiovascular disease, which is the most common cause of death worldwide [58]. This group of diseases includes stroke, which is one of the most common causes of death. Annually, there are about twelve million cases of stroke worldwide, of which about 62% are ischemic in origin [58,59]. About 87% of ischemic stroke cases are associated with the presence of modifiable risk factors, such as lipid levels, as one of the most common causes of stroke is atherosclerotic disease, usually affecting the proximal portion of the internal carotid arteries [59]. This is why early diagnosis and treatment of pathological conditions that can easily improve the prevention of atherosclerosis is so important.

Undoubtedly, an unprecedented achievement is the development of methods in the field of intravascular imaging diagnostics represent a major advance in terms of assessing the composition and morphology of atherosclerotic plaque [57,60]. Previous studies have reported that accurate diagnosis of plaque rupture, plaque erosion, or calcified nodule (the three most common causes for the onset of coronary thrombosis [61]) can be helpful in choosing appropriate therapy specific to unstable lesion types in acute coronary syndromes [60,62,63]. Coronary thrombosis based on plaque rupture more often results in no-flow and distal embolization after percutaneous coronary intervention and larger myocardial infarct size [64]. Acute coronary syndromes occurring from coronary thrombosis based on plaque erosion have a better clinical prognosis compared to those with plaque rupture and, in addition, are potentially stabilizable without stent implantation, only with anticoagulant treatment [63,65]. In the studies described so far, acute coronary syndromes due to calcified nodules have been associated with incidents of incomplete stent expansion, resulting in an increased risk of restenosis and stent thrombosis [66].

With the development of novel imaging methods for atherosclerotic plaque, the expected prognostically significant endpoints can be identified with increasing precision. This now makes it possible not only to assess the burden of atherosclerosis, but also to accurately determine the composition of the plaque. With these advances, the effectiveness of the anti-atherosclerotic treatment used can be accurately assessed and the progression of the disease can be controlled. The need for further development of these imaging techniques is dictated by the constant effort to improve the resolution and technical quality of examinations, which will enable increasingly accurate assessment of atherosclerotic plaque composition [67]. Subsequent studies are becoming more precise in determining the effectiveness and seeking optimal sensitivity and specificity of particular imaging techniques [57,67]. Yabushita et al. were the first to show that the accuracy of OCT in diagnosing necrotic lipid plaques was suboptimal [68], Di Vito et al. confirmed these observations and noted the greater precision of a technique combining IVUS and NIRS [69]. Many studies have used the imaging techniques discussed above to evaluate and prove the reversibility of the atherosclerotic process through pharmacological anti-atherosclerotic therapy [70–73]. Nicholls et al. used IVUS to assess the inhibition of atherosclerosis progression when statins were used as well as a proprotein convertase subtilisin kexin type 9 (PCSK9) inhibitor. The availability of coronary imaging has also allowed studies to identify patients with atherosclerotic plaque erosion amenable to stabilization with antithrombotic therapy without stent implantation [65]. There are an increasing number of reports available regarding the effectiveness of treatment with Inclisiran and monoclonal antibodies against PCSK9. According to the literature, Inclisiran has a good safety profile and can reduce even 50% of the LDL-C level when compared to placebo [74].

Further research is needed to develop the clinical application of imaging studies in diagnosing the status of atherosclerosis, especially within the coronary arteries. Previous reports confirm the sense of intensive therapy focused on reducing risk factors in slowing the progression of the disease. Thanks to imaging studies, it is possible to control not only the volume, but also the composition of atherosclerotic plaques that play a key role in their stabilization, and on which the impact of anti-atherosclerotic therapies still remains to be clarified [67]. Achieving effective therapies to stabilize plaque will better control the increasing prevalence of atherogenic risk factors and reduce the incidence of their cardiovascular complications.

5. Conclusions

To summarize, in our manuscript we attempted to overview different methods used to diagnose atherosclerotic plaque. We found literature supporting the usage of an ultrasound examination of plaque but with limitations to shallowly placed vessels, we covered intravascular ultrasound examination and contrast-enhanced with assessments of microbubbles. Furthermore, we described the computed tomography assessment of plaque with their most important patterns: angiography and calcium scoring and with their limitations. We described optimal coherence tomography with its accuracy in assessing the thickness of fibrous cap and limitations in distinctions between calcium and lipids. In the last part, we introduced magnetic resonance imaging and nuclear medicine imaging with its strengths of assessing the density of plaque macrophages and its possibility to predict progression in the calcification score. We also briefly described legal challenges that the introduction of artificial intelligence imaging brings to this field, such as data protection problems and the analysis of different scenarios of diagnostic errors liability. We conclude that both the assessment of quantity and the composition of plaque are important, which can be achieved by further improvement of resolution and quality of examinations.

Author Contributions: Conceptualization, A.J.-M., W.H., P.G.; writing, P.G., W.H., A.J.-M., D.Ż., A.Ż.; writing—review and editing, T.M. and R.P.; supervision, P.G. and R.P. All authors have read and agreed to the published version of the manuscript.

Funding: This research received no external funding.

Institutional Review Board Statement: Not applicable.

Informed Consent Statement: Not applicable.

Data Availability Statement: Not applicable.

Conflicts of Interest: The authors declare no conflicts of interest.

References

1. Townsend, N.; Kazakiewicz, D.; Lucy Wright, F.; Timmis, A.; Huculeci, R.; Torbica, A.; Gale, C.P.; Achenbach, S.; Weidinger, F.; Vardas, P.I. Epidemiology of cardiovascular disease in Europe. *Nat. Rev. Cardiol.* **2022**, *19*, 133–143. [CrossRef] [PubMed]
2. Eurostat Causes of Death Statistics. 2024. Available online: https://ec.europa.eu/eurostat/statistics-explained/index.php?title=Causes_of_death_statistics (accessed on 31 July 2024).
3. Visseren, F.L.J.; Mach, F.; Smulders, Y.M.; Carballo, D.; Koskinas, K.C.; Bäck, M.; Benetos, A.; Biffi, A.; Boavida, J.M.; Capodanno, D. 2021 ESC Guidelines on cardiovascular disease prevention in clinical practice. *Eur. Heart J.* **2021**, *42*, 3227–3337. [CrossRef]
4. Mughal, M.M.; Khan, M.K.; DeMarco, J.K.; Majid, A.; Shamoun, F.; Abela, G.S. Symptomatic and asymptomatic carotid artery plaque. *Expert. Rev. Cardiovasc. Ther.* **2011**, *9*, 1315–1330. [CrossRef]
5. Byrne, R.A.; Rossello, X.; Coughlan, J.J.; Barbato, E.; Berry, C.; Chieffo, A.; Claeys, M.J.; Dan, G.A.; Dweck, M.R.; Galbraith, M. 2023 ESC Guidelines for the management of acute coronary syndromes. *Eur. Heart J.* **2023**, *44*, 3720–3826. [CrossRef]
6. Vrints, C.; Andreotti, F.; Koskinas, K.C.; Rossello, X.; Adamo, M.; Ainslie, J.; Banning, A.P.; Budaj, A.; Buechel, R.R.; Chiariello, G.A. 2024 ESC Guidelines for the management of chronic coronary syndromes. *Eur. Heart J.* **2024**, *45*, 3415–3537.
7. Hackett, D.; Verwilghen, J.; Davies, G.; Maseri, A. Coronary stenoses before and after acute myocardial infarction. *Am. J. Cardiol.* **1989**, *63*, 1517–1518. [CrossRef]

8. Dawson, L.P.; Lum, M.; Nerleker, N.; Nicholls, S.J.; Layland, J. Coronary Atherosclerotic Plaque Regression. *J. Am. Coll. Cardiol.* **2022**, *79*, 66–82. [CrossRef]
9. Ahmadi, A.; Argulian, E.; Leipsic, J.; Newby, D.E.; Narula, J. From Subclinical Atherosclerosis to Plaque Progression and Acute Coronary Events. *J. Am. Coll. Cardiol.* **2019**, *74*, 1608–1617. [CrossRef]
10. Stary, H.C.; Chandler, A.B.; Dinsmore, R.E.; Fuster, V.; Glagov, S.; Insull, W., Jr.; Rosenfeld, M.E.; Schwartz, C.J.; Wagner, W.D.; Wissler, R.W. A Definition of Advanced Types of Atherosclerotic Lesions and a Histological Classification of Atherosclerosis. *Circulation* **1995**, *92*, 1355–1374. [CrossRef]
11. Fayad, Z.A.; Fuster, V. Clinical Imaging of the High-Risk or Vulnerable Atherosclerotic Plaque. *Circ. Res.* **2001**, *89*, 305–316. [CrossRef]
12. Poznyak, A.V.; Sukhorukov, V.N.; Eremin, I.I.; Nadelyaeva, I.I.; Orekhov, A.N. Diagnostics of atherosclerosis: Overview of the existing methods. *Front. Cardiovasc. Med.* **2023**, *10*, 1134097. [CrossRef] [PubMed]
13. Flohr, T.; Petersilka, M.; Henning, A.; Ulzheimer, S.; Ferda, J.; Schmidt, B. Photon-counting CT review. *Phys. Medica* **2020**, *79*, 126–136. [CrossRef] [PubMed]
14. Ibañez, B.; Badimon, J.J.; Garcia, M.J. Diagnosis of Atherosclerosis by Imaging. *Am. J. Med.* **2009**, *122*, S15–S25. [CrossRef]
15. Balu, N.; Wang, J.; Dong, L.; Baluyot, F.; Chen, H.; Yuan, C. Current Techniques for MR Imaging of Atherosclerosis. *Top. Magn. Reson. Imaging* **2009**, *20*, 203–215. [CrossRef]
16. Noguchi, T.; Yamada, N.; Kawasaki, T.; Tanaka, A.; Yasuda, S. Detection of High-Risk Atherosclerotic Plaques by Magnetic Resonance Imaging. *Circ. J.* **2013**, *77*, 1975–1983. [CrossRef]
17. Touboul, P.J.; Hennerici, M.G.; Meairs, S.; Adams, H.; Amarenco, P.; Bornstein, N.; Csiba, L.; Desvarieux, M.; Ebrahim, S.; Hernandez Hernandez, R. Mannheim Carotid Intima-Media Thickness and Plaque Consensus (2004–2006–2011). *Cerebrovasc. Dis.* **2012**, *34*, 290–296. [CrossRef]
18. Yang, C.W.; Guo, Y.C.; Li, C.I.; Liu, C.S.; Lin, C.H.; Liu, C.H.; Wang, M.C.; Yang, S.Y.; Li, T.C.; Lin, C.C. Subclinical Atherosclerosis Markers of Carotid Intima-Media Thickness, Carotid Plaques, Carotid Stenosis, and Mortality in Community-Dwelling Adults. *Int. J. Environ. Res. Public Health* **2020**, *17*, 4745. [CrossRef]
19. Johri, A.M.; Nambi, V.; Naqvi, T.Z.; Feinstein, S.B.; Kim, E.S.H.; Park, M.M.; Becher, H.; Sillesen, H. Recommendations for the Assessment of Carotid Arterial Plaque by Ultrasound for the Characterization of Atherosclerosis and Evaluation of Cardiovascular Risk: From the American Society of Echocardiography. *J. Am. Soc. Echocardiogr.* **2020**, *33*, 917–933. [CrossRef] [PubMed]
20. Knuuti, J.; Wijns, W.; Saraste, A.; Capodanno, D.; Barbato, E.; Funck-Brentano, C.; Prescott, E.; Storey, R.F.; Deaton, C.; Cuisset, T. 2019 ESC Guidelines for the diagnosis and management of chronic coronary syndromes. *Eur. Heart J.* **2020**, *41*, 407–477. [CrossRef]
21. Sicari, R.; Nihoyannopoulos, P.; Evangelista, A.; Kasprzak, J.; Lancellotti, P.; Poldermans, D.; Voigt, J.U.; Zamorano, J.L.; European Association of Echocardiography. Stress echocardiography expert consensus statement: European Association of Echocardiography (EAE) (a registered branch of the ESC). *Eur. J. Echocardiogr.* **2008**, *9*, 415–437. [CrossRef]
22. Owen, D.R.J.; Lindsay, A.C.; Choudhury, R.P.; Fayad, Z.A. Imaging of Atherosclerosis. *Annu. Rev. Med.* **2011**, *62*, 25–40. [CrossRef] [PubMed]
23. Owen, D.R.; Shalhoub, J.; Miller, S.; Gauthier, T.; Doryforou, O.; Davies, A.H.; Leen, E.L. Inflammation within Carotid Atherosclerotic Plaque: Assessment with Late-Phase Contrast-enhanced US. *Radiology* **2010**, *255*, 638–644. [CrossRef] [PubMed]
24. Schinkel, A.F.L.; Kaspar, M.; Staub, D. Contrast-enhanced ultrasound: Clinical applications in patients with atherosclerosis. *Int. J. Cardiovasc. Imaging* **2016**, *32*, 35–48. [CrossRef] [PubMed]
25. Sidhu, P.S.; Cantisani, V.; Dietrich, C.F.; Gilja, O.H.; Saftoiu, A.; Bartels, E.; Bertolotto, M.; Calliada, F.; Clevert, D.A.; Cosgrove, D. The EFSUMB Guidelines and Recommendations for the Clinical Practice of Contrast-Enhanced Ultrasound (CEUS) in Non-Hepatic Applications: Update 2017 (Short Version). *Ultraschall Der Med.-Eur. J. Ultrasound* **2018**, *39*, 154–180.
26. Piscaglia, F.; Bolondi, L. The safety of Sonovue® in abdominal applications: Retrospective analysis of 23,188 investigations. *Ultrasound Med. Biol.* **2006**, *32*, 1369–1375. [CrossRef]
27. Miele, V.; Piccolo, C.L.; Galluzzo, M.; Ianniello, S.; Sessa, B.; Trinci, M. Contrast-enhanced ultrasound (CEUS) in blunt abdominal trauma. *Br. J. Radiol.* **2016**, *89*, 20150823. [CrossRef]
28. Dietrich, C.F.; Averkiou, M.; Nielsen, M.B.; Barr, R.G.; Burns, P.N.; Calliada, F.; Cantisani, V.; Choi, B.; Chammas, M.C.; Clevert, D.A.; et al. How to perform Contrast-Enhanced Ultrasound (CEUS). *Ultrasound Int. Open* **2018**, *4*, E2–E15. [CrossRef]
29. López-Melgar, B.; Fernández-Friera, L.; Oliva, B.; García-Ruiz, J.M.; Peñalvo, J.L.; Gómez-Talavera, S.; Sánchez-González, J.; Mendiguren, J.M.; Ibáñez, B.; Fernández-Ortiz, A. Subclinical Atherosclerosis Burden by 3D Ultrasound in Mid-Life. *J. Am. Coll. Cardiol.* **2017**, *70*, 301–313. [CrossRef]
30. López-Melgar, B.; Mass, V.; Nogales, P.; Sánchez-González, J.; Entrekin, R.; Collet-Billon, A.; Rossello, X.; Fernández-Friera, L.; Fernández-Ortiz, A.; Sanz, J. New 3-Dimensional Volumetric Ultrasound Method for Accurate Quantification of Atherosclerotic Plaque Volume. *JACC Cardiovasc. Imaging* **2022**, *15*, 1124–1135. [CrossRef]
31. Mushenkova, N.V.; Summerhill, V.I.; Zhang, D.; Romanenko, E.B.; Grechko, A.V.; Orekhov, A.N. Current Advances in the Diagnostic Imaging of Atherosclerosis: Insights into the Pathophysiology of Vulnerable Plaque. *Int. J. Mol. Sci.* **2020**, *21*, 2992. [CrossRef]
32. Schulte-Altedorneburg, G.; Droste, D.W.; Felszeghy, S.; Kellermann, M.; Popa, V.; Hegedüs, K.; Hegedüs, C.; Schmid, M. Accuracy of In Vivo Carotid B-Mode Ultrasound Compared With Pathological Analysis. *Stroke* **2001**, *32*, 1520–1524. [CrossRef] [PubMed]

33. Saba, L.; Yuan, C.; Hatsukami, T.S.; Balu, N.; Qiao, Y.; DeMarco, J.K.; Saam, T.; Moody, A.R. Carotid Artery Wall Imaging: Perspective and Guidelines from the ASNR Vessel Wall Imaging Study Group and Expert Consensus Recommendations of the American Society of Neuroradiology. *Am. J. Neuroradiol.* **2018**, *39*, E9–E31. [CrossRef] [PubMed]
34. Sangiorgi, G.; Rumberger, J.A.; Severson, A.; Edwards, W.D.; Gregoire, J.; Fitzpatrick, L.A.; Schwartz, R.S. Arterial Calcification and Not Lumen Stenosis Is Highly Correlated with Atherosclerotic Plaque Burden in Humans: A Histologic Study of 723 Coronary Artery Segments Using Nondecalcifying Methodology. *J. Am. Coll. Cardiol.* **1998**, *31*, 126–133. [CrossRef]
35. Andrews, J.P.M.; Fayad, Z.A.; Dweck, M.R. New methods to image unstable atherosclerotic plaques. *Atherosclerosis* **2018**, *272*, 118–128. [CrossRef]
36. Soeda, T.; Uemura, S.; Morikawa, Y.; Ishigami, K.; Okayama, S.; Hee, S.J.; Nishida, T.; Onoue, K.; Somekawa, S.; Takeda, Y. Diagnostic accuracy of dual-source computed tomography in the characterization of coronary atherosclerotic plaques: Comparison with intravascular optical coherence tomography. *Int. J. Cardiol.* **2011**, *148*, 313–318. [CrossRef] [PubMed]
37. Nehra, A.K.; Rajendran, K.; Baffour, F.I.; Mileto, A.; Rajiah, P.S.; Horst, K.K.; Inoue, A.; Johnson, T.F.; Diehn, F.E.; Glazebrook, K.N. Seeing More with Less: Clinical Benefits of Photon-counting Detector CT. *RadioGraphics* **2023**, *43*, e220158. [CrossRef]
38. Tarkin, J.M.; Dweck, M.R.; Evans, N.R.; Takx, R.A.; Brown, A.J.; Tawakol, A.; Fayad, Z.A.; Rudd, J.H. Imaging Atherosclerosis. *Circ. Res.* **2016**, *118*, 750–769. [CrossRef]
39. Jang, I.K.; Bouma, B.E.; Kang, D.H.; Park, S.J.; Park, S.W.; Seung, K.B.; Choi, K.B.; Shishkov, M.; Schlendorf, K.; Pomerantsev, E. Visualization of coronary atherosclerotic plaques in patients using optical coherence tomography: Comparison with intravascular ultrasound. *J. Am. Coll. Cardiol.* **2002**, *39*, 604–609. [CrossRef] [PubMed]
40. Noguchi, T.; Nakao, K.; Asaumi, Y.; Morita, Y.; Otsuka, F.; Kataoka, Y.; Hosoda, H.; Miura, H.; Fukuda, T.; Yasuda, S. Noninvasive Coronary Plaque Imaging. *J. Atheroscler. Thromb.* **2018**, *25*, 281–293. [CrossRef]
41. Guimarães, J.; de Almeida, J.; Mendes, P.L.; Ferreira, M.J.; Gonçalves, L. Advancements in non-invasive imaging of atherosclerosis: Future perspectives. *J. Clin. Lipidol.* **2024**, *18*, e142–e152. [CrossRef]
42. Nelson, A.J.; Ardissino, M.; Psaltis, P.J. Current approach to the diagnosis of atherosclerotic coronary artery disease: More questions than answers. *Ther. Adv. Chronic. Dis.* **2019**, *10*, 204062231988481. [CrossRef] [PubMed]
43. Colacchio, E.C.; Berton, M.; Squizzato, F.; Menegolo, M.; Piazza, M.; Grego, F.; Antonello, M. The role of multimodal imaging in emergency vascular conditions: The journey from diagnosis to hybrid operating rooms. *Semin. Vasc. Surg.* **2023**, *36*, 355–362. [CrossRef]
44. Li, J.; Montarello, N.J.; Hoogendoorn, A.; Verjans, J.W.; Bursill, C.A.; Peter, K.; Nicholls, S.J.; McLaughlin, R.A.; Psaltis, P.J. Multimodality Intravascular Imaging of High-Risk Coronary Plaque. *JACC Cardiovasc. Imaging* **2022**, *15*, 145–159. [CrossRef]
45. Michail, M.; Serruys, P.W.; Stettler, R.; Crake, T.; Torii, R.; Tenekecioglu, E.; Zeng, Y.; Onuma, Y.; Mathur, A.; Bourantas, C.V. Intravascular multimodality imaging: Feasibility and role in the evaluation of coronary plaque pathology. *Eur. Heart J. Cardiovasc. Imaging* **2017**, *18*, 613–620. [CrossRef] [PubMed]
46. Silvera, S.S.; Aidi, H.E.; Rudd, J.H.; Mani, V.; Yang, L.; Farkouh, M.; Fuster, V.; Fayad, Z.A. Multimodality imaging of atherosclerotic plaque activity and composition using FDG-PET/CT and MRI in carotid and femoral arteries. *Atherosclerosis* **2009**, *207*, 139–143. [CrossRef] [PubMed]
47. Cau, R.; Flanders, A.; Mannelli, L.; Politi, C.; Faa, G.; Suri, J.S.; Saba, L. Artificial intelligence in computed tomography plaque characterization: A review. *Eur. J. Radiol.* **2021**, *140*, 109767. [CrossRef]
48. Föllmer, B.; Williams, M.C.; Dey, D.; Arbab-Zadeh, A.; Maurovich-Horvat, P.; Volleberg, R.H.J.A.; Rueckert, D.; Schnabel, J.A.; Newby, D.E.; Dweck, M.R. Roadmap on the use of artificial intelligence for imaging of vulnerable atherosclerotic plaque in coronary arteries. *Nat. Rev. Cardiol.* **2024**, *21*, 51–64. [CrossRef]
49. Motwani, M.; Dey, D.; Berman, D.S.; Germano, G.; Achenbach, S.; Al-Mallah, M.H.; Andreini, D.; Budoff, M.J.; Cademartiri, F.; Callister, T.Q. Machine learning for prediction of all-cause mortality in patients with suspected coronary artery disease: A 5-year multicentre prospective registry analysis. *Eur. Heart J.* **2016**, *38*, 500–507. [CrossRef] [PubMed]
50. Lin, A.; van Diemen, P.A.; Motwani, M.; McElhinney, P.; Otaki, Y.; Han, D.; Kwan, A.; Tzolos, E.; Klein, E.; Kuronuma, K. Machine Learning from Quantitative Coronary Computed Tomography Angiography Predicts Fractional Flow Reserve–Defined Ischemia and Impaired Myocardial Blood Flow. *Circ. Cardiovasc. Imaging* **2022**, *15*, e014369. [CrossRef]
51. European Parliament and Council Regulation (EU) 2017/745 of April 5, 2017, on Medical Devices. Available online: https://eur-lex.europa.eu/legal-content/EN/TXT/?uri=CELEX:32017R0745 (accessed on 16 July 2024).
52. General Data Protection Regulation (GDPR) (EU) 2016/679. Available online: https://eur-lex.europa.eu/legal-content/EN/TXT/?uri=CELEX:32016R0679 (accessed on 16 July 2024).
53. Brynjolfsson, E.; Rock, D.; Syverson, C. *Artificial Intelligence and the Modern Productivity Paradox: A Clash of Expectations and Statistics*; University of Chicago Press: Chicago, IL, USA, 2017. [CrossRef]
54. World Health Organization. *Ethics and Governance of Artificial Intelligence for Health*; WHO: Geneva, Switzerland, 2021; Available online: https://www.who.int/publications/i/item/9789240029200 (accessed on 31 July 2024).
55. Feig, J.E.; Feig, J.L.; Dangas, G.D. The role of HDL in plaque stabilization and regression. *Coron. Artery Dis.* **2016**, *27*, 592–603. [CrossRef]
56. Basiak, M.; Hachula, M.; Kosowski, M.; Machnik, G.; Maliglowka, M.; Dziubinska-Basiak, M.; Krysiak, R.; Okopien, B. The Effect of PCSK9 Inhibition on the Stabilization of Atherosclerotic Plaque Determined by Biochemical and Diagnostic Imaging Methods. *Molecules* **2023**, *28*, 5928. [CrossRef] [PubMed]

57. Biondi-Zoccai, G.; Mastrangeli, S.; Romagnoli, E.; Peruzzi, M.; Frati, G.; Roever, L.; Giordano, A. What We Have Learned from the Recent Meta-analyses on Diagnostic Methods for Atherosclerotic Plaque Regression. *Curr. Atheroscler. Rep.* **2018**, *20*, 2. [CrossRef] [PubMed]
58. Cardiovascular Diseases (CVDs). Available online: https://www.who.int/news-room/fact-sheets/detail/cardiovascular-diseases-(cvds) (accessed on 16 July 2024).
59. World Stroke Organization (WSO): Global Stroke Fact Sheet. 2022. Available online: https://ghdx.healthdata.org/gbd-results-tool (accessed on 16 July 2024).
60. Theofilis, P.; Vlachakis, P.K.; Papanikolaou, A.; Karakasis, P.; Oikonomou, E.; Tsioufis, K.; Tousoulis, D. Coronary Plaque Erosion: Epidemiology, Diagnosis, and Treatment. *Int. J. Mol. Sci.* **2024**, *25*, 5786. [CrossRef] [PubMed]
61. Terada, K.; Kubo, T.; Kameyama, T.; Matsuo, Y.; Ino, Y.; Emori, H.; Higashioka, D.; Katayama, Y.; Khalifa, A.K.M.; Takahata, M. NIRS-IVUS for Differentiating Coronary Plaque Rupture, Erosion, and Calcified Nodule in Acute Myocardial Infarction. *JACC Cardiovasc. Imaging* **2021**, *14*, 1440–1450. [CrossRef]
62. Alfonso, F.; Virmani, R. The coronary substrate determines prognosis in acute coronary syndromes: The kaleidoscope has been shaken... again! *Eur. Heart J.* **2015**, *36*, 1357–1360. [CrossRef]
63. Niccoli, G.; Montone, R.A.; Di Vito, L.; Gramegna, M.; Refaat, H.; Scalone, G.; Leone, A.M.; Trani, C.; Burzotta, F.; Porto, I. Plaque rupture and intact fibrous cap assessed by optical coherence tomography portend different outcomes in patients with acute coronary syndrome. *Eur. Heart J.* **2015**, *36*, 1377–1384. [CrossRef]
64. Satogami, K.; Ino, Y.; Kubo, T.; Tanimoto, T.; Orii, M.; Matsuo, Y.; Ota, S.; Yamaguchi, T.; Shiono, Y.; Shimamura, K. Impact of Plaque Rupture Detected by Optical Coherence Tomography on Transmural Extent of Infarction After Successful Stenting in ST-Segment Elevation Acute Myocardial Infarction. *JACC Cardiovasc. Interv.* **2017**, *10*, 1025–1033. [CrossRef]
65. Xing, L.; Yamamoto, E.; Sugiyama, T.; Jia, H.; Ma, L.; Hu, S.; Wang, C.; Zhu, Y.; Li, L.; Xu, M. EROSION Study (Effective Anti-Thrombotic Therapy Without Stenting: Intravascular Optical Coherence Tomography–Based Management in Plaque Erosion). *Circ. Cardiovasc. Interv.* **2017**, *10*, e005860. [CrossRef]
66. Higuma, T.; Soeda, T.; Abe, N.; Yamada, M.; Yokoyama, H.; Shibutani, S.; Vergallo, R.; Minami, Y.; Ong, D.S.; Lee, H. A Combined Optical Coherence Tomography and Intravascular Ultrasound Study on Plaque Rupture, Plaque Erosion, and Calcified Nodule in Patients With ST-Segment Elevation Myocardial Infarction. *JACC Cardiovasc. Interv.* **2015**, *8*, 1166–1176. [CrossRef]
67. Kataoka, Y.; Uno, K.; Puri, R.; Nicholls, S.J. Current imaging modalities for atherosclerosis. *Expert. Rev. Cardiovasc. Ther.* **2012**, *10*, 457–471. [CrossRef]
68. Yabushita, H.; Bouma, B.E.; Houser, S.L.; Aretz, H.T.; Jang, I.K.; Schlendorf, K.H.; Kauffman, C.R.; Shishkov, M.; Kang, D.H.; Halpern, E.F. Characterization of Human Atherosclerosis by Optical Coherence Tomography. *Circulation* **2002**, *106*, 1640–1645. [CrossRef] [PubMed]
69. Di Vito, L.; Imola, F.; Gatto, L.; Romagnoli, E.; Limbruno, U.; Marco, V.; Picchi, A.; Micari, A.; Albertucci, M.; Prati, F. Limitations of OCT in identifying and quantifying lipid components: An in vivo comparison study with IVUS-NIRS. *EuroIntervention* **2017**, *13*, 303–311. [CrossRef] [PubMed]
70. Worthley, S.G.; Helft, G.; Fuster, V.; Zaman, A.G.; Fayad, Z.A.; Fallon, J.T.; Badimon, J.J. Serial In Vivo MRI Documents Arterial Remodeling in Experimental Atherosclerosis. *Circulation* **2000**, *101*, 586–589. [CrossRef] [PubMed]
71. Kamal-Bahl, S.J.; Burke, T.; Watson, D.; Wentworth, C. Discontinuation of Lipid Modifying Drugs Among Commercially Insured United States Patients in Recent Clinical Practice. *Am. J. Cardiol.* **2007**, *99*, 530–534. [CrossRef]
72. Hibi, K.; Kimura, T.; Kimura, K.; Morimoto, T.; Hiro, T.; Miyauchi, K.; Nakagawa, Y.; Yamagishi, M.; Ozaki, Y.; Saito, S. Clinically evident polyvascular disease and regression of coronary atherosclerosis after intensive statin therapy in patients with acute coronary syndrome: Serial intravascular ultrasound from the Japanese assessment of pitavastatin and atorvastatin in acute coronary syndrome (JAPAN-ACS) trial. *Atherosclerosis* **2011**, *219*, 743–749.
73. Nicholls, S.J.; Puri, R.; Anderson, T.; Ballantyne, C.M.; Cho, L.; Kastelein, J.J.; Koenig, W.; Somaratne, R.; Kassahun, H.; Yang, J. Effect of Evolocumab on Progression of Coronary Disease in Statin-Treated Patients. *JAMA* **2016**, *316*, 2373. [CrossRef]
74. Di Fusco, S.A.; Maggioni, A.P.; Bernelli, C.; Perone, F.; De Marzo, V.; Conte, E.; Musella, F.; Uccello, G.; Luca, L.; Gabrielli, D. Inclisiran: A New Pharmacological Approach for Hypercholesterolemia. *Rev. Cardiovasc. Med.* **2022**, *23*, 375. [CrossRef]

Journal of
Cardiovascular Development and Disease

MDPI

Article

Impact of Baseline Hypoalbuminemia on Long-Term Survival Following Acute Myocardial Infarction According to Body Mass Index

Alon Shechter [1,2,3], Shani Dahan [4,5,6], Arthur Shiyovich [2,3,7], Harel Gilutz [6] and Ygal Plakht [8,9,*]

1 Department of Cardiology, Smidt Heart Institute, Cedars-Sinai Medical Center, Los Angeles, CA 90048, USA; alonshechter@gmail.com
2 Department of Cardiology, Rabin Medical Center, Petach Tikva 4941492, Israel; arthur.shiyovich@gmail.com
3 Faculty of Medical and Health Sciences, Tel Aviv University, Tel Aviv 6997801, Israel
4 Division of Cardiology, Massachusetts General Hospital, Boston, MA 02114, USA; shish.dahan@gmail.com
5 Department of Cardiology, Assuta Medical Center, Ashdod 7747629, Israel
6 Goldman Medical School, Faculty of Health Sciences, Ben-Gurion University of the Negev, Beer Sheva 8410501, Israel; gilutz@bgu.ac.il
7 Cardiovascular Division, Department of Medicine, Harvard Medical School, Boston, MA 02115, USA
8 Department of Nursing, Recanati School for Community Health Professions, Faculty of Health Sciences, Ben-Gurion University of the Negev, Beer Sheva 84105, Israel
9 Department of Emergency Medicine, Soroka University Medical Center, Beer Sheva P.O. Box 151, Israel
* Correspondence: plakht@bgu.ac.il; Tel.: +972-86477725

Abstract: Serum albumin and body mass index (BMI, kg/m^2) have been associated with outcomes following acute myocardial infarction (AMI). Aiming to assess whether the mortality risk inflicted by hypoalbuminemia (<3.5 g/dL) in this context is influenced by BMI, we conducted a retrospective analysis of AMI survivors hospitalized during 2004–2017. Stratified by admission-time albumin level and BMI, eligible cases were evaluated for all-cause mortality up to 10 years after discharge. A total of 6283 individuals (74.1% males, mean age 64.1 ± 13.1 years, 44.3% with ST-elevation MI) were included. Of them, 22.7% had hypoalbuminemia and 1.2%, 41.0%, and 28.6% were underweight (BMI < 18.5), overweight (BMI 25–30), and obese (BMI ≥ 30), respectively. Over a median of 7.9 (IQR, 4.8–10.0) years of follow-up, 42.5% of patients died. Hypoalbuminemia was independently associated with a heightened mortality risk overall (AdjHR = 1.54, 95%CI 1.42–1.67, $p < 0.001$), accounted for by the normal weight (AdjHR = 1.73, 95%CI 1.50–1.99, $p < 0.001$), overweight (AdjHR = 1.55, 95%CI 1.35–1.79, $p < 0.001$), and class 1 obesity (BMI 30–35) (AdjHR = 1.37, 95%CI 1.12–1.68, $p = 0.002$) subgroups. Upon interaction analysis, the mortality risk imposed by hypoalbuminemia was most pronounced among individuals with normal BMI. In conclusion, hypoalbuminemia constituted a negative prognostic marker for long-term survival in AMI patients with normal or mildly elevated but not reduced or severely increased BMI. Pending further research, addressing hypoalbuminemia based on BMI range may prove beneficial.

Keywords: albumin; body mass index; myocardial infarction; survival

1. Introduction

Over the last decades, significant improvement in survival after acute myocardial infarction (AMI) has led to an extensive search for prognostic indicators to further enhance disease management and outcomes. Among the numerous factors explored, serum albumin and body mass index (BMI) have emerged as particularly intriguing variables with potential impact on the post-MI course [1,2]. Albumin, a vital component of plasma, which plays a multifaceted role in various physiological processes [3], has been shown to mark nutritional status, inflammation extent, organ (e.g., kidneys, liver) function, and numerous illnesses severity [4]. Accordingly, low serum albumin levels have been linked to a higher risk of incident AMI and chronic coronary artery disease (CAD) [5,6]. Furthermore, among AMI patients, decreased serum albumin upon admission has been associated with worse in-hospital outcomes (death included) and long-term survival as well as no-reflow in those with ST-elevation MI who had undergone primary percutaneous intervention [7–9]. BMI, an anthropometric measure representing the ratio of weight (in kg) to height (in m squared) [10], has demonstrated contradicting implications in cardiac patients—collectively referred to as the "obesity paradox"—in which higher values denote elevated risk of cardiovascular morbidity but also improved prognosis among patients with the established disease [11–15]. Acknowledging the possible modifying effect of BMI on outcomes, we aimed to assess whether the prognostic implication of hypoalbuminemia among AMI survivors is indeed altered by BMI.

2. Materials and Methods

2.1. Study Population and Outcomes

Our study represents a retrospective analysis of the Soroka University Medical Center (SUMC) registry of consecutive AMI hospitalizations occurring between 1 June 2004 and 31 October 2017. Included in the study were adult (i.e., ≥18-year-old) Israeli citizens who were hospitalized with AMI as the primary/main diagnosis and survived the index event and for whom there were available data regarding serum albumin level and BMI at admission. For subjects with multiple AMI admissions at SUMC, only the first one was considered. The study outcome was all-cause mortality up to 10 years after hospital discharge or 31 July 2023, whichever occurred first.

This project conformed to the Declaration of Helsinki and was approved by Soroka's Institutional Review Board (approval number SOR-0319-16), which waived the need for informed consent in view of the investigation's retrospective nature.

2.2. Data Collection and Definitions

Clinical data were retrieved from a web-based medical chart platform, in which baseline comorbidities were identified by the International Classification of Diseases, Ninth Revision, Clinical Modification (ICD-9-CM) [16] codes, as documented in real time by the treating medical team and according to the prespecified criteria outlined below. Death events were obtained from the Israeli Ministry of the Interior Population Registry.

AMI diagnosis was based on the constellation of ischemic signs and/or symptoms coupled with an abrupt rise and fall in cardiac biomarkers levels consistent with acute myocardial injury, as dictated by the Universal Definition of Myocardial Infarction at the time [17]. Obstructive CAD required the presence of a ≥70% vessel stenosis, as assessed by angiography.

Hypoalbuminemia was defined as a serum albumin level of <3.5 g/dL [18]. BMI classification followed the Centers for Disease Control and Prevention's scheme [19], resulting in six distinct categories: underweight—<18.5 kg/m^2; normal weight—18.5 to <25 kg/m^2; overweight—25 to <30 kg/m^2; class 1 obesity—30 to <35 kg/m^2; class 2 obesity—35 to <40 kg/m^2; and class 3 (or morbid) obesity—≥40 kg/m^2. Importantly, only the first measurements reported within the initial 24 h of admission were taken into consideration. The presence of diabetes mellitus and dyslipidemia was ascertained by HbA1c and low-density lipoprotein levels of ≥6.5% and ≥100 mg/dL, respectively, at any timepoint during a 12-month period starting 6 months before the hospitalization.

Echocardiographic diagnoses followed the American Society of Echocardiography guidelines. Specifically, severe left ventricular (LV) dysfunction was defined by an LV ejection fraction (LVEF) of <30% on the first in-hospital echocardiogram. Pulmonary hypertension was declared upon a pulmonary arterial systolic pressure of ≥37 mmHg on the same exam.

2.3. Statistical Analysis

The study cohort was analyzed in its entirety and according to hypoalbuminemia status and BMI category at admission. Variables were reported as frequencies and percentages, medians and interquartile ranges (IQRs), or means and standard deviations, and compared using Pearson's Chi-Square, Fisher's exact, Student's t, and analysis of variance (ANOVA) tests. Predictors for hypoalbuminemia in the total cohort were identified using a binary logistic regression multivariable analysis, which incorporated baseline variables demonstrating a p-value of <0.1 at the univariate stage.

The time-dependent probability and cumulative incidence of mortality as a function of hypoalbuminemia and various BMI ranges were assessed by the Kaplan–Meier method and compared using the Log-Rank test. Independent associations with the risk for all-cause death, both in the total cohort and in each of the BMI categories subgroups, were evaluated by a Cox proportional hazard multivariable analysis, using a stepwise approach as described above. Lastly, an interaction analysis was undertaken to determine the relative prognostic value of hypoalbuminemia in relation to a BMI range other than normal.

Cases with missing values were censored from the relevant calculations. Statistical significance required a two-sided p-value of <0.05. All analyses were performed using Statistical Package for the Social Sciences (SPSS), version 29 (IBM Corporation, Armonk, NY, USA).

3. Results

3.1. Baseline Characteristics of the Study Population

Out of 15,329 AMI hospitalizations identified at SUMC between 2004 and 2017, 6283 (41.0%) were first-time admissions of Israeli citizens who survived to discharge and had documented albumin and BMI values during the first 24 h of hospital stay (Supplemental Figure S1). Among these, hypoalbuminemia was observed in 1425 (22.7%) (Table 1). Concurrently, underweight was diagnosed in 77 (1.2%) subjects, normal weight in 1825 (29.1%), overweight in 2578 (41.0%), class 1 obesity in 1303 (20.7%), class 2 obesity in 372 (5.9%), and class 3 obesity in 128 (2.0%). Overall, the serum albumin level increased and the prevalence of hypoalbuminemia decreased as the BMI was higher—from 50.6% in underweight patients to 23.4% in those with class 3 obesity (p for trend < 0.001) (Supplemental Figure S2 and Table S1). BMI, on its part, was lower among hypoalbuminemic compared to normoalbuminemic patients, at 26.9 ± 5.3 vs. 28.1 ± 4.8 kg/m^2 ($p < 0.001$). Notably, higher odds for hypoalbuminemia were associated with older age, female sex, non-Jewish minority, comorbidities (other than overweight/obesity and dyslipidemia), lack of prior revascularization, and an ST-elevation MI presentation (Supplemental Table S2).

Both patients with hypoalbuminemia and those exhibiting a lower BMI were older and more likely to be male and to exhibit a greater burden of non-CV comorbidities compared to non-hypoalbuminemic and higher-range BMI patients, respectively (Table 1 and Supplemental Table S1). By contrast, the CV risk factors and comorbidities distribution was more heterogenous.

The trends associated with hypoalbuminemia in the total cohort were largely maintained within the normal to moderately elevated BMI categories (i.e., normal weight to class 2 obesity) subgroups. Among patients at BMI extremes (i.e., with underweight or class 3 obesity), however, CV morbidity—rather than general demographics and non-CV conditions—was related to serum albumin status, demonstrating a higher frequency in hypoalbuminemic individuals (Supplemental Tables S3 and S4).

Table 1. Baseline clinical characteristics according to serum albumin status.

	Total Cohort (n = 6283)	Serum Albumin Status		*p*-Value *
		Normal (n = 4858)	Low (n = 1425)	
Demographic Details				
Age (years)	64.1 ± 13.1	62.8 ± 13.0	68.6 ± 12.5	**<0.001 †**
Sex Male	4657 (74.1)	3753 (77.3)	904 (63.4)	**<0.001**
Non-Jewish Minority	1123 (17.9)	842 (17.3)	281 (19.7)	**<0.001**
Cardiovascular Risk Factors				
Diabetes Mellitus	2782 (44.3)	2040 (42.0)	742 (52.1)	**<0.001**
Dyslipidemia	5304 (84.4)	4202 (86.5)	1102 (77.3)	**<0.001**
Hypertension	3477 (55.3)	2683 (55.2)	794 (55.7)	0.743
Smoking History	2999 (47.7)	2446 (50.3)	553 (38.8)	**<0.001**
Family History of IHD	725 (11.5)	627 (12.9)	98 (6.9)	**<0.001**
Cardiovascular Morbidity				
Ischemic Heart Disease	5476 (87.2)	4328 (89.1)	1148 (80.6)	**<0.001**
History of MI	989 (15.7)	739 (15.2)	250 (17.5)	**0.034**
Prior Revascularization				
PCI	1102 (17.5)	869 (17.9)	233 (16.4)	0.180
CABG	592 (9.4)	456 (9.4)	136 (9.5)	0.858
Peripheral Arterial Disease	767 (12.2)	518 (10.7)	249 (17.5)	**<0.001**
Atrial Fibrillation/Flutter	958 (15.2)	642 (13.2)	316 (22.2)	**<0.001**
Atrioventricular Block	259 (4.1)	181 (3.7)	78 (5.5)	**0.004**
Clinical Heart Failure	1040 (16.6)	657 (13.5)	383 (26.9)	**<0.001**
Non-Cardiovascular Morbidity				
COPD	533 (8.5)	355 (7.3)	178 (12.5)	**<0.001**
Stage ≥ III CKD	577 (9.2)	322 (6.6)	255 (17.9)	**<0.001**
Anemia	3043 (48.4)	2066 (42.5)	977 (68.6)	**<0.001**
Neurological Disorders	949 (15.1)	624 (12.8)	325 (22.8)	**<0.001**
Malignancy	603 (9.8)	412 (8.5)	191 (13.4)	**<0.001**
Psychotic Disorders	86 (1.4)	56 (1.2)	30 (2.1)	**0.007**
Alcohol/Drug Abuse	140 (2.2)	108 (2.2)	32 (2.2)	0.960
Serum Albumin				
Mean Level (g/dL)	3.7 ± 0.5	3.9 ± 0.3	3.1 ± 0.3	**<0.001 †**
Body Mass Index				
Mean Value (kg/m^2)	27.8 ± 5.0	28.1 ± 4.8	26.9 ± 5.3	**<0.001 †**
Category				**<0.001**
Underweight	77 (1.2)	38 (0.8)	39 (2.7)	
Normal Weight	1825 (29.1)	1296 (26.7)	529 (37.1)	
Overweight	2578 (41.0)	2073 (42.7)	505 (35.4)	
Class 1 Obesity	1303 (20.7)	1047 (21.6)	256 (18.0)	
Class 2 Obesity	372 (5.9)	306 (6.3)	66 (4.6)	
Class 3 Obesity	128 (2.0)	98 (2.0)	30 (2.1)	

Data are presented as number (percent) or mean ± standard deviation. Figures in bold denote statistical significance. * Chi-square test unless stated otherwise; † Student's *t*-test. CABG = coronary artery bypass grafting; CKD = chronic kidney disease; COPD = chronic obstructive pulmonary disease; IHD = ischemic heart disease; MI = myocardial infarction; PCI = percutaneous coronary intervention.

3.2. Acute Event Aspects

Mirroring baseline characteristics, patients with vs. those without hypoalbuminemia and those with a lower BMI presented more often with cardiogenic shock and non-ST-elevation MI (Table 2 and Supplemental Table S5). Such patients were also more likely to display severe LV dysfunction, pulmonary hypertension, and significant valvular regurgitation upon admission, and their coronary angiograms revealed a greater extent of obstructive CAD. Notably, echocardiographic and angiographic assessment as well as revascularization therapy were employed less frequently among subjects with hypoalbuminemia and lower BMI. The hospitalization course in these patients was lengthier and more complex, involving higher rates of sepsis, mechanical ventilation, and blood transfusion.

Table 2. Acute event aspects according to serum albumin status.

	Total Cohort (n = 6283)	Serum Albumin Status		*p*-Value *
		Normal (n = 4858)	Low (n = 1425)	
Clinical Presentation				
Cardiac Arrest	28 (0.4)	15 (0.3)	13 (0.9)	**0.003**
Cardiogenic Shock	106 (1.7)	48 (1.0)	58 (4.1)	**<0.001**
ST-Elevation MI	2784 (44.3)	2187 (45.0)	597 (41.9)	**0.037**
Echocardiographic Parameters				
Echocardiogram Performed	5186 (82.5)	4094 (84.3)	1092 (76.6)	**<0.001**
Severe LV Dysfunction	620 (12.0)	396 (9.7)	224 (20.5)	**<0.001**
LV Hypertrophy	300 (5.8)	224 (5.5)	76 (7.0)	0.061
Mitral Regurgitation	319 (6.2)	196 (4.8)	123 (11.3)	**<0.001**
Tricuspid Regurgitation	189 (3.6)	113 (2.8)	76 (7.0)	**<0.001**
Pulmonary Hypertension	398 (7.7)	252 (6.2)	146 (13.4)	**<0.001**
Angiographic Parameters				
Angiogram Performed	4793 (76.3)	3880 (79.9)	913 (64.1)	**<0.001**
Vessels Significantly Involved				**<0.001**
0	168 (3.5)	132 (3.4)	36 (3.9)	
1	1106 (23.1)	929 (23.9)	177 (19.4)	
2	1284 (26.8)	1062 (27.4)	222 (24.3)	
3/Left Main	2235 (46.6)	1757 (45.3)	478 (52.4)	
Hospital Course				
Revascularization Approach				**<0.001**
No/Conservative Treatment	1063 (16.9)	646 (13.3)	417 (29.3)	
PCI	3737 (59.5)	3047 (62.7)	690 (48.4)	
CABG	1483 (23.6)	1165 (24.0)	318 (22.3)	
Intra-Aortic Balloon Pulsation	172 (2.7)	82 (1.7)	90 (6.3)	**<0.001**
Any Form of Pacing	136 (2.2)	83 (1.7)	53 (3.7)	**<0.001**
Mechanical Ventilation	246 (4.2)	122 (2.5)	142 (10.0)	**<0.001**
Gastrointestinal Bleeding	147 (2.3)	76 (1.6)	71 (5.0)	**<0.001**
Blood Transfusion	1019 (16.2)	649 (13.4)	370 (26.0)	**<0.001**
Sepsis	84 (1.3)	23 (0.5)	61 (4.3)	**<0.001**
Intensive Care Unit Stay	4675 (74.4)	3727 (76.7)	948 (66.5)	**<0.001**
Hospitalization Length (days)	11.3 ± 9.9	10.4 ± 8.5	14.3 ± 13.0	**<0.001** †

Data are presented as number (percent) or mean ± standard deviation, as appropriate. Figures in bold denote statistical significance. * Chi-square test unless stated otherwise; † Student's *t*-test. CABG = coronary artery bypass grafting; LV = left ventricular; MI = myocardial infarction; PCI = percutaneous coronary intervention.

Once again, most findings associated with hypoalbuminemia were observed only among patients with either normal weight, overweight, or class 1–2 obesity (Supplemental Tables S6 and S7). Accordingly, within the underweight and class 3 obesity subgroups, patients with normal and low serum albumin experienced a more comparable course.

3.3. Outcome

By a median of 7.9 (IQR, 4.8–10.0) years of follow-up, a total of 2669 (42.5%) patients died (Supplemental Table S8). The mortality rates were higher in the presence of hypoalbuminemia (66.2%) and BMI extremes (77.9% and 53.9% among underweight and class 3 obese patients, respectively)—compared to normoalbuminemia (35.5%) and normal-range BMI (47.5%) (all $p < 0.001$). Likewise, cumulative survival was reduced in the low vs. normal serum albumin and lower BMI subgroups (Supplemental Figure S3).

The increased rate and cumulative incidence of mortality associated with hypoalbuminemia in the total cohort were also observed in each of the BMI categories subgroups. Concurrently, the univariate (i.e., unadjusted) hazard ratios imposed by hypoalbuminemia demonstrated a somewhat U-shape trend, reaching a peak within the normal to mildly elevated BMI (i.e., normal weight to class 1 obesity) subgroups. The excess mortality linked to BMI extremes was evident regardless of hypoalbuminemia status (Supplemental Table S8 and Figure 1).

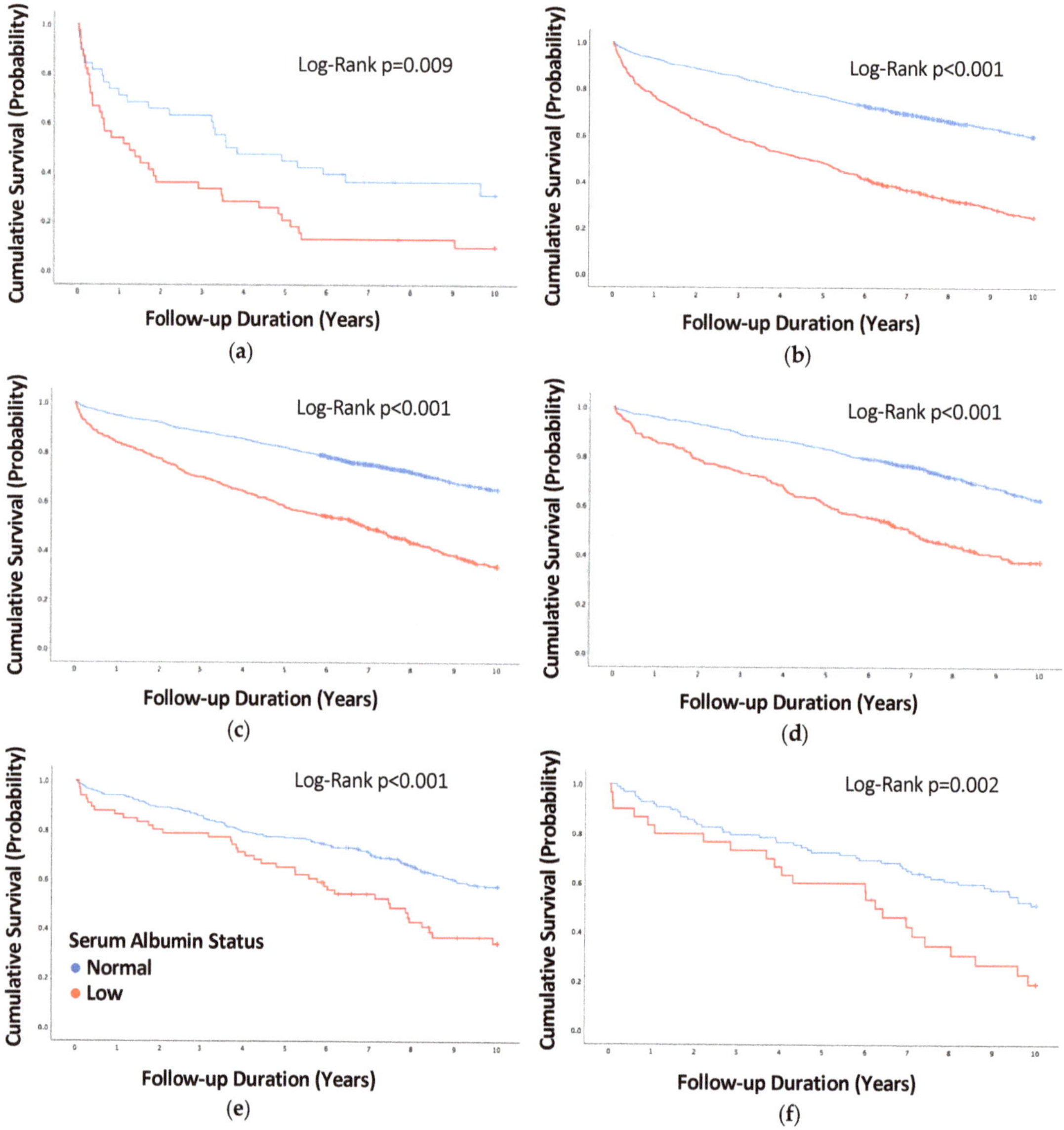

Figure 1. Cumulative survival according to serum albumin status and body mass index category: (**a**) underweight; (**b**) normal weight; (**c**) overweight; (**d**) class 1 obesity; (**e**) class 2 obesity; (**f**) class 3 obesity. BMI = body mass index.

Per multivariable analysis, both decreasing albumin level (as a continuous variable), hypoalbuminemia (vs. normoalbuminemia), and below-normal (vs. normal) BMI independently conferred a higher 10-year mortality risk (AdjHR for 1 g/dL-decrease 1.61, 95% CI

1.48–1.75, AdjHR 1.54, 95% CI 1.42–1.67, and AdjHR 1.98, 95% CI 1.52–2.58, respectively, all $p < 0.001$) (Table 3). Notably, there was a steep rise in the risk at a serum albumin level of around 3.5 g/dL, corresponding to the cutoff level used to define hypoalbuminemia (Supplemental Figure S4). Contrasting the afore-mentioned, an above-normal (compared with normal) BMI was associated with either a reduced risk (overweight to class 2 obesity) (AdjHR 0.74 to 0.83, $p < 0.001$ to 0.037) or a similar risk (class 3 obesity) (AdjHR 1.10, 95% CI 0.86–1.41, $p = 0.464$).

Table 3. Multivariable Cox proportional hazard model for the outcome of all-cause mortality at 10 years and interaction analysis.

Parameter	AdjHR (95% CI)	*p*-Value *
Age (vs. <65 years)		
65–74 years	1.97 (1.77–2.18)	**<0.001**
≥75 years	3.14 (2.83–3.49)	**<0.001**
Diabetes Mellitus	1.38 (1.27–1.50)	**<0.001**
Dyslipidemia	0.91 (0.83–1.01)	0.076
Family History of Ischemic Heart Disease	0.64 (0.52–0.79)	**<0.001**
History of Myocardial Infarction	1.18 (1.07–1.30)	**<0.001**
Peripheral Arterial Disease	1.32 (1.19–1.45)	**<0.001**
Atrial Fibrillation/Flutter	1.37 (1.26–1.51)	**<0.001**
Clinical Heart Failure	1.24 (1.13–1.36)	**<0.001**
Chronic Obstructive Pulmonary Disease	1.65 (1.48–1.85)	**<0.001**
Stage ≥ III Chronic Kidney Disease	1.70 (1.53–1.89)	**<0.001**
Anemia	1.39 (1.27–1.51)	**<0.001**
Neurological Disorders	1.54 (1.40–1.68)	**<0.001**
Malignancy	1.77 (1.53–2.06)	**<0.001**
Alcohol/Drug abuse	1.62 (1.27–2.07)	**<0.001**
Non-ST Elevation vs. ST-Elevation Myocardial Infarction	1.24 (1.14–1.36)	**<0.001**
Severe Left Ventricular Dysfunction	1.44 (1.28–1.62)	**<0.001**
Left Ventricular Hypertrophy	1.37 (1.17–1.61)	**<0.001**
Tricuspid Regurgitation	1.28 (1.07–1.54)	**0.007**
Pulmonary Hypertension	1.27 (1.11–1.45)	**<0.001**
Revascularization Approach (vs. Conservative):		
Percutaneous Coronary Intervention	0.57 (0.52–0.63)	**<0.001**
Coronary Artery Bypass Grafting	0.42 (0.37–0.47)	**<0.001**
Serum Albumin Status and Body Mass Index Category		
Decreasing Serum Albumin Level (continuous, per 1 g/dL decrease)	1.61 (1.48–1.75)	**<0.001**
Low vs. Normal Serum Albumin Level	1.54 (1.42–1.67)	**<0.001**
Abnormal vs. Normal Weight		
Underweight	1.98 (1.52–2.58)	**<0.001**
Overweight	0.80 (0.73–0.88)	**<0.001**
Class 1 Obesity	0.74 (0.67–0.83)	**<0.001**
Class 2 Obesity	0.83 (0.70–0.99)	**0.037**
Class 3 Obesity	1.10 (0.86–1.41)	0.464
Interaction Analysis: Abnormal Weight x Hypoalbuminemia		
Underweight x Hypoalbuminemia	0.69 (0.40–1.17)	0.167
Overweight x Hypoalbuminemia	0.91 (0.75–1.10)	0.322
Class 1 Obesity x Hypoalbuminemia	0.73 (0.58–0.92)	**0.008**
Class 2 Obesity x Hypoalbuminemia	0.63 (0.43–0.92)	**0.017**
Class 3 Obesity x Hypoalbuminemia	0.67 (0.40–1.14)	0.139

Figures in bold denote statistical significance. * Cox regression analysis. AdjHR = adjusted hazard ratio; CI = confidence interval.

The hazard imposed by low serum albumin status was only manifested in patients presenting at hospitalization with either a normal BMI (AdjHR 1.73, 95% CI 1.50–1.99, $p < 0.001$), overweight (AdjHR 1.55, 95% CI 1.35–1.79, $p < 0.001$), or class 1 obesity (AdjHR 1.37, 95% CI 1.12–1.68, $p = 0.002$)—but not with underweight (AdjHR 0.84, 95% CI 0.35–2.00, $p = 0.698$), class 2 obesity (AdjHR 1.17, 95% CI 0.77–1.75, $p = 0.465$), or class 3 obesity (AdjHR 1.70, 95% CI 0.84–3.42, $p = 0.137$) (Supplemental Tables S9 and S10, and Figure 2). Likewise, a 1 g/dL decrease in serum albumin level independently conferred an increased mortality risk only within the normal weight to class 1 obesity subgroups (Supplemental Figure S5). Upon interaction analysis, hypoalbuminemia demonstrated a weaker association with mortality among patients with abnormal vs. normal BMI, reaching statistical significance in the class 1–2 obesity subgroups (Table 3 and Figure 2).

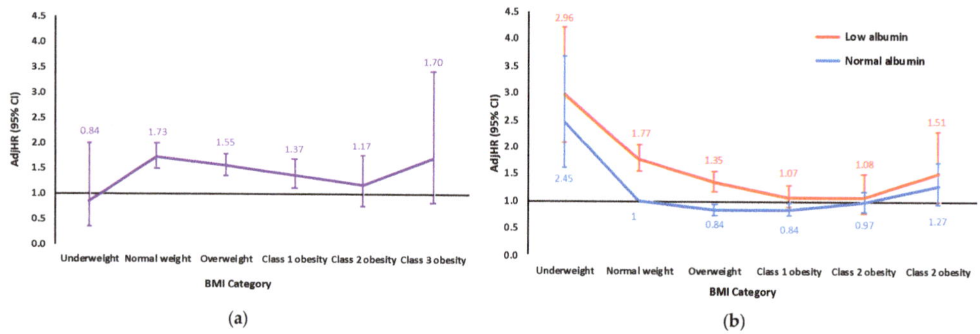

Figure 2. Hypoalbuminemia-associated risk of all-cause mortality at 10 years after acute myocardial infarction according to body mass index category: (**a**) per multivariable analysis in each of the BMI categories' subgroups; (**b**) per interaction analysis in the total cohort. AdjHR = adjusted hazard ratio; BMI = body mass index; CI = confidence interval.

4. Discussion

Our study examined the long-term mortality effect of admission-time hypoalbuminemia, defined as a serum albumin level of <3.5 g/dL, according to BMI range among 6283 AMI survivors. Its main findings were as follows: 1. averaging 22.7% in the total cohort, the prevalence of hypoalbuminemia was overall inversely proportional to BMI value and highest at 50.6% (or lowest at 24.3%) among underweight (or morbidly obese) subjects; 2. compared to normal albumin, hypoalbuminemia was accompanied by a greater burden of comorbidities at baseline, a more complex presentation and hospitalization course and, ultimately, a reduced 10-year survival following the index event; however this was only evident within the normal weight to class 2 obesity (i.e., 18.5 to <40 kg/m^2) subgroups; and 3. the independent association between hypoalbuminemia and increased risk for mortality was confined to patients with normal to mildly increased BMI (i.e., 18.5 to <35 kg/m^2), and the hazardous impact of hypoalbuminemia was generally most pronounced in normal weight individuals.

To our knowledge, the current study is the first to report on the interplay between albumin and BMI in the setting of AMI. Stemming from a relatively large registry that incorporated patient-level data and a long follow-up period, the study's observations are supported by comprehensive regression models, all reinforcing the validity and applicability to the constantly growing population of AMI survivors. Taken together, and in view of the concomitantly expanding obesity pandemic, we believe the study is timely and addresses an important and widely relevant topic in the acute coronary syndrome arena that may carry actionable implications, as outlined below.

Two main 'take-home' messages may be offered by our study. The first is that a higher-risk profile and more adverse outcomes that classically accompany hypoalbuminemia may not apply to underweight and moderately to extremely obese individuals recovering from AMI. Despite the small representation of these BMI subgroups in the study's cohort (n = 577, 9.2%), our results arguably suggest a genuine modifying effect of BMI on the prognostic implications of hypoalbuminemia nonetheless, as the mortality rate was nominally highest within the aforementioned subgroups as well. One possible explanation relating to the lower BMI extreme is that a higher comorbid state (and, presumably, malnutrition) associated with underweight may have dictated a less favorable outcome irrespective of albumin level. As for the above-normal BMI extreme, hypoalbuminemia may have been less reflective of poor nutrition and any associated phenomena (e.g., energy crisis, infections) in patients with pronounced obesity. Alternatively, it could be that a greater endothelial dysfunction, previously shown to characterize obese patients [20], played a more decisive prognostic role, somewhat overshadowing the effect of hypoalbuminemia. Still further, one may speculate about the well-documented and poorly understood obesity paradox that led to hypoalbuminemia being less prognostically meaningful in patients with obesity. As suggested by prior works [21], it could be that secondary preventive measures, not explicitly explored in our database, were more extensive among obese subjects, thus counteracting the deleterious effects of hypoalbuminemia. Due to the study's retrospective nature and lack of information on death causes and hypoalbuminemia etiologies, we were not able to determine causality and reliably identify the mechanisms underlying our results. Accordingly, these may best be attested by future prospective research.

The second, more practical notion arising from our study is that consideration of both albumin status and BMI range, as opposed albumin status alone, could allow for a more personalized risk stratification both before and after AMI, which in turn may translate to a more targeted management and surveillance scheme and, potentially, improved resource utilization and patient outcome. Theoretically, as hypoalbuminemia demonstrated an independent predictive capacity for death among AMI patients with normal weight to mild obesity only, it seems rational to focus diagnostic, preventive, and corrective measures of a low serum albumin level (e.g., dietary consultation, nutritional support, and albumin replacement) in this subset of individuals. In the same sense, the presence of hypoalbuminemia in AMI patients at BMI extremes may be regarded as less prognostically alarming on its own, thereby emphasizing the importance of addressing these BMI deviations while sparing the potential cost and hazards (e.g., allergic reactions, volume overload, and infections) associated with (parenteral) hypoalbuminemia treatment, the efficacy of which has yet to be established in CV patients, particularly in terms of primary and secondary prevention of ACS [22]. This implication of specifically targeting normal weight to mildly obese subjects—rather than moderately to severely obese ones—may apply to primary prevention pathways (not assessed in the current study) as well and provide an interesting perspective to practice guidelines [23], which at present mainly focus on the more obese patients. Once again, further, preferentially multi-center, studies are needed to evaluate the above-mentioned hypotheses and their application in actual clinical practice.

Limitations

First, our study is the product of a single-center, retrospective analysis that did not employ external adjudication and in which more than half of patients were excluded (mostly due to the absence of data regarding baseline BMI), all of which could lead to selection bias and hamper the generalizability of the results. However, we relied on one of the largest cohorts reported thus far, which represents a population of close to 1 million and whose baseline characteristics resembled those of prior real-world publications. Secondly, some complications (e.g., sepsis) were rather uncommon, thereby altering statistical power and possibly the final multivariable models. Thirdly, the protracted timeframe of enrollment may have led to inconsistencies in medical definitions and treatment approaches, which could have affected the interpretation of the findings. Nevertheless, all patients were exposed to similarly evolving diagnostic criteria and practices. Fourthly, hypoalbuminemia was mainly analyzed as a dichotomous variable, using a cutoff value that has been defined according to a steady-state scenario. While potentially introducing misclassification bias by disregarding the fluctuating nature of serum albumin level, we believe this approach a. is more practical in an acute setting and b. may possess greater clinical relevance compared to a continuous variable-centered analysis, the limited results of which further suggested the 3.5 g/dL cutoff used to define hypoalbuminemia as the most significant prognostically. Fifthly, we were not aware of hypoalbuminemia and abnormal BMI causes (e.g., metabolic, inflammatory, nutritional, pharmacologic, etc.) and durations, which by themselves could affect outcomes. Similarly, our database did not include information on markers of inflammation, medical therapies (other than blood transfusion), or specific measures of hemodynamic status and MI type (most importantly type 2 MI). Consequently, we could not determine the pathophysiologic basis accounting for our observations or rule out confounding by non-coronary-related phenomena. These setbacks were addressed by a. deliberately excluding patients whose primary admission diagnosis was not AMI (e.g., acute illness, infection, etc.) and b. performing extensive multivariable analyses that controlled for baseline and acute event characteristics as well as hospitalization parameters. Lastly, we did not have data on cardiac biomarkers levels. Yet, we believe this knowledge gap did not alter the study's findings, as a. such levels are highly dependent upon testing timing, accompanying disease states (e.g., renal failure), and the kits used, all of which could differ substantially between patients, and b. we did consider paralleling aspects of MI severity, including the presence of severe LV dysfunction, the number of diseased vessels on angiography, and cardiogenic shock presentation.

5. Conclusions

In our large single-center experience, hypoalbuminemia constituted an adverse prognostic marker for long-term survival in AMI patients with normal or mildly elevated—but not with reduced or severely increased—BMI. Pending future research, tailoring the management of hypoalbuminemia in these cases based on BMI range may prove beneficial.

Supplementary Materials: The following supporting information can be downloaded at https://www.mdpi.com/article/10.3390/jcdd11120378/s1, Figure S1: Study flow chart; Figure S2: Hypoalbuminemia prevalence and serum albumin level according to body mass index category; Figure S3: Cumulative survival: (a) according to serum albumin status; (b) according to body mass index category; Figure S4: Serum albumin decrease-associated risk of all-cause mortality at 10 years after acute myocardial infarction per multivariable analysis in the total cohort; Figure S5: Serum albumin decrease-associated risk of all-cause mortality at 10 years after acute myocardial infarction per multivariable analysis in each of the body mass index categories subgroups; Table S1: Baseline clinical characteristics according to body mass index category; Table S2: Multivariable binary logistic regression model for admission-time hypoalbuminemia in the total cohort; Table S3: Baseline clinical characteristics of patients with underweight, normal weight, and overweight, stratified by serum albumin status; Table S4: Baseline clinical characteristics of patients with obesity, stratified by serum albumin status; Table S5: Acute event aspects by body mass index category; Table S6: Acute event aspects in patients with underweight, normal weight, and overweight, stratified by serum albumin status; Table S7: Acute event aspects in patients with obesity, stratified by serum albumin status; Table S8: Ten-year all-cause mortality; Table S9: Multivariable Cox proportional hazard models for the outcome of all-cause mortality at 10 years in patients with underweight, normal weight, and overweight; Table S10: Multivariable Cox proportional hazard models for the outcome of all-cause mortality at 10 years in patients with obesity.

Author Contributions: Conceptualization, A.S. (Alon Shechter), S.D., A.S. (Arthur Shiyovich), H.G. and Y.P.; Methodology, A.S. (Alon Shechter) and Y.P.; Data curation, Y.P.; Writing—original draft, A.S. (Alon Shechter); Writing—review & editing, S.D., A.S. (Arthur Shiyovich), H.G. and Y.P.; Supervision, H.G. All authors have read and agreed to the published version of the manuscript.

Funding: This research received no external funding.

Institutional Review Board Statement: The study was conducted in accordance with the Declaration of Helsinki and approved by Soroka's Institutional Review Board (approval number SOR-0319-16), for studies involving humans.

Informed Consent Statement: Patient consent was waived due to the investigation's retrospective nature.

Data Availability Statement: The data underlying this article will be shared upon reasonable request to the corresponding author.

Conflicts of Interest: The authors declare no conflicts of interest.

References

1. Sujino, Y.; Tanno, J.; Nakano, S.; Funada, S.; Hosoi, Y.; Senbonmatsu, T.; Nishimura, S. Impact of Hypoalbuminemia, Frailty, and Body Mass Index on Early Prognosis in Older Patients ($\geq$ 85 years) with ST-Elevation Myocardial Infarction. *J. Cardiol.* **2015**, *66*, 263–268. [CrossRef] [PubMed]
2. Herrmann, J.; Gersh, B.J.; Goldfinger, J.Z.; Witzenbichler, B.; Guagliumi, G.; Dudek, D.; Kornowski, R.; Brener, S.J.; Parise, H.; Fahy, M.; et al. Body Mass Index and Acute and Long-Term Outcomes After Acute Myocardial Infarction (from the Harmonizing Outcomes with Revascularization and Stents in Acute Myocardial Infarction Trial). *Am. J. Cardiol.* **2014**, *114*, 9–16. [CrossRef] [PubMed]
3. Margarson, M.P.; Soni, N. Serum Albumin: Touchstone or Totem? *Anaesthesia* **1998**, *53*, 789–803. [CrossRef] [PubMed]
4. Covinsky, K.E.; Covinsky, M.H.; Palmer, R.M.; Sehgal, A.R. Serum Albumin Concentration and Clinical Assessments of Nutritional Status in Hospitalized Older People: Different Sides of Different Coins? *J. Am. Geriatr. Soc.* **2002**, *50*, 631–637. [CrossRef] [PubMed]
5. Nelson, J.J.; Liao, D.; Sharrett, A.R.; Folsom, A.R.; Chambless, L.E.; Shahar, E.; Szklo, M.; Eckfeldt, J.; Heiss, G. Serum Albumin Level as a Predictor of Incident Coronary Heart Disease: The Atherosclerosis Risk in Communities (ARIC) Study. *Am. J. Epidemiol.* **2000**, *151*, 468–477. [CrossRef] [PubMed]
6. Djoussé, L.; Rothman, K.J.; Cupples, L.A.; Levy, D.; Ellison, R.C. Serum Albumin and Risk of Myocardial Infarction and All-Cause Mortality in the Framingham Offspring Study. *Circulation* **2000**, *2106*, 2919–2924. [CrossRef] [PubMed]
7. Biccirè, F.G.; Pastori, D.; Tanzilli, A.; Pignatelli, P.; Viceconte, N.; Barillà, F.; Versaci, F.; Gaudio, C.; Violi, F.; Tanzilli, G. Low Serum Albumin Levels and In-Hospital Outcomes in Patients with ST Segment Elevation Myocardial Infarction. *Nutr. Metab. Cardiovasc. Dis.* **2021**, *31*, 2904–2911. [CrossRef] [PubMed]
8. Plakht, Y.; Gilutz, H.; Shiyovich, A. Decreased Admission Serum Albumin Level is an Independent Predictor of Long-Term Mortality in Hospital Survivors of Acute Myocardial Infarction. Soroka Acute Myocardial Infarction II (SAMI-II) project. *Int. J. Cardiol.* **2016**, *219*, 20–24. [CrossRef] [PubMed]
9. Liu, H.; Zhang, F.; Li, Y.; Liu, L.; Song, X.; Wang, J.; Dang, Y.; Qi, X. The HALP Score Predicts No-Reflow Phenomenon and Long-Term Prognosis in Patients with ST-Segment Elevation Myocardial Infarction after Primary Percutaneous Coronary Intervention. *Coron. Artery Dis.* **2024**. *ahead of print*. [CrossRef]
10. Keys, A.; Fidanza, F.; Karvonen, M.J.; Kimura, N.; Taylor, H.L. Indices of Relative Weight and Obesity. *Int. J. Epidemiol.* **2014**, *43*, 655–665. [CrossRef] [PubMed]
11. Gelber, R.P.; Gaziano, J.M.; Orav, E.J.; Manson, J.E.; Buring, J.E.; Kurth, T. Measures of Obesity and Cardiovascular Risk Among Men and Women. *J. Am. Coll. Cardiol.* **2008**, *52*, 605–615. [CrossRef] [PubMed]
12. Kosuge, M.; Kimura, K.; Kojima, S.; Sakamoto, T.; Ishihara, M.; Asada, Y.; Tei, C.; Miyazaki, S.; Sonoda, M.; Tsuchihashi, K.; et al. Impact of Body Mass Index on In-Hospital Outcomes after Percutaneous Coronary Intervention for ST Segment Elevation Acute Myocardial Infarction. *Circ. J.* **2007**, *72*, 521–525. [CrossRef] [PubMed]
13. Mehta, L.; Devlin, W.; McCullough, P.A.; O'Neill, W.W.; Skelding, K.A.; Stone, G.W.; Boura, J.A.; Grines, C.L. Impact of Body Mass Index on Outcomes After Percutaneous Coronary Intervention in Patients with Acute Myocardial Infarction. *Am. J. Cardiol.* **2007**, *99*, 906–910. [CrossRef] [PubMed]
14. Nikolsky, E.; Stone, G.W.; Grines, C.L.; Cox, D.A.; Garcia, E.; Tcheng, J.E.; Griffin, J.J.; Guagliumi, G.; Stuckey, T.; Turco, M.; et al. Impact of Body Mass Index on Outcomes After Primary Angioplasty in Acute Myocardial Infarction. *Am. Heart J.* **2006**, *151*, 168–175. [CrossRef] [PubMed]
15. Kang, W.Y.; Jeong, M.H.; Ahn, Y.K.; Kim, J.H.; Chae, S.C.; Kim, Y.J.; Hur, S.H.; Seong, I.W.; Hong, T.J.; Choi, D.H.; et al. Obesity Paradox in Korean Patients Undergoing Primary Percutaneous Coronary Intervention in ST-Segment Elevation Myocardial Infarction. *J. Cardiol.* **2010**, *55*, 84–91. [CrossRef] [PubMed]
16. Centers for Disease Control. 2014. Available online: https://www.cms.gov/Medicare/Coding/ICD9ProviderDiagnosticCodes/codes (accessed on 1 November 2022).
17. Thygesen, K.; Alpert, J.S.; Jaffe, A.S.; Chaitman, B.R.; Bax, J.J.; Morrow, D.A.; White, H.D. Executive Group on behalf of the Joint European Society of Cardiology (ESC)/American College of Cardiology (ACC)/American Heart Association (AHA)/World Heart Federation (WHF) Task Force for the Universal Definition of Myocardial Infarction. Fourth Universal Definition of Myocardial Infarction (2018). *J. Am. Coll. Cardiol.* **2018**, *72*, 2231–2264.
18. Weaving, G.; Batstone, G.F.; Jones, R.G. Age and Sex Variation in Serum Albumin Concentration: An Observational Study. *Ann. Clin. Biochem.* **2016**, *53*, 106–111. [CrossRef] [PubMed]
19. Centers for Disease Control and Prevention. Defining Adult Overweight and Obesity. Available online: https://www.cdc.gov/obesity/basics/adult-defining.html#:~:text=If%20your%20BMI%20is%2018.5,falls%20within%20the%20obesity%20range (accessed on 1 November 2022).

20. Mauricio, M.D.; Aldasoro, M.; Ortega, J.; Vila, J.M. Endothelial Dysfunction in Morbid Obesity. *Curr. Pharm. Des.* **2013**, *19*, 5718–5729. [CrossRef] [PubMed]
21. Diercks, D.B.; Roe, M.T.; Mulgund, J.; Pollack, C.V., Jr.; Kirk, J.D.; Gibler, W.B.; Ohman, E.M.; Smith, S.C., Jr.; Boden, W.E.; Peterson, E.D. The Obesity Paradox in Non-ST-Segment Elevation Acute Coronary Syndromes: Results from the Can Rapid Risk Stratification of Unstable Angina Patients Suppress Adverse Outcomes with Early Implementation of the American College of Cardiology/American Heart Association Guidelines Quality Improvement Initiative. *Am. Heart J.* **2006**, *152*, 140–148. [PubMed]
22. Manolis, A.A.; Manolis, T.A.; Melita, H.; Mikhailidis, D.P.; Manolis, A.S. Low Serum Albumin: A neglected Predictor in Patients with Cardiovascular Disease. *Eur. J. Intern. Med.* **2022**, *102*, 24–39. [CrossRef] [PubMed]
23. Visseren, F.L.; Mach, F.; Smulders, Y.M.; Carballo, D.; Koskinas, K.C.; Bäck, M.; Benetos, A.; Biffi, A.; Boavida, J.M.; Capodanno, D.; et al. ESC National Cardiac Societies; ESC Scientific Document Group. 2021 ESC Guidelines on Cardiovascular Disease Prevention in Clinical Practice. *Eur. Heart J.* **2021**, *42*, 3227–3337. [CrossRef] [PubMed]

Journal of
Cardiovascular Development and Disease

MDPI

Article

Retrospective Study on Short-Term Reverse Cardiac Remodeling in Obese Patients Undergoing Sleeve Gastrectomy

Carmine Izzo [1,*,†], Valeria Visco [1,†], Alessandra Cirillo [1], Davide Bonadies [1], Giuseppe Caliendo [1], Maria Rosaria Rusciano [1], Nicola Virtuoso [2], Francesco Loria [1], Alessia Bramanti [1], Eleonora Venturini [3], Paola Di Pietro [1], Vincenzo Pilone [4], Luigi Schiavo [1], Albino Carrizzo [1,3], Carmine Vecchione [1,3] and Michele Ciccarelli [1]

1 Department of Medicine, Surgery and Dentistry, University of Salerno, 84081 Salerno, Italy; vvisco@unisa.it (V.V.); alessandra.cirillo167@gmail.com (A.C.); d.bonadies1@gmail.com (D.B.); giuseppecaliendo1995@gmail.com (G.C.); mrusciano@unisa.it (M.R.R.); francescoloria94@gmail.com (F.L.); abramanti@unisa.it (A.B.); pdipietro@unisa.it (P.D.P.); lschiavo@unisa.it (L.S.); acarrizzo@unisa.it (A.C.); cvecchione@unisa.it (C.V.); mciccarelli@unisa.it (M.C.)

2 Cardiology Unit, University Hospital "San Giovanni di Dio e Ruggi d'Aragona", 84081 Salerno, Italy; n1virtuoso@hotmail.it

3 Vascular Physiopathology Unit, IRCCS Neuromed Mediterranean Neurological Institute, 86077 Pozzilli, Italy; ele.venturini94@gmail.com

4 Public Health Department, Naples "Federico II" University, AOU "Federico II", Via S. Pansini 5, 80131 Naples, Italy; vincenzo.pilone@unina.it

* Correspondence: carmine.izzo93@gmail.com; Tel.: +39-3480774351

† These authors equally contributed to this work.

Abstract: Severe obesity is closely associated with an increased risk of comorbidities and alterations in cardiac structure and function. The primary objective of this study was to investigate cardiovascular (CV) risk factors and ventricular remodeling in individuals from an obese population eligible for bariatric surgery. The secondary objective was to evaluate changes in anthropometric, clinical laboratory, and echocardiographic measurements 12 weeks after surgery compared to baseline values. This retrospective observational cohort study involved patients from a single specialized bariatric surgery center. A total of 35 patients were included (mean age 41.5 ± 10.3 years; BMI 43.4 ± 6.6 kg/m^2), of whom 34.2% had a family history of coronary artery disease (CAD), 5.7% had a prior history of CAD, 8 had essential hypertension, 11.4% had dyslipidemia, 20% were smokers, and 8.6% were former smokers. Approximately 57% of the patients exhibited concentric left ventricular remodeling, and 14% had grade I diastolic dysfunction. At 12 weeks post-surgery, with an average weight loss of 25 kg and a mean BMI reduction of 8.5 kg/m^2, 14% of the patients still exhibited concentric left ventricular remodeling, and about 11% had grade I diastolic dysfunction. Bariatric surgery contributes to the improvement of cardiac function and structure over time as a result of significant weight loss.

Keywords: obesity; echocardiography; cardiac remodeling; cardiology; cardiovascular risk factors; bariatric surgery; sleeve gastrectomy; weight loss

1. Introduction

1.1. Obesity

Obesity, defined by the World Health Organization (WHO) as excessive body fat accumulation, arises from genetic, environmental, and lifestyle factors, including the adoption of a sedentary "Western lifestyle" and high-calorie diets. This global public health challenge has arisen in recent decades due to socioeconomic and behavioral shifts [1,2].

The Body Mass Index (BMI) is the standard tool for classifying obesity, with thresholds of 18.5–24.9 kg/m^2 for normal weight, over 25 kg/m^2 for overweight, and over 30 kg/m^2

for obesity. Severe obesity is marked by a BMI exceeding 40 kg/m^2. However, BMI has limitations, as it fails to account for differences in body composition, such as muscle mass and fat distribution, potentially misclassifying individuals [3,4].

Advanced methods like Dual-Energy X-ray Absorptiometry (DEXA), Bioelectrical Impedance Analysis (BIA), and imaging techniques provide more precise assessments but are rarely used clinically due to complexity. Instead, simpler measurements like waist circumference and metabolic indicators (e.g., blood glucose and cholesterol levels) are preferred to evaluate health risks more comprehensively [5].

This nuanced approach acknowledges the rising global prevalence of obesity driven by decreased physical activity and dietary changes, personalized lifestyle modifications to address associated health risks effectively [4,6].

1.2. Obesity and Left Ventricular Remodeling

The heart exhibits remarkable adaptability, remodeling itself in response to physiological and pathological conditions. Physiological remodeling occurs during physical exercise, pregnancy, or growth, whereas pathological remodeling, such as left ventricular hypertrophy (LVH), arises from chronic conditions like hypertension. LVH involves molecular and cellular changes, including myocyte enlargement and extracellular matrix restructuring. Initially compensatory, these adaptations may become maladaptive, contributing to cardiovascular complications [7,8].

Hypertension is a primary driver of cardiac remodeling, triggering mechanical stress on ventricular walls, collagen turnover, and calcium transport dysfunction in myocytes. Elevated intracellular calcium activates calcineurin, leading to hypertrophic signaling. Echocardiography remains the gold standard for assessing left ventricular structure, with left ventricular mass index (LVMI) and relative wall thickness (RWT) used to classify remodeling patterns into concentric or eccentric hypertrophy and concentric remodeling [9,10].

Obesity is strongly linked to left ventricular remodeling and heart failure risk. Excess weight imposes hemodynamic and metabolic burdens, leading to structural and functional changes in the heart. Bariatric surgery, particularly sleeve gastrectomy (SG), has emerged as an effective treatment for severe obesity, offering not only significant weight loss but also cardiovascular benefits. Studies indicate that weight loss achieved through bariatric surgery can reverse cardiac remodeling, reducing left ventricular mass, wall thickness, and improving systolic and diastolic functions.

Research by Frea et al. and Karason et al. demonstrates that bariatric surgery alleviates concentric hypertrophy and improves diastolic filling by lowering hemodynamic load and enhancing metabolic health. Systematic reviews and meta-analyses corroborate these findings, highlighting reductions in LV wall thickness and improvements in ventricular compliance and function after surgery. The mechanisms of reverse remodeling are multifactorial, involving hemodynamic, inflammatory, and metabolic changes [10–12].

Bariatric surgery reduces preload and afterload on the left ventricle, alleviating myocardial wall stress. It also decreases systemic inflammation and oxidative stress, as evidenced by reductions in inflammatory markers like C-reactive protein (CRP) and interleukin-6 (IL-6), both associated with LV hypertrophy and fibrosis. Enhanced glucose metabolism and insulin sensitivity following surgery further support cardiac function by reducing myocardial fat infiltration, which is linked to impaired relaxation and compliance [13].

Moreover, weight loss lowers circulating levels of leptin and other adipokines that activate the sympathetic nervous system, potentially reducing heart rate, blood pressure, and myocardial workload. These suggest improvements that bariatric surgery not only promotes weight reduction but also improves cardiac health, particularly for individuals with obesity-related left ventricular remodeling [14].

The clinical significance of addressing LVH lies in its association with increased risks of heart failure, arrhythmias, myocardial infarction, and sudden cardiac death. By mitigating these risks, bariatric surgery emerges as a transformative approach for both obesity and cardiovascular health, offering hope for improved outcomes in patients with obesity-related cardiac remodeling [15,16].

1.3. Obesity Therapy and Treatment Options

Managing obesity is a persistent challenge, with lifestyle modifications like a healthy diet and regular exercise serving as the cornerstone of treatment. A weight loss of at least 5% from baseline is associated with significant improvements in cardiometabolic risk factors. However, long-term adherence to lifestyle changes is difficult, with most individuals regaining weight within five years. While medical therapies offer limited success, bariatric surgery remains the most effective long-term treatment for sustainable weight loss and the alleviation of obesity-related complications [17].

Bariatric surgery is recommended for individuals with a BMI ≥ 40 kg/m^2 or those with a BMI ≥ 35 kg/m^2 accompanied by comorbidities such as type 2 diabetes, hypertension, dyslipidemia, non-alcoholic fatty liver disease, or severe sleep apnea. Candidates must demonstrate prior failure with conventional treatments and undergo comprehensive evaluations to ensure readiness and commitment to postoperative care [18,19].

Surgical techniques are categorized as malabsorptive, which limit nutrient absorption, or restrictive, which reduce stomach capacity to promote satiety. Common procedures include Roux-en-Y gastric bypass, sleeve gastrectomy, and adjustable gastric banding, which lead to substantial weight loss sustained over a decade [20]. Beyond weight reduction, bariatric surgery improves cardiovascular health by mitigating risk factors and reversing structural cardiac changes [21].

This study evaluates cardiovascular risk factors and echocardiographic alterations in obese individuals, exploring how these parameters are modified after bariatric surgery to advance understanding of its benefits for obesity-related cardiovascular health.

2. Materials and Methods

2.1. Study Design and Population

This is a retrospective observational cohort study involving obese patients who were indicated for bariatric surgery via sleeve gastrectomy (SG) at the Azienda Ospedaliera Universitaria San Giovanni di Dio e Ruggi d'Aragona in Salerno. The patients were recruited between June 2022 and April 2023 in accordance with the guidelines of the Italian Society of Surgery (SIC) and the Italian Society of Obesity Surgery (SICOB). The enrolled patients were referred from the Azienda Ospedaliera Universitaria San Giovanni di Dio e Ruggi d'Aragona in Salerno. All patients referred were included in the study regardless of age if they fell within previously mentioned guidelines. Exclusion criteria included previous major cardiovascular disease or other concomitant/previous major disease (e.g., oncological disease).

Data were collected during the preoperative assessment, which was conducted on a day-hospital basis at the Azienda Ospedaliera Universitaria San Giovanni di Dio e Ruggi d'Aragona. The collected data included anthropometric measurements, resting vital signs, instrumental parameters, electrocardiographic readings, and transthoracic echocardiographic assessments. Hematochemical values were retrieved through the hospital's online information system.

2.2. Clinical Examination, Laboratory Testing, and Instrumental Testing

All patients had the following measurements recorded: age, sex, height, weight, waist and hip circumference, and BMI. Height was measured using a wall-mounted tape measure with patients standing barefoot and with feet together. Weight was measured using a KERN platform scale (model MPO 300k-1LM, Frankfurt am Main, Germany) with patients wearing light clothing and no shoes. Waist circumference was measured with a non-flexible tape measure placed midway between the lower rib margin and the iliac crest, encircling the entire waist. Hip circumference was measured with a standard non-flexible tape measure placed around the widest part of the hips, encircling the entire circumference. BMI was calculated as weight (kg) divided by the square of height (m^2). Blood pressure was measured three times within a 10–20-min interval using the same aneroid sphygmomanometer (ERKA, model 1-tube EN 1060 Kobold Smart Rapid with a size 6 Adult Large cuff 34–43 cm, Bad Tölz, Germany). Measurements were taken with the cuff covering two-thirds of the left arm while the patient was seated. The average of the results was calculated. Systolic blood pressure was defined as the value at which the sound begins, and diastolic pressure as the fifth Korotkoff phase. Values were recorded in mmHg.

ECG was performed to assess cardiac electrical activity using standard 12-lead methods with the MAC2000 (GE Healthcare, Waukesha, WI, USA) and was interpreted by experienced operators. Echocardiographic assessments were conducted to evaluate ventricular structure and function using standard methods [16]. Two of the same expert operators, both medical director cardiologists, not blinded, performed the echocardiograms using the Vivid E9 scanner (GE Healthcare, Waukesha, WI, USA) with offline analysis to ensure consistency (EchoPac version 201, GE Healthcare, Waukesha, WI, USA), equipped with a 4.6 MHz transducer (GE-M5Sc-D XDClear, GE Medical Systems, Waukesha WI, USA). Measurements were performed according to the guidelines and recommendation.

Echocardiography enables accurate assessment of left ventricular remodeling in patients. The study of ventricular geometry begins with the measurement of interventricular septum thickness (IVS), posterior wall thickness (PW), and left ventricular end-diastolic diameter (LVEDd). These measurements allow for the calculation of ventricular volume and mass using specific formulas. Currently, left ventricular mass (LVM) is calculated according to the recommendations of the American Society of Echocardiography (ASE) [22].

Normal values for left ventricular mass indexed to body surface area (BSA) should be less than 95 g/m^2 for women and 115 g/m^2 for men, according to linear methods. Left ventricular hypertrophy (LVH) is defined when left ventricular mass index (LVMI) values exceed 115 g/m^2 for men and 95 g/m^2 for women. The calculation of relative wall thickness (RWT) allows for the classification of hypertrophy as concentric (RWT > 0.42) or eccentric (RWT $\leq$ 0.42) and helps identify concentric remodeling without hypertrophy (normal LVMI with increased RWT). This method identifies four geometric patterns: normal (LVMI $\leq$ 115 g/m^2 for men and $\leq$95 g/m^2 for women; RWT $\leq$ 0.42); concentric ventricular remodeling (LVMI $\leq$ 115 g/m^2 for men and $\leq$95 g/m^2 for women; RWT > 0.42); eccentric ventricular hypertrophy (LVMI > 115 g/m^2 for men and >95 g/m^2 for women; RWT $\leq$ 0.42); and concentric ventricular hypertrophy (LVMI > 115 g/m^2 for men and >95 g/m^2 for women; RWT > 0.42) [22].

Laboratory tests in fasting venous blood samples were analyzed for triglycerides (TGs), low-density lipoproteins (LDLs), high-density lipoproteins (HDLs), total cholesterol, glucose, glycated hemoglobin (HbA1c), complete blood count, hemoglobin, C-reactive protein (CRP), erythrocyte sedimentation rate (ESR), N-terminal pro b-type natriuretic peptide (NT-proBNP), albumin, creatinine, urea, uric acid, sodium, potassium, calcium, aspartate aminotransferase (AST), alanine aminotransferase (ALT), and total bilirubin. The analyses were performed at the laboratory of the Gaetano Fucito Hospital in Mercato San Severino (SA).

3. Statistical Analysis

The statistical analysis of the collected data was performed using both parametric and non-parametric tests as appropriate. Specifically, the Student's t-test and Mann–Whitney test were used for continuous variables, while Fisher's exact test was employed to compare frequencies and categorical variables. Before applying the appropriate tests, a Kolmogorov–Smirnov (K–S) "Goodness of Fit" test was conducted to assess whether the continuous variables followed a normal distribution. Simple linear regression was used to estimate the relationship between one independent quantitative variable and one dependent quantitative variable of interest. Measures of central tendency and dispersion were calculated, including means, standard deviations, and medians. Additionally, inferential statistics were employed to determine the probability of obtaining observed differences by chance alone. Statistical analyses were carried out using GraphPad® version 9.5.5 (La Jolla, CA,

USA) for Macintosh®. Statistical significance was defined as $p < 0.05$ in a two-tailed test with a 95% confidence interval.

4. Results

Thirty-five obese patients were evaluated at baseline (T0) and 12 weeks post-bariatric surgery (T1). At T0, the mean age was 41.5 years, with a mean weight of 124.1 kg, BMI of 43.5 kg/m^2, waist circumference of 127.7 cm, and hip circumference of 136.5 cm. By T1, these values improved significantly, with mean weight at 99.6 kg, BMI at 35.03 kg/m^2, waist circumference at 108.5 cm, and hip circumference at 118.2 cm. Patients showed an average weight loss of 24.46 kg, equivalent to a BMI reduction of 8.47 kg/m^2 (Table 1).

Table 1. Anthropometric and hemodynamic data at baseline (T0) and 12 weeks (T1).

	T0 (n = 35)	T1 (n = 35)	*p*-Value
Female	20 (57%)	=	ns
Age (years)	41.5 ± 10.3	41.8 ± 10.3	ns
Hip circumference (cm)	136.5 ± 19.13	118.2 ± 14.34	<0.0001 *
Waist circumference (cm)	127.7 ± 20.04	108.5 ± 14.51	<0.0001 *
Height (m)	1.68 ± 0.12	1.68 ± 0.12	ns
Weight (kg)	124.1 ± 23.47	99.6 ± 18.71	<0.0001 *
BMI (kg/m^2)	43.5 ± 6.67	35.03 ± 5.91	<0.0001 *
BSA (m^2)	2.29 ± 0.27	2.08 ± 0.24	<0.0001 *
Systolic blood pressure (mmHg)	126.5 ± 13	119.9 ± 11.41	0.0027 *
Diastolic blood pressure (mmHg)	82.29 ± 9.28	78.34 ± 5.98	0.0055 *
Heart rate (bpm)	78.26 ± 11.36	64.6 ± 8.51	<0.0001 *

"*" stands for statistically significant, "ns" stands for non significant.

At baseline, 34% of patients reported a family history of coronary artery disease (CAD), 22% had hypertension, and 11% had mixed dyslipidemia. Smoking was reported by 20% (current) and 8.5% (former). Additionally, 57% had undiagnosed dyslipidemia, 29% had elevated blood pressure, and 28.5% met metabolic syndrome criteria. By T1, only one patient had elevated blood pressure, and dyslipidemia persisted in four patients, reflecting significant improvements in cardiovascular risk factors (Table 2).

Table 2. Medical history and risk factors.

	T0 (n = 35)	T1 (n = 35)
Family history of cardiovascular disease, n (%)	12 (34%)	-
Chronic coronary artery disease, n (%)	2 (5.7%)	-
Hypertension (mmHg)	8 (22%)	-
Elevated blood pressure values, n (%)	10 (29%)	1 (2.85%)
Total dyslipidemia, n (%)	24 (68.6%)	8 (22.8%)
Known dyslipidemia, n (%)	4 (11%)	-
Unknown dyslipidemia, n (%)	20 (57%)	4 (11%)
Type II diabetes mellitus, n (%)	0	0
High risk for diabetes mellitus, n (%)	12 (35.28%)	0
Hyperuricemia, n (%)	12 (34%)	0
Smokers, n (%)	7 (20%)	-
Ex-smokers, n (%)	3 (8.5%)	-

Laboratory findings demonstrated notable improvements in lipid profiles, glucose metabolism, and inflammatory markers. LDL levels reduced significantly, while HbA1c and uric acid levels improved, supporting metabolic benefits from weight loss. Echocardiographic measures, including lateral E′ wave and E/e′ ratio, indicated enhanced diastolic function. Importantly, no patients exhibited impaired glucose tolerance or metabolic syndrome at follow-up (Table 3).

Table 3. Laboratory tests at T0 and T1.

	T0 (n = 35)	T1 (n = 35)	*p*-Value
Albumin (gr/dL)	4.29 ± 0.15	4.11 ± 0.46	ns
C-reactive protein (mg/L)	1.47 ± 1.11	5.41 ± 6.58	0.0105 *
Vitamin D (UI)	13.02 ± 5.06	14.18 ± 8.28	ns
Glycated hemoglobin (%)	5.92 ± 0.53	5.45 ± 0.44	0.002 *
Glucose (mg/dL)	98.77 ± 20.93	88.56 ± 12.67	0.0312 *
Blood urea nitrogen (mg/dL)	29.33 ± 6.41	29.21 ± 8.23	ns
Uric acid (mg/dL)	6.47 ± 1.27	5.89 ± 1.26	0.0307 *
Estimated glomerular filtration rate (mL/min)	131.3 ± 32.94	101.3 ± 20.44	ns
Creatinine (mg/mL)	0.77 ± 0.15	0.75 ± 0.18	ns
Sodium (mEq/L)	138 ± 1.35	141.6 ± 2.25	0.0002 *
Potassium (mEq/L)	4.22 ± 0.22	4.14 ± 0.31	ns
Bilirubin	0.67 ± 0.43	0.81 ± 0.33	ns
AST (aspartate aminotransferase) (U/L)	20.75 ± 8.18	19.25 ± 3.77	ns
ALT (alanine aminotransferase) (U/L)	24.33 ± 14.43	16.67 ± 4.51	ns
Calcium (mg/dL)	9.38 ± 0.29	9.77 ± 0.40	ns
BNP (B-type natriuretic peptide) (pg/mL)	19.78 ± 12.47	24.42 ± 8.9	ns
Total cholesterol (mg/dL)	191.9 ± 31.9	179.8 ± 24.64	ns
HDL-C (high-density lipoprotein cholesterol)	48.67 ± 9.55	53.67 ± 16.62	ns
LDL-C (low-density lipoprotein cholesterol)	124.2 ± 25.82	108.5 ± 21.69	0.0127 *
Triglycerides	95.8 ± 27.99	89.4 ± 25.36	ns
White blood cell count (WBC) (n/μL)	6.87 ± 1.75	6.45 ± 1.81	ns
Hemoglobin (g/dL)	13.46 ± 1.26	13.14 ± 0.89	ns
Platelets (n/μL)	254.9 ± 54.31	239.6 ± 54	ns

"*" stands for statistically significant, "ns" stands for non significant.

Echocardiographic findings revealed that 57% of patients had concentric LV remodeling, and 14% had grade I diastolic dysfunction at T0 (Figure 1). These rates improved to 14% and 11.4%, respectively, at T1. Reductions in LVMI, RWT, and lateral E′ wave values indicated reverse remodeling and improved diastolic function (Table 4).

Analysis showed BMI correlated positively with RWT, suggesting an impact of body weight on LV geometry. Age also moderately influenced RWT, though less significantly than BMI. However, BMI did not correlate with LVMI/BSA, indicating it was not a primary factor in LV hypertrophy (Figures 2–4).

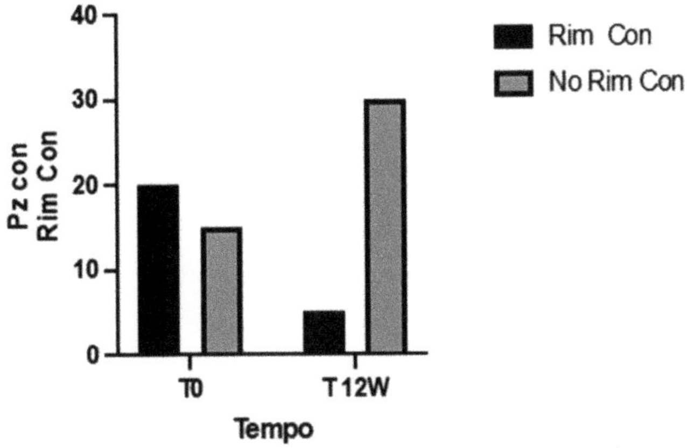

Figure 1. Contingency retrospective data (Fisher's exact test).

Table 4. Diastolic and systolic function in obese patients assessed by standard and advanced echocardiographic parameters.

	T0 (n = 35)	T1 (n = 35)	*p*
Ejection fraction (%)	61.99 ± 6.74	63.74 ± 5.81	ns
Ascending aorta (mm)	31.37 ± 3.18	30.86 ± 3.02	ns
PAPs (mmHg)	17.36 ± 5.52	18.68 ± 5.74	ns
IVSd (mm)	10.4 ± 1.19	9.48 ± 1.06	ns
LVPWd (mm)	8.97 ± 1.15	8.05 ± 1.55	0.0034 *
dVStd (mm)	47.63 ± 5.58	47.6 ± 5.55	ns
RA area (cm^2)	13.7 ± 3.33	14.2 ± 3.34	ns
RWT	0.41 ± 0.05	0.37 ± 0.06	0.0023 *
E wave (m/s)	0.76 ± 15.45	0.75 ± 16.24	ns
A wave (m/s)	0.69 ± 18.12	0.66 ± 14.07	ns
E/A	1.16 ± 0.38	1.18 ± 0.31	ns
Deceleration time (ms)	213.5 ± 50.46	217 ± 51.67	ns
E/e′	6.74 ± 1.005	6.16 ± 1.54	0.0443 *
LAVi (ml/m^2)	24 ± 6.13	24.61 ± 7.73	ns
TAPSE (mm)	24.43 ± 3.02	24.97 ± 3.16	ns
RVs′ (cm/s)	13.34 ± 1.86	13.17 ± 1.93	ns
LVMI/BSA	72.17 ± 13.07	69.45 ± 12.57	ns
LVESV (mL)	43.69 ± 15.89	40.91 ± 16.04	ns
LVEDV (mL)	113.7 ± 32.46	111.3 ± 36.33	ns
E′l wave (cm/s)	13.26 ± 3.56	15.14 ± 4.24	0.0002 *
E′s wave (cm/s)	9.8 ± 2.16	10.34 ± 2.66	ns
RVd1 (mm)	32.26 ± 3.49	30.86 ± 3.78	0.0080 *
LVMI (g/m^2)	166 ± 38.98	145.7 ± 36.13	0.0002 *

LVEDV: left ventricular end-diastolic volume; LVESV: left ventricular end-systolic volume; IVSd: interventricular septum at end-diastole; LVPWd: left ventricular posterior wall at end-diastole; LV: left ventricle; RWT: relative wall thickness; LAVi: indexed left atrial volume; TAPSE: tricuspid annular plane systolic excursion; RV: right ventricle; LVMI: left ventricular mass index. "*" stands for statistically significant, "ns" stands for non significant.

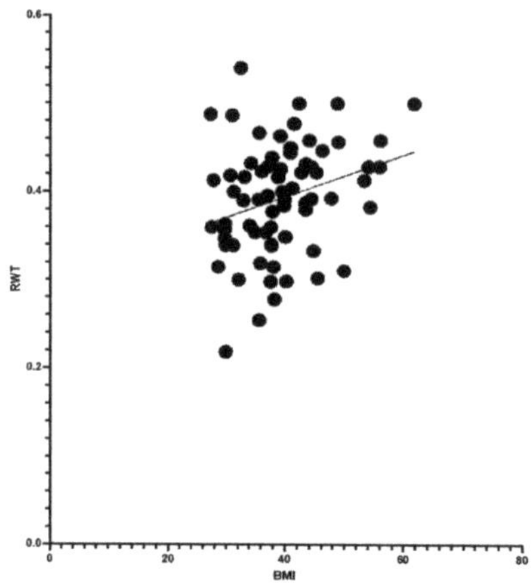

Figure 2. BMI and RWT with simple linear regression (p-value 0.0179 * and Pearson R 0.2822). "*" stands for statistically significant.

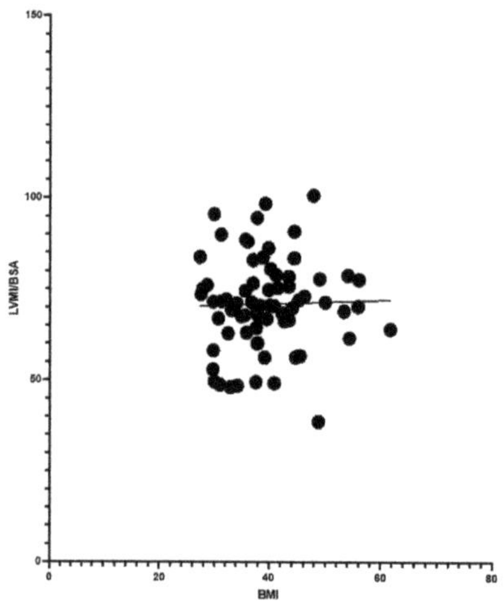

Figure 3. BMI and LVMI/BSA with simple linear regression (p-value 0.803 and Pearson R 0.030).

These results emphasize the rapid cardiovascular benefits of bariatric surgery, particularly in reversing concentric LV remodeling and improving metabolic health. However, the 12-week follow-up limits conclusions about long-term outcomes.

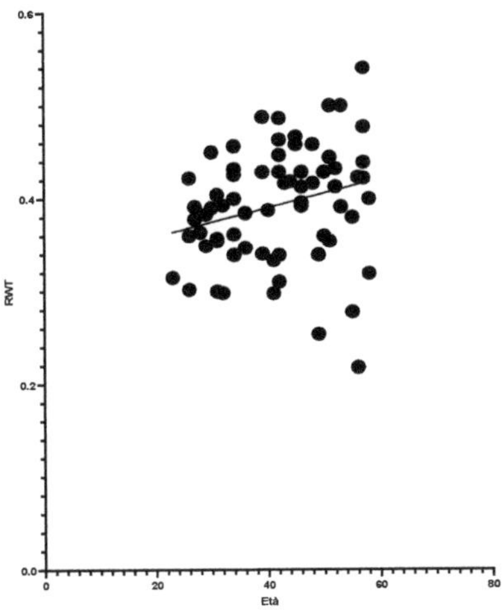

Figure 4. Age and RWT with simple linear regression (p-value 0.037 * and Pearson R 0.249). "*" stands for statistically significant.

5. Discussion

Severe obesity is a major risk factor for cardiovascular diseases (CVDs), contributing to changes in cardiac structure and function even in individuals without a history of cardiovascular conditions. In this study, 71.4% of participants had undiagnosed cardiovascular conditions, while 82.8% had unidentified risk factors, such as elevated blood pressure (29%) and dyslipidemia (57%). Obesity-related lipid imbalances were evident, with 22.8% of patients exhibiting low HDL levels (<40 mg/dL) and 82.8% having elevated LDL levels (>100 mg/dL). These findings emphasize the importance of early cardiovascular screening in obese individuals [15,23,24].

Obesity-induced left ventricular (LV) remodeling often presents as concentric remodeling without hypertrophy, driven by increased preload, afterload, and myocardial dysfunction. At baseline, 57% of patients had concentric remodeling, and 14% showed grade I diastolic dysfunction. Weight loss following bariatric surgery, specifically sleeve gastrectomy, significantly improved cardiac structure and function. After 12 weeks, only 14% exhibited concentric remodeling, and diastolic dysfunction decreased to 11.4%. Significant reductions in interventricular septum thickness, posterior wall thickness, LV mass index (LVMI), and relative wall thickness (RWT) were observed, indicating reverse remodeling [25,26].

The mechanisms underlying these improvements include decreased mechanical load, improved metabolic flexibility, and reduced systemic inflammation. Weight loss alleviates myocardial stress, decreases plasma volume, and mitigates sympathetic activation. It also reduces levels of inflammatory cytokines like TNF-α and IL-6, oxidative stress, and myocardial fibrosis, enhancing myocardial compliance and diastolic function [27]. Improvements in insulin sensitivity further restore cardiomyocyte function, reducing lipid accumulation and improving calcium cycling for efficient myocardial contraction and relaxation [26,28,29].

Despite these benefits, the study's short 12-week follow-up limits its ability to confirm whether these structural improvements lead to sustained cardiovascular benefits, such as reduced incidence of heart failure or CVD mortality. Longer-term studies are needed to evaluate these outcomes and understand the relationship between short-term reverse remodeling and long-term cardiovascular health [30].

This study's findings emphasize the effectiveness of bariatric surgery not only for weight loss but also for cardiovascular health [31]. The observed reductions in blood pressure, heart rate, and lipid profiles highlight the procedure's role in mitigating obesity-related CVD risk. However, the retrospective nature of the study and its small sample size limit broader applicability. Future research should involve larger patient cohorts with extended follow-up periods, potentially incorporating myocardial biopsies and advanced imaging to further elucidate the molecular mechanisms of reverse remodeling.

This study's findings have important clinical implications, especially given the short-term nature of the 12-week follow-up. The observed improvements in left ventricular (LV) remodeling, including reductions in left ventricular mass index (LVMI) and relative wall thickness (RWT), suggest that even within a brief period, bariatric surgery can initiate meaningful reverse cardiac remodeling. This aligns with prior studies demonstrating that reductions in hemodynamic load can lead to structural and functional cardiac improvements. However, the short duration of follow-up limits the ability to fully evaluate whether these changes will translate into sustained long-term benefits, such as reduced incidence of heart failure or cardiovascular mortality.

Bariatric surgery provides substantial cardiovascular benefits in obese individuals, initiating meaningful reverse cardiac remodeling even in the short term. These findings highlight the systemic advantages of significant weight loss and emphasize the need for early cardiovascular assessment and long-term monitoring to optimize outcomes for patients undergoing bariatric surgery.

6. Limitations

While this study provides valuable insights into the effects of sleeve gastrectomy on obese patients, it is essential to acknowledge several limitations that may affect the generalizability and robustness of the findings.

The study's retrospective and observational nature and the relatively small sample size of 35 patients limits the statistical power of the analysis. The study period of 12 weeks post-surgery, although useful for observing short-term effects, is insufficient to assess the long-term sustainability of weight loss and cardiovascular improvements. Although, the anthropometric changes in the study population are of great significance, the lack of a control group represents a further limitation. Furthermore, the study was conducted at a single center in Italy.

7. Conclusions and Future Perspective

Obesity is a chronic condition closely tied to cardiovascular risk factors and cardiac alterations. Bariatric surgery, particularly sleeve gastrectomy (SG), offers a powerful approach for mitigating these risks by achieving significant weight loss. This study demonstrates the potential of SG to improve anthropometric and cardiovascular parameters within a short 12-week follow-up, highlighting reductions in weight, BMI, and waist and hip circumferences, alongside better blood pressure, heart rate, and lipid profiles. Importantly, the reversal of concentric left ventricular remodeling and improvements in echocardiographic parameters, such as reduced left ventricular mass index (LVMI) and relative wall thickness (RWT), emphasize the cardiac benefits of weight loss.

Future research should focus on longer follow-up periods to confirm the durability of these benefits and their impact on cardiovascular outcomes, such as heart failure or myocardial infarction. Studies exploring additional cardiac parameters, including myocardial strain and diastolic function, are also needed. Investigating the molecular mechanisms behind these changes, such as neurohormonal modulation, inflammatory reduction, and metabolic improvements, could provide deeper insights.

In conclusion, SG facilitates substantial weight loss and meaningful cardiovascular improvements, establishing its critical role in managing obesity and its complications. Further research is essential to expand our understanding of the long-term benefits and mechanisms driving these outcomes.

Author Contributions: Conceptualization, C.I., V.V., C.V. and M.C.; methodology, V.P., L.S. and A.C. (Albino Carrizzo); validation, M.R.R., N.V. and F.L.; data curation, D.B., G.C., A.B. and E.V.; writing—original draft preparation, C.I. and A.C. (Alessandra Cirillo); writing—review and editing, P.D.P., M.C., A.C. (Albino Carrizzo) and C.V. All authors have read and agreed to the published version of the manuscript.

Funding: This research received no external funding.

Institutional Review Board Statement: The study was conducted in accordance with the Declaration of Helsinki. In accordance with the research purposes as declared by the Italian Data Protection Authority (G.U. No. 72 26 March 2012), this study does not require an Ethics Committee due to its anonymous, observational, and retrospective nature without personalized impact on the data subjects.

Informed Consent Statement: Informed consent was obtained from all subjects involved in the study.

Data Availability Statement: The data presented in this study are available on request from the corresponding author due to privacy.

Conflicts of Interest: The authors declare no conflicts of interest.

References

1. Vecchie, A.; Dallegri, F.; Carbone, F.; Bonaventura, A.; Liberale, L.; Portincasa, P.; Fruhbeck, G.; Montecucco, F. Obesity phenotypes and their paradoxical association with cardiovascular diseases. *Eur. J. Intern. Med.* **2018**, *48*, 6–17. [CrossRef] [PubMed]
2. Bluher, M. Obesity: Global epidemiology and pathogenesis. *Nat. Rev. Endocrinol.* **2019**, *15*, 288–298. [CrossRef]
3. Dietz, W.H. The response of the US Centers for Disease Control and Prevention to the obesity epidemic. *Annu. Rev. Public Health* **2015**, *36*, 575–596. [CrossRef]
4. Muscogiuri, G.; Verde, L.; Colao, A. Body Mass Index (BMI): Still be used? *Eur. J. Intern. Med.* **2023**, *117*, 50–51. [CrossRef] [PubMed]
5. Heymsfield, S.B.; Wadden, T.A. Mechanisms, Pathophysiology, and Management of Obesity. *N. Engl. J. Med.* **2017**, *376*, 254–266. [CrossRef] [PubMed]
6. Flegal, K.M.; Kit, B.K.; Orpana, H.; Graubard, B.I. Association of all-cause mortality with overweight and obesity using standard body mass index categories: A systematic review and meta-analysis. *JAMA* **2013**, *309*, 71–82. [CrossRef]
7. Stencel, J.; Alai, H.R.; Dhore-Patil, A.; Urina-Jassir, D.; Le Jemtel, T.H. Obesity, Preserved Ejection Fraction Heart Failure, and Left Ventricular Remodeling. *J. Clin. Med.* **2023**, *12*, 3341. [CrossRef]
8. Ciccarelli, M.; Giallauria, F.; Carrizzo, A.; Visco, V.; Silverio, A.; Cesaro, A.; Calabro, P.; De Luca, N.; Mancusi, C.; Masarone, D.; et al. Artificial intelligence in cardiovascular prevention: New ways will open new doors. *J. Cardiovasc. Med.* **2023**, *24*, e106–e115. [CrossRef]
9. Shi, K.; Huang, S.; Li, X.; Xu, H.Y.; Yang, M.X.; Li, Y.; Guo, Y.K.; Yang, Z.G. Effect of Obesity on Left Ventricular Remodeling and Clinical Outcome in Chinese Patients with Hypertrophic Cardiomyopathy: Assessed by Cardiac MRI. *J. Magn. Reson. Imaging* **2023**, *57*, 800–809. [CrossRef]
10. Frea, S.; Andreis, A.; Scarlatta, V.; Rovera, C.; Vairo, A.; Pistone, E.; Anselmino, M.; Golzio, P.G.; Toppino, M.; Giustetto, C.; et al. Subclinical Left Ventricular Dysfunction in Severe Obesity and Reverse Cardiac Remodeling after Bariatric Surgery. *J. Cardiovasc. Echogr.* **2020**, *30*, 22–28. [CrossRef]
11. Karason, K.; Wallentin, I.; Larsson, B.; Sjostrom, L. Effects of obesity and weight loss on left ventricular mass and relative wall thickness: Survey and intervention study. *BMJ* **1997**, *315*, 912–916. [CrossRef] [PubMed]
12. Esparham, A.; Shoar, S.; Kheradmand, H.R.; Ahmadyar, S.; Dalili, A.; Rezapanah, A.; Zandbaf, T.; Khorgami, Z. The Impact of Bariatric Surgery on Cardiac Structure, and Systolic and Diastolic Function in Patients with Obesity: A Systematic Review and Meta-analysis. *Obes. Surg.* **2023**, *33*, 345–361. [CrossRef] [PubMed]
13. Kindel, T.L.; Strande, J.L. Bariatric surgery as a treatment for heart failure: Review of the literature and potential mechanisms. *Surg. Obes. Relat. Dis.* **2018**, *14*, 117–122. [CrossRef] [PubMed]
14. Kardassis, D.; Bech-Hanssen, O.; Schonander, M.; Sjostrom, L.; Petzold, M.; Karason, K. Impact of body composition, fat distribution and sustained weight loss on cardiac function in obesity. *Int. J. Cardiol.* **2012**, *159*, 128–133. [CrossRef]
15. Aryee, E.K.; Ozkan, B.; Ndumele, C.E. Heart Failure and Obesity: The Latest Pandemic. *Prog. Cardiovasc. Dis.* **2023**, *78*, 43–48. [CrossRef]
16. Fucile, I.; Mancusi, C.; Visco, V.; De Luca, C.; Ambrosino, P.; Bianco, A.; Ciccarelli, M.; Iaccarino, G.; Morisco, C.; De Luca, N. Serum parathormone, vitamin D and cardiovascular risk factors and markers: A pilot study. *Nutr. Metab. Cardiovasc. Dis.* **2024**, *34*, 2298–2304. [CrossRef]
17. Ballo, P.; Motto, A.; Mondillo, S.; Faraguti, S.A. Impact of obesity on left ventricular mass and function in subjects with chronic volume overload. *Obesity* **2007**, *15*, 2019–2026. [CrossRef]
18. Buchwald, H. The evolution of metabolic/bariatric surgery. *Obes. Surg.* **2014**, *24*, 1126–1135. [CrossRef]

19. Phillips, B.T.; Shikora, S.A. The history of metabolic and bariatric surgery: Development of standards for patient safety and efficacy. *Metabolism* **2018**, *79*, 97–107. [CrossRef]
20. Brunaud, L. Bariatric surgery: Are we responsible but not guilty? *J. Visc. Surg.* **2017**, *154*, 225–226. [CrossRef]
21. Gould, J.C.; Garren, M.J.; Gutowski, K.A. Bariatric surgery. *Clin. Obstet. Gynecol.* **2006**, *49*, 375–388. [CrossRef] [PubMed]
22. Lang, R.M.; Badano, L.P.; Mor-Avi, V.; Afilalo, J.; Armstrong, A.; Ernande, L.; Flachskampf, F.A.; Foster, E.; Goldstein, S.A.; Kuznetsova, T.; et al. Recommendations for cardiac chamber quantification by echocardiography in adults: An update from the American Society of Echocardiography and the European Association of Cardiovascular Imaging. *J. Am. Soc. Echocardiogr.* **2015**, *28*, 1–39.e14. [CrossRef] [PubMed]
23. Koskinas, K.C.; Van Craenenbroeck, E.M.; Antoniades, C.; Bluher, M.; Gorter, T.M.; Hanssen, H.; Marx, N.; McDonagh, T.A.; Mingrone, G.; Rosengren, A.; et al. Obesity and cardiovascular disease: An ESC clinical consensus statement. *Eur. Heart J.* **2024**, *45*, 4063–4098. [CrossRef] [PubMed]
24. Wong, C.; Marwick, T.H. Obesity cardiomyopathy: Diagnosis and therapeutic implications. *Nat. Clin. Pract. Cardiovasc. Med.* **2007**, *4*, 480–490. [CrossRef]
25. Wang, Q.; Li, H.; Xie, H.; Fu, M.; Guo, B.; Ding, Y.; Li, W.; Yu, H. 25-Hydroxyvitamin D3 attenuates experimental periodontitis through downregulation of TLR4 and JAK1/STAT3 signaling in diabetic mice. *J. Steroid Biochem. Mol. Biol.* **2013**, *135*, 43–50. [CrossRef]
26. Kolwicz, S.C., Jr.; Purohit, S.; Tian, R. Cardiac metabolism and its interactions with contraction, growth, and survival of cardiomyocytes. *Circ. Res.* **2013**, *113*, 603–616. [CrossRef]
27. Cuspidi, C.; Rescaldani, M.; Tadic, M.; Sala, C.; Grassi, G. Effects of bariatric surgery on cardiac structure and function: A systematic review and meta-analysis. *Am. J. Hypertens.* **2014**, *27*, 146–156. [CrossRef]
28. Sorimachi, H.; Obokata, M.; Omote, K.; Reddy, Y.N.V.; Takahashi, N.; Koepp, K.E.; Ng, A.C.T.; Rider, O.J.; Borlaug, B.A. Long-Term Changes in Cardiac Structure and Function Following Bariatric Surgery. *J. Am. Coll. Cardiol.* **2022**, *80*, 1501–1512. [CrossRef]
29. Preda, A.; Carbone, F.; Tirandi, A.; Montecucco, F.; Liberale, L. Obesity phenotypes and cardiovascular risk: From pathophysiology to clinical management. *Rev. Endocr. Metab. Disord.* **2023**, *24*, 901–919. [CrossRef]
30. Hruby, A.; Hu, F.B. The Epidemiology of Obesity: A Big Picture. *Pharmacoeconomics* **2015**, *33*, 673–689. [CrossRef]
31. Alpert, M.A.; Lavie, C.J.; Agrawal, H.; Kumar, A.; Kumar, S.A. Cardiac Effects of Obesity: Pathophysiologic, clinical, and prognostic consequences—A review. *J. Cardiopulm. Rehabil. Prev.* **2016**, *36*, 1–11. [CrossRef]

Journal of
Cardiovascular Development and Disease

MDPI

Article

Compliance Behaviour After a Coronary Ischaemic Event: A Quasi-Experimental Study of Adherence to a Protocolised Follow-Up in Primary Care

Ángel Lizcano-Álvarez [1,2], Laura Carretero-Julián [2,3], Ana Talavera-Sáez [1,2], Almudena Alameda-Cuesta [1], Rocío Rodríguez-Vázquez [1], Beatriz Cristobal-Zárate [2,4] and María-Gema Cid-Expósito [1,*,†]
on behalf of the REccAP Group (Cardiovascular Care Nursing Network in Primary Care)

1 Faculty of Health Sciences, Department of Nursing and Stomatology, Rey Juan Carlos University, Alcorcón, 28922 Madrid, Spain; angel.lizcano@urjc.es (Á.L.-Á.); ana.talavera@urjc.es (A.T.-S.); almudena.alameda@urjc.es (A.A.-C.); rocio.vazquez@urjc.es (R.R.-V.)
2 Nursing Research Group Cardiovascular Care, Madrid Society of Family and Community Nursing (SEMAP), 28007 Madrid, Spain; mcarre20@ucm.es (L.C.-J.); bea_zafiro@hotmail.com (B.C.-Z.)
3 Faculty of Nursing, Physiotherapy and Podiatry, Department of Nursing, Complutense University, 28040 Madrid, Spain
4 Barcelona Healthcare Centre, Primary Care Assistance Management, Madrid Health Service, Móstoles, 28933 Madrid, Spain
* Correspondence: gema.cid@urjc.es
† Collaborators of the REccAP Group (Cardiovascular Care Nursing Network in Primary Care) are indicated in Acknowledgments.

Abstract: Following a coronary ischaemic event, it is essential to promote empowerment in self-care decision making. Primary care nursing is crucial for intensive follow-up to promote adherence to the therapeutic regimen. Objective: To ascertain whether adherence to a protocolised follow-up programme, with the support of a patient notebook, improves compliance behaviours in terms of physical activity, prescribed diet and medication. This is a quasi-experimental multicentre pre/post study. Population: Individuals aged 40–70 years, diagnosed with cardiac ischaemia in the last 18 months with a follow-up from March 2017 to January 2019, were included in a protocolised follow-up programme consisting of 11 visits over 12 months. A total of 194 patients started the programme and 132 completed it. Of these, 67.4% exhibited good adherence to follow-up, 31.8% exhibited medium adherence, and 0.8% exhibited poor adherence. Therefore, the patients were recoded into two variables: Medium–Low Adherence and High. The Nursing Outcomes Classification variables were significantly different between the Poor–Medium and Good Adherence groups and were always higher in the Good Adherence group (p-values < 0.05 t-student). There was a significant relationship between level of adherence and compliance behaviour. Good adherence to a follow-up plan led by primary care nurses improves compliance behaviours in terms of prescribed diet, physical activity, and medication. Early, intensive and protocolised follow-up by primary care nurses is essential to improve adherence to the therapeutic regimen and compliance behaviour among individuals with cardiac ischaemia. The use of a cardiovascular self-care notebook promotes adherence.

Keywords: cardiovascular diseases; myocardial infarction; patient compliance; cardiovascular risk factors; primary health care; nursing; self care

1. Introduction

The onset of cardiovascular disease (CVD) can be prevented, and the consequences of the disease may be minimized by the management of cardiovascular risk factors, many of which are behavioural in nature [1]. However, the EUROASPIRE V study, conducted in 27 European countries, shows that the vast majority of individuals with CVD lead unhealthy lives in terms of smoking, diet, sedentary lifestyle, and poor adherence to their treatment plans [2]. Early initiation and long-term maintenance of secondary prevention programmes are required to improve adherence to the treatment plan and to achieve lifestyle changes [3].

Adherence to the treatment plan involves a set of individual actions and behaviours in line with professional recommendations, such as adherence to medication, dietary regimen, or a follow-up plan. However, individuals with CVD have difficulty in maintaining adherence, which decreases considerably six months after discharge from hospital [3–6].

Amongst patients, the underlying causes can be attributed to low self-efficacy, a lack of motivation to learn about the prevention and control of CVD, a limited understanding of the subject matter, and beliefs about the health-disease process [4,7]. Therefore, continuous assessment of patient compliance behaviour is required. The Nursing Outcomes Classification (NOC) [8] is a standardised terminology for practice-sensitive outcomes in nursing. NOC outcomes include Compliance Behaviour: Prescribed Diet (1622), Compliance Behaviour: Prescribed Medication (1623) and Compliance Behaviour: Prescribed Activity (1632), which are fundamental axes in the follow-up of individuals with cardiac ischaemia. The NOC defines these outcomes as voluntary personal actions to follow a therapeutic regimen prescribed by health professionals.

Consequently, the individual should abandon the typical passive role and adopt an active role, with a good level of self-care and self-management of their health-disease process, participating in decision making and committing themselves to their own health [5,9,10]. Hence the importance of the role of accountability in adherence programmes. There is a link between adherence and accountability, as intensive follow-up during the first months after an ischaemic event improves the therapeutic relationship given that patients are accountable to their healthcare professional [11].

Primary care nurses are responsible and referents for the secondary cardiovascular prevention of patients with cardiac ischemia after hospital discharge. The primary care model in Spain has a structure based on health centres, each with a multidisciplinary team made up of general practitioners, paediatricians and nurses. Through health education and continuous follow-up, primary care nurses support the empowerment of patients regarding their cardiovascular self-care [9,12,13].

To improve shared decision making, primary care nursing care is based on the use of taxonomies such as NANDA-International [14], NOC [8], and NIC (Nursing Interventions Classification) [15]. In addition, an individual and family approach is adopted, favouring an integrated and holistic approach to the patient. Furthermore, the assessment of M. Gordon's functional patterns [16] helps nurses to systematise the nursing care they provide to patients with CVD [17–19].

A number of studies have demonstrated the superior efficacy of nurse-led cardiovascular prevention programmes, both for patients with established CVD and for high-risk individuals, in comparison to the conventional approach [20]. However, it is important that secondary cardiovascular prevention is implemented as soon as possible after hospital discharge, as it improves quality of life and reduces readmissions and mortality [21].

To foster compliance behaviours among CVD patients, it is necessary to support them with tools to motivate them and facilitate follow-up in primary care nursing consultations. The Madrid Society of Family and Community Nursing (SEMAP), along with six Spanish nursing societies, developed the Patient's Notebook in heart-healthy self-care [22]. This notebook is intended to improve communication between nurses and patients, to foster patient and family involvement in the self-management of risk factors through self-reporting, to increase patient knowledge, and to facilitate the follow-up plan and communication between professionals in healthcare facilities and those in the hospital setting. It also promotes patient empowerment and follow-up by primary care professionals [23].

Consequently, our objective was to ascertain whether good adherence of patients with cardiac ischaemia to a protocolised therapeutic follow-up, led by primary care nurses and with the support of the cardiovascular self-care notebook, could improve the following NOC outcomes: Compliance Behaviour: Prescribed Diet (1622), Compliance Behaviour: Prescribed Activity (1632), and Compliance Behaviour: Prescribed Medication (1623).

2. Materials and Methods

2.1. Design

This is a quasi-experimental multicentre pre/post study without a control group. The results of the study are reported in compliance with the Transparent Reporting of Evaluations with Non-randomised Designs (TREND) statement [24].

2.2. Setting and Participants

The study was conducted from March 2017 to January 2019 in nurses' offices of 40 healthcare facilities in Madrid (Spain). The inclusion criteria were patients between 40 and 70 years old who were diagnosed in the previous six months with one of the following ICPC diagnoses: K74 (Ischaemic heart disease with angina); K75 (Acute myocardial infarction); or K76 (Ischaemic heart disease without angina) [25]. Along with the informed consent, patients signed an agreement to attend all appointments for the duration of the programme. Patients with a life expectancy below one year, with problems travelling independently, and with comprehension difficulties due to cognitive impairment or language barriers were excluded from the programme.

2.3. Recruitment

An informative e-mail was sent to 320 primary care nurses inviting them to participate in the study. Of these, 59 nurses showed interest in participating in the study by signing a research commitment document. This group of nurses was referred to as the Clinical Care Group.

A non-probability purposive sampling technique was used by selecting patients who attended consultations at their healthcare facilities and met the inclusion criteria. Each nurse was asked to select at least three patients for follow-up. The recruitment period lasted five months (from February to June 2017).

The sample size required to estimate an unknown prevalence from a finite population size with 50% variance, 95% confidence and 5% precision was set at 341 patients. Due to time constraints during the recruitment period, the study was ultimately initiated with a sample of 209 patients (Figure 1).

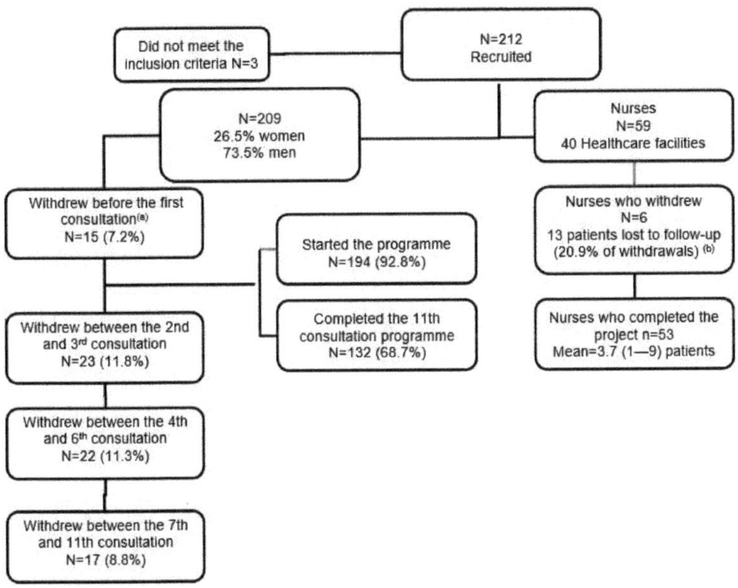

Figure 1. Flow chart showing the study population and recruited nurses. [a] Patients who dropped out of the study after signing the informed consent form at consultation 0 and did not attend the first consultation; [b] percentage of the 62 patients who dropped out once the programme had started.

2.4. Variables

Data on sociodemographic and clinical variables were recorded. The sub-variables relating to the level of adherence to the protocol were based on the register made by the nurses at the beginning of each consultation and were as follows: (1) whether or not the patient attended the new appointment in accordance with the protocol; (2) whether or not the patient self-recorded data and used the self-care notebook; and (3) whether or not the patient complied with the recommendations provided to them at the previous visit. Each was awarded between 1 and 3 points, from lowest to highest compliance or adherence. The three sub-variables were recoded into one main variable: overall adherence to the monitoring plan (OAMP). To calculate the OAMP, the three sub-variables were measured during ten of the eleven visits of the follow-up protocol (2nd to 11th), making the OAMP range 30–90 points.

Therefore, the outcome variables were the OAMP and the following NOC outcome indicators: Compliance Behaviour: Prescribed Medication (1623), Compliance Behaviour: Prescribed Activity (1632) and Compliance Behaviour: Prescribed Diet (1622) (Table 1). Each indicator was rated on a Likert scale ranging from 1 (never demonstrated) to 5 (always demonstrated).

Table 1. Outcome indicators selected for each Nursing Outcomes Classification (NOC) outcome.

NOC Outcome	Outcome Indicators
1632 Compliance Behaviour: Prescribed Activity	Identifies expected benefits of physical activity.
	Identifies barriers to implement prescribed physical activity.
	Sets achievable short-term activity goals with health professional.
	Participates in prescribed physical activity (3–5 days per week, 30–45 min per day, or 150 min per week with intensity specific to each patient).
	Seeks external reinforcement for performance of health behaviours.
	Identifies and reports symptoms experienced during activity to health professional.
	Knows and monitors target heart rate set by health professional.
1622 Compliance Behaviour: Prescribed Diet	Plans and prepares heart-healthy meals consistent with activity and tastes.
	Knows what food to eat when eating out.
	Uses nutritional information on labels to guide selections.
	Close relatives are aware of the agreed diet.
	Participates in setting achievable dietary goals with health professional.
1623 Compliance Behaviour: Prescribed Medication	Keeps a list of all medication with dose and frequency.
	Obtains required medication.
	Takes all medication at intervals prescribed (assessed using the Morinsky–Green test).
	Knows and monitors medication therapeutic effects (why and for what purpose it is being taken).
	Knows and monitors medication side effects.
	Knows and informs health professional of all medication being taken (name, dosage, frequency, and how it is being taken).

2.5. Ethical Considerations

The current study was conducted after receiving ethical approval from the Institutional Review Board of the Clinical Research Ethics Committee of the Ramón y Cajal University Hospital (protocol code 139/16) and followed the ethical principles contained in the Declaration of Helsinki [26].

Each nurse was responsible for ensuring that participating patients were adequately informed about the nature, purpose, risks and benefits of the study. Prior to the commencement of data collection, informed consent was obtained and signed by both nurses and patients.

The data were entered into a database and used exclusively by the research team in accordance with Spanish legislation (Organic Law 15/1999 of 13 December for Protection of Personal Data; and Law 14/2007 of 3 July for Biomedical Research).

2.6. Intervention and Data Collection Procedures

To optimize the standardization of the intervention and the use of the cardiovascular self-care notebook, nurses were taught to standardize the recording of data and intervention procedures through a manual that protocolised the actions to be carried out in each nursing consultation. This was recorded in the patient's medical record.

The organizational structure (Figure S1) was nodal and consisted of three levels. The first level, the Technical Research Group (TRG), was made up of two main researchers and two coordinators. These coordinators were responsible for monitoring four nodes of nurses. In each of these four nodes, there were nurses who would form the second level, called the Clinical Research Group (CRG). Each of these eight nurses was responsible for the follow-up of one node, the third level, formed between seven and eight nurses, who, as mentioned above, constituted the Clinical Care Group (CCG).

Patients who were initially interested were scheduled for the recruitment appointment or informative consultation. The study was explained to them and those interested signed the informed consent form and were then given the cardiovascular self-care notebook.

Eleven interventions were performed in nursing consultations over a period of 12–15 months. For all patients, each consultation was assigned a frequency, the first ones being more frequent (15 days) to favour the therapeutic relationship, while the last ones were at an interval of between 30 and 45 days. The estimated duration of each consultation was between 30 and 60 min.

There were actions common to each intervention including the three sub-variables of the overall adherence to the monitoring plan (OAMP):

- Assessment of adherence to the follow-up plan and self-care plan from the previous consultation (whether or not the patient attended the new appointment in accordance with the protocol and complied with the recommendations provided to them at the previous visit).
- Actions with the patient. Assessment and data collection on the NOC indicators linked to the corresponding M. Gordon's functional health pattern.
- Actions with the patient's notebook, including a self-monitoring section and a cardiovascular risk factor (CVRF) self-care information section (whether or not the patient self-recorded data and used the self-care notebook).
- Recording of information on the data collection platform and the medical record.
- Explaining heart-healthy actions and self-care to the patient for the next consultation.

The structure of the follow-up protocol in each nursing consultation followed M. Gordon's functional health patterns. This was as follows:

- Consultation 0: Recruitment consultation. Signing the informed consent form.
- Consultation 1: History. Heart-healthy lifestyle.
- Consultation 2: Assessment of the health perception/health management pattern and the cognitive-perceptual pattern.
- Consultation 3: Assessment of the nutritional-metabolic pattern.
- Consultation 4: Assessment of the nutritional-metabolic pattern.
- Consultation 5: Assessment of the physical activity/exercise pattern.
- Consultation 6: Assessment of the self-perception/self-concept pattern.
- Consultation 7: Assessment of the role-relationship pattern and sexuality-reproductive pattern.
- Consultation 8: Assessment of the coping/stress tolerance pattern and value-belief pattern.
- Consultation 9: Assessment of the elimination pattern and sleep-rest pattern.
- Consultation 10: Family assessment.

- Consultation 11: Final assessment. Expert Patient Diploma.

During each consultation, both the OAMP and the assessments of the NOC indicators associated with each of M. Gordon's functional patterns were documented [16]. In the final consultation, a final assessment of all the NOC indicators was made. To minimise the bias of feeling observed and evaluated, which could influence the final assessment, the nurse could not see the assessments or scores assigned to the indicators in previous consultations.

2.7. Data Analysis

To analyse the potential pre-post variation in the NOC dimensions and whether they varied similarly depending on the level of adherence, a general linear model of repeated measures was applied.

To verify the reliability of the NOC indicators, Cronbach's α internal consistency model [27] was used, considering values $\geq$0.7 as optimal. To confirm the one-dimensionality of the NOC indicators and the validity of the scales, an exploratory factor analysis of principal components with Varimax rotation was applied using the criterion of eigenvalues greater than 1. Significance was ensured using the Kaiser–Meyer–Olkin test and Bartlett's test of sphericity.

The Student's t-test for two independent samples (parametric) and the one-way ANOVA for more than two independent samples (parametric) were also used. Pearson's correlation was used for continuous variables. Given the adequate sample size in each group (n > 30), normality of the main variables was assumed by applying the central limit theorem [28]. The statistical significance threshold was set at 5% (α = 0.05). The data were processed and analysed using SPSS (version 25) software by IBM.3. Results

Of the 209 patients who signed the consent form, 194 started the programme (92.8%) and 132 (68.7%) completed the 11 consultations. The follow-up between the first consultation (PRE) and the last (POST) was on average 356.10 days (SD 25.4). The interval between each consultation was 32.37 days (SD 2.3).

Of these 132 patients, 73.5% were male, with a mean age of 58.2 (SD = 9.7) years; the mean age of the women was 61.4 years (SD = 16.2). The percentage of men between 40 and 55 years old was 35.1%, while the percentage of women in this premenopausal and menopause range was lower at 28.6%. In addition, 52.3% had completed secondary or tertiary education. Their cardiovascular risk factors included the following: hypertension (58.3%); dyslipidaemia (65.2%); diabetes (24.2%); obesity (32.1%); and tobacco use (10.6%).

The mean adherence for the OAMP variable was 80.8% (SD = 10.9). This level of adherence was divided into quartiles, resulting in three levels: less than 50 points (poor adherence), between 50 and 75 points (moderate adherence), and between 76 and 100 points (good adherence). Thus, 67.4% had good adherence, 31.8% had moderate adherence and only 0.8% had poor adherence. This led to a recording of the levels into two variables: Moderate–Low Adherence and High Adherence.

Regarding the relationship between sociodemographic and clinical variables with the OAMP (Table 2), the only variable with statistical significance was tobacco use (** $p < 0.001$). Individuals who smoked at the time of the study had a lower OAMP than ex-smokers and non-smokers. On analysis of the relationship between sociodemographic and clinical variables with adherence by levels (Moderate–Low Adherence and High Adherence) (Table 3), high adherence seems to be linked to patients who do not currently smoke (** $p < 0.001$). There was a tendency for men to have better adherence than women (* $p < 0.052$). The remaining variables did not have a significant relationship with the various adherence levels.

With the exception of the post value of Compliance Behaviour: Prescribed Medication (close to the threshold of 0.7), the criteria for reliability as a measurement scale can be considered to be met. An exploratory factor analysis was performed on all results to assess their one-dimensionality, both pre and post. All results were valid (KMO > 0.6 and Bartlett's sphericity $p < 0.05$) and one-dimensional (one single factor with eigenvalue > 1), while the percentage of variance explained was greater than 40% [29,30]. To assess the relationship between the OAMP and the three compliance behaviour outcomes (medication, diet, and physical activity), we analysed whether there were variations between pre and post, and whether these variations occurred in line with the level of adherence (Table 4).

Table 2. Relationship of variables to Overall Adherence Level (OAMP).

Variables		Overall Adherence Level (OAMP)		
		N (%)	M ± SD	(p-Value) *
Gender	Total	132 (100)	80.86 ± 10.99	0.167 [1]
	Men	97 (73.5)	81.66 ± 10.92	
	Women	35 (26.5)	78.66 ± 11.05	
Level of education	Total	132 (100)	80.86 ± 10.99	0.969 [2]
	Primary education	63 (47.7)	80.78 ± 11.68	
	Secondary education	49 (37.1)	81.14 ± 10.22	
	University education	20 (15.2)	80.45 ± 11.11	
ICPC	Total	132 (100)	80.86 ± 10.99	0.904 [2]
	K74	47 (35.6)	80.70 ± 11.68	
	K75	82 (62.1)	80.85 ± 10.78	
	K76	3 (2.3)	83.67 ± 7.57	
High blood pressure	Total	132 (100)	80.86 ± 10.99	0.392 [1]
	No	55 (41.7)	81.84 ± 10.53	
	Yes	77 (58.3)	80.17 ± 11.33	
Tobacco use	Total	132 (100)	80.86 ± 10.99	0.001 ***[2]
	Smoker	14 (10.6)	71.14 ± 10.47	
	Ex-smoker	58 (43.9)	80.53 ± 10.87	
	Non-smoker	60 (45.5)	83.45 ± 10.03	
Dyslipidaemia	Total	132(100)	80.86 ± 10.99	0.652 [1]
	No	46 (34.8)	81.46 ± 10.76	
	Yes	86 (65.2)	80.55 ± 11.16	
Diabetes	Total	132 (100)	80.86 ± 10.99	0.624 [1]
	No	100 (75.8)	81.13 ± 10.84	
	Yes	32 (24.2)	80.03 ± 11.60	
Body Mass Index	Total	132 (100)	80.86 ± 10.99	0.197 [2]
	Normal (18.5–24.9)	23 (17.4)	77.83 ± 14.21	
	Overweight (25–29.9)	68 (51.5)	82.26 ± 10.60	
	Obese I (30–34.9)	27 (20.5)	81.85 ± 8.61	
	Obese II (35–39.9)	14 (10.6)	77.14 ± 10.22	

SD: standard deviation; ICPC: International Classification of Primary Care; K74: Ischaemic heart disease with angina; K75: Acute myocardial infarction; K76: Ischaemic heart disease without angina. [1] (Student's t); [2] (one-way ANOVA) *** $p < 0.001$, two-tailed.

Our results reflect a significant change in the adherence indicators throughout follow-up (pre-post). The two levels of adherence were the same for adherence to diet (mean +0.45) and for adherence to physical activity (mean +0.33). By contrast, compliance with medication showed a greater increase in the group with lower adherence (0.88 points) than in the group with high adherence (0.64 points).

Table 3. Relationship of variables to Overall Adherence (OAMP) by levels.

Variables		Overall Adhesion (OAMP) by Levels			
		Total	Moderate–Low Adherence	High Adherence	(p-Value) *
		N	n (%)	n (%)	
Gender	Total	132	43 (32.6)	89 (67.4)	
	Men	97	27 (27.8)	70 (72.2)	0.052 [1]
	Women	35	16 (45.7)	19 (54.3)	
Level of education	Total	132	43 (32.6)	89 (67.4)	
	Primary education	63	26 (41.3)	37 (58.7)	0.110 [2]
	Secondary education	49	13 (26.5)	36 (73.5)	
	University education	20	4 (20.0)	16 (80.0)	
High blood pressure	Total	132	43 (32.6)	89 (67.4)	
	No	55	16 (29.1)	39 (70.9)	0.472 [1]
	Yes	77	27 (35.1)	50 (64.9)	
Tobacco use	Total	132	43 (32.6)	89 (67.4)	
	Smoker	14	10 (71.4)	4 (28.6)	0.001 ***[2]
	Ex-smoker	58	20 (34.5)	38 (65.5)	
	Non-smoker	60	13 (21.7)	47 (78.3)	
ICPC	Total	132	43 (32.6)	89 (67.4)	
	K74	47	17 (36.2)	30 (63.8)	0.803 [2]
	K75	82	25 (30.5)	57 (69.5)	
	K76	3	1 (33.3)	2 (66.7)	
Alcohol consumption	Total	132	43 (32.6)	89 (67.4)	
	No	7	3 (42.9)	4 (57.1)	0.551 [1]
	Yes	125	40 (32.0)	85 (68.0)	
Dyslipidaemia	Total	132	43 (32.6)	89 (67.4)	
	No	46	14 (30.4)	32 (69.6)	0.701 [1]
	Yes	86	29 (33.7)	57 (66.3)	
Diabetes	Total	132	43 (32.6)	89 (67.4)	
	No	100	30 (30.0)	70 (70.0)	0.264 [1]
	Yes	32	13 (40.6)	19 (59.4)	
Body Mass Index	Total	132	43 (32.6)	89 (67.4)	
	Normal (18.5–24.9)	23	10 (43.5)	13 (56.5)	0.223 [2]
	Overweight (25–29.9)	68	21 (30.9)	47 (69.1)	
	Obese I (30–34.9)	27	5 (18.5)	22 (81.5)	
	Obese II (35–39.9)	14	7 (50.0)	7 (50.0)	

ICPC: International Classification of Primary Care; K74: Ischaemic heart disease with angina; K75: Acute myocardial infarction; K76: Ischaemic heart disease without angina. [1] (Student's t); [2] (one-way ANOVA) *** $p < 0.001$, two-tailed.

Table 4. Variation in adherence behaviour per adherence levels at the beginning (Pre) and end (Post) of the monitoring plan.

Compliance Behaviour	Level of Adherence	Pre	Post	Pre-Post Difference	
		M ± SD	M ± SD	M ± SD	*p*-Value *
Prescribed Medication	Total	3.98 ± 0.59	4.70 ± 0.37	0.71 ± 0.62	0.000 ***
	Moderate–Low Adherence	3.70 ± 0.66	4.58 ± 0.44	0.87 ± 0.68	0.039
	High Adherence	4.11 ± 0.50	4.75 ± 0.31	0.63 ± 0.58	
Prescribed Diet	Total	3.70 ± 0.68	4.14 ± 0.76	0.44 ± 0.83	0.000 ***
	Moderate–Low Adherence	3.30 ± 0.70	3.76 ± 0.80	0.46 ± 0.86	0.863
	High Adherence	3.89 ± 0.57	4.33 ± 0.67	0.43 ± 0.82	
Prescribed Activity	Total	3.99 ± 0.75	4.32 ± 0.67	0.33 ± 0.73	0.000 ***
	Moderate–Low Adherence	3.56 ± 0.78	3.89 ± 0.70	0.33 ± 0.82	0.962
	High Adherence	4.20 ± 0.64	4.53 ± 0.55	0.33 ± 0.69	

SD: standard deviation; Pre-post difference: at the beginning (Pre) and end (Post) of the monitoring plan. *** $p < 0.001$, two-tailed.

3. Discussion

Adherence to treatment regimens is one of the most influential factors in chronic diseases. Indicators of adherence include patient attendance to scheduled appointments with healthcare professionals, compliance with the recommendations made by these professionals, and their assessment of the implementation of these recommendations. Given that accountability favours responsible behaviour in adherence programmes [31], and that most adherence interventions occur during visits to professionals, we found that the use and evaluation of the notebook as a health education tool at the beginning of each of the 11 consultations favoured follow-up and promoted shared decision making. The use of patient self-management guidelines and improved cardiovascular care skills among PHC nurses are also influential factors in improving adherence [32].

Adherence may have a multifactorial influence. Firstly, it is important to consider the role of sex/gender as predictors of higher adherence in men and lower adherence in women in secondary prevention. These determinants should be taken into account in our clinical practice [32–34].

The observed correlation between male sex and enhanced adherence is corroborated by the findings of the studies conducted by Huber et al. [35] and Moreno et al. [36], where female sex was identified as a predictor of non-adherence to medication, diet and physical activity. It is notable that female sex itself was not identified as a biological predictor of non-adherence; rather, it was aspects related to gender inequalities, such as family care burden, depression or smoking, that emerged as significant factors [34].

Educating cardiovascular patients through structured education with telephone follow-up and monitoring has a statistically significant positive effect on self-care, self-efficacy and quality of life and thus adherence to the treatment plan [37]. Our data on improved self-care in association with intensive nurse-led follow-up among patients with ischaemic heart disease are consistent with other studies [38]. In the RESPONSE-2 trial, the effect of comprehensive primary care nursing programmes on lifestyle was assessed [39]. Similarly, in a scoping review, Freeley et al. [32] confirm that there is a sustained improvement over time when health professionals provide care in a person-centred manner.

The higher overall adherence to intensive follow-up of our patients in both diet and physical activity, and consequently their improvement, correlates with the results of a meta-analysis concluding that educational interventions for secondary prevention are effective in improving healthy behaviours at short- and long-term follow-up, with longer duration programmes being more effective [40].

It is quite possible that a long-term relationship between nurse and patient, an involvement of nursing with continuous follow-up, improves adherence to diet, physical activity [41], and medication as a result of mutual trust and a better understanding of the disease [4,35].

Regarding diet and physical activity, as reported in the clinical trials by Zakeri et al. [4] and Köhler et al. [9], there is a clear emphasis on the significance of nurse-led educational programs in empowering patients to navigate their disease process and to adhere to dietary and physical activity regimens. In our study, as in the trial by Westland et al. [42], the support of primary care nurses promotes the effectiveness of engaging patients in heart-healthy physical activity and avoiding sedentary lifestyles [2].

One striking result of our study was a major change in compliance behaviour with prescribed medication in the Moderate–Low adherence group when compared with adherence to diet and physical activity. This could be due to a social preconception and certain coping behaviours of the individual in the face of a new infarction, as they perceive medication to be more important than following lifestyle recommendations or attending nurse's appointments. Other studies link the benefits of joint decision making in an established patient–professional relationship to improved medication adherence [43].

Poor adherence to prescribed medication is one of the most recurrent themes in morbidity and mortality studies in cardiovascular prevention, as reflected in the results of the Euroaspire V study [2]. A strategy that would supplement our follow-up intervention in the future would be reinforcing adherence to the therapeutic plan by means of telephone or internet follow-up [44]. Although studies on the presence of accountability in digital interventions are still lacking [45], research has shown improvement in terms of adherence to prescribed diet and medication among patients with myocardial infarction [35]. In the study by Shim and Hwang, conducted with older people with acute myocardial infarction, it was found that there was an increase in patients' quality of life after one year of telephone follow-up [12].

Improvements in this type of intervention may be required, which may include training primary care nurses in the development of skills for follow-up after a coronary event [23] or developing innovative programmes by interdisciplinary teams that address all aspects of lifestyle and CVRF management [2].

Our study supports the statement of the Association of Cardiovascular Nursing and Allied Professions of the European Society of Cardiology, which reaffirms the need for integrated and holistic cardiovascular care involving patients and families to ensure that the person is at the centre of care [45].

Limitations: the exclusion criteria used in this study were based on age and having a life expectancy of less than one year. As a result, our sample may be biased in favour of healthier patients. As this was a quasi-experimental study, there was no control group or randomisation. Although there was a training seminar for nurses and a data collection manual was made available, inter- and intra-observer variability may have been present. The OAMP variable and its levels were designed based on the experiential criteria of the researchers. In this study, as recommended by the NOC taxonomy itself, the indicators for each outcome were selected according to the care setting and the characteristics of the individuals. Nevertheless, this selection could have been validated on the basis of relevance to the primary care setting, the estimated duration of patient care, conceptual clarity, and understandability. Similarly, there may have been a drop-out bias due to the abandonment of the follow-up programme, which could be taken into account by other authors wishing to carry out similar research with such intensive and prolonged follow-up.

Therefore, our study shows that primary care nurses can undertake an intensive, protocolised and comprehensive follow-up of patients during the first months after a coronary ischemic event. The role of the primary care nurse enhances adherence to the therapeutic regimen, self-management of heart disease, and compliance with the prescribed diet, physical activity, and medication. The use of self-care-based health education tools improves the empowerment and self-efficacy of people with chronic cardiovascular disease and their family members.

Whether a limitation or a strength, we were unable to find any studies on the effects of an educational tool such as our patient notebook on improving follow-up, compliance and empowerment in patients with cardiac ischaemia. Finally, the follow-up period was one year, which means that we do not know whether the results obtained were maintained afterwards.

4. Conclusions

The results of this study suggest that a good level of adherence to a follow-up plan led by primary care nurses leads to improved compliance with self-care in terms of prescribed diet, physical activity, and medication. Furthermore, our results highlight the importance of secondary cardiovascular prevention programmes in primary care focusing on the interaction between patients and nurses, as this is considered to be one of the most important factors in improving the health of patients with chronic diseases such as CVD. The educational support of a cardiovascular self-care notebook leads to improved adherence to the therapeutic regimen.

Supplementary Materials: The following supporting information can be downloaded at: https://www.mdpi.com/article/10.3390/jcdd11120407/s1. Figure S1: Clinical Investigators group ReccAP.

Author Contributions: Conceptualization, Á.L.-Á. and L.C.-J.; methodology, Á.L.-Á. and A.A.-C.; software, Á.L.-Á., L.C.-J. and A.A.-C.; validation, Á.L.-Á., L.C.-J., A.A.-C. and M.-G.C.-E.; formal analysis, L.C.-J. and A.A.-C.; investigation, Á.L.-Á., L.C.-J. and A.A.-C.; resources, Á.L.-Á. and L.C.-J.; data curation, Á.L.-Á., L.C.-J., M.-G.C.-E., A.T.-S., R.R.-V. and B.C.-Z.; writing—original draft preparation, Á.L.-Á.; writing—review and editing, L.C.-J., M.-G.C.-E., A.T.-S. and R.R.-V.; visualization, M.-G.C.-E.; supervision, Á.L.-Á., L.C.-J., M.-G.C.-E., A.T.-S., R.R.-V. and B.C.-Z.; funding acquisition, Á.L.-Á. and L.C.-J. All authors have read and agreed to the published version of the manuscript.

Funding: Funding was provided by the Gregorio Marañón General University Hospital in Madrid, as this research was granted the first national prize for the best nursing research project in 2017.

Institutional Review Board Statement: The study was conducted in accordance with the Declaration of Helsinki, and approved by the Clinical Research Ethics Committee of the Ramón y Cajal University Hospital (Madrid) (protocol code 139/16, 27 July 2016). Each nurse was responsible for fully informing participating patients about the nature, purpose, risks, and benefits of the study. Informed consent was obtained and signed by nurses and patients alike before commencing data collection. The data were entered into a database and used exclusively by the research team in accordance with Spanish legislation (Organic Law 15/1999 of 13 December for Protection of Personal Data, and Law 14/2007, of 3 July for Biomedical Research).

Informed Consent Statement: Informed consent was obtained from all subjects involved in the study. Written informed consent has been obtained from the patients to publish this paper. The authors confirm that all patient/person identifiers have been removed or disguised so that the patient(s)/person(s) described are not identifiable and cannot be identified through the details of their clinical records.

Data Availability Statement: The data presented in this study are available on request from the corresponding author. The data are not publicly available due to legal restrictions.

Acknowledgments: We thank all the patients and nurses of the primary care teams involved. We also thank the Clinical and Assistance Research Group of the Cardiovascular Nursing Network in Primary Care (REccAP), which belongs to the SEMAP (Madrid Society of Family and Community Nursing), for making this study possible. (Lead Clinical Investigators Group, REccAP: Cristina Gómez Menor; José Dionisio Benito; Lobato; Juana Mª Gómez Puente; Laura López Köllmer; Sergio Belmonte Sánchez; Teresa Villar Espejo; Laura Iglesias Rus; Gemma Ferrero García, Milagros Rico Blazquez, María Gálvez Fernandez. Clinical Investigators at primary care facilities: Adoración Ortega Temiño, Ángeles Álvarez Hermida, Carmen Yegler Velasco, Carolina Guerrero Mártir, Carolina Regacho Ramírez, Encarnación Tornay Muñoz, Eva María Rey Camacho, Eva Molina Alén, Inmaculada Moreno Gª-Herrera, Leonor Molina Alameda, Leticia Gómez Chacón, Mª Ángeles de Francisco

Casado, Mª Beatriz Pérez Vallejo, Mª del Mar Garcia Navarro, Mª José Barras Bermejo, Mª Rosario Campo Martínez, Mª Sonsoles Molina Herráez, Maria Belén Pose García, Maria Luisa Merino Cuesta, Mónica Costumero García, Montserrat Jurado Sueiro, Rosa Cayetano Díaz, Rosa Mª Martínez Ortega, Sagrario Sancha Canales, Vanesa Gonzalez Alonso, Ana Rosa León Casquete, Arancha Martin Belinchón, Aránzazu Ramos Martín, Irene Díaz Jimenez, Mª José Muñoz Cátedra, Adoración Ortega Temiño, Ana Isabel Palacios Calle, Ana María Polo González, Amalia Domínguez González, Concepción Espariz Campano, Esther Blázquez Hernández, Mª Pilar Escudero Socorro, Mª Sandra Hernández Rodríguez, Margarita Ortiz Sánchez, Margarita Vázquez Asenjo, Nieves López Yunquera, Olga Brezo García del Pino, Tania Casasola Gutierrez).

Conflicts of Interest: The authors declare that they have no conflicts of interest.

References

1. Visseren, F.L.J.; Mach, F.; Smulders, Y.M.; Carballo, D.; Koskinas, K.C.; Bäck, M.; Benetos, A.; Biffi, A.; Boavida, J.-M.; Capodanno, D.; et al. 2021 ESC Guidelines on Cardiovascular Disease Prevention in Clinical Practice: Developed by the Task Force for Cardiovascular Disease Prevention in Clinical Practice with Representatives of the European Society of Cardiology and 12 Medical Societies With the Special Contribution of the European Association of Preventive Cardiology (EAPC). *Rev. Española Cardiol.* **2022**, *75*, 429. [CrossRef]
2. Kotseva, K.; De Backer, G.; De Bacquer, D.; Rydén, L.; Hoes, A.; Grobbee, D.; Maggioni, A.; Marques-Vidal, P.; Jennings, C.; Abreu, A.; et al. Lifestyle and Impact on Cardiovascular Risk Factor Control in Coronary Patients across 27 Countries: Results from the European Society of Cardiology ESC-EORP EUROASPIRE V Registry. *Eur. J. Prev. Cardiol.* **2019**, *26*, 824–835. [CrossRef] [PubMed]
3. Schwalm, J.D.; Ivers, N.M.; Natarajan, M.K.; Taljaard, M.; Rao-Melacini, P.; Witteman, H.O.; Zwarenstein, M.; Grimshaw, J.M. Cluster Randomized Controlled Trial of Delayed Educational Reminders for Long-Term Medication Adherence in ST-Elevation Myocardial Infarction (DERLA-STEMI). *Am. Heart J.* **2015**, *170*, 903–913. [CrossRef]
4. Zakeri, M.A.; Khoshnood, Z.; Dehghan, M.; Abazari, F. The Effect of the Continuous Care Model on Treatment Adherence in Patients with Myocardial Infarction: A Randomised Controlled Trial. *J. Res. Nurs.* **2020**, *25*, 54–65. [CrossRef]
5. Polsook, R.; Aungsuroch, Y.; Thongvichean, T. The Effect of Self-Efficacy Enhancement Program on Medication Adherence among Post-Acute Myocardial Infarction. *Appl. Nurs. Res.* **2016**, *32*, 67–72. [CrossRef]
6. Lizcano Álvarez, A. Conocimientos, Actitudes y Grado de Aplicación de Cuidados Integrales En La Prevención Cardiovascular Por Parte de La Enfermera En El Ámbito de La Atención Primaria. Dotoral Thesis, Facultad Ciencias de la Salud, Universidad Rey Juan Carlos, Madrid, Spain, 2015.
7. Lei, H.; Yang, J.; Kong, L.; Liu, N.; Liu, S.; Yu, N.; Peng, Y.; Wen, Y.; Tang, J. Correlations among Psychological Resilience, Self-Efficacy, and Negative Emotion in Acute Myocardial Infarction Patients after Percutaneous Coronary Intervention. *Front. Psychiatry* **2018**, *9*, 1. [CrossRef]
8. Moorhead, S.; Swanson, E.; Johnson, M.; Maas, M. *Nursing Outcomes Classification (NOC)*, 6th ed.; Elsevier: Amsterdam, The Netherlands, 2018; ISBN 9780323497640.
9. Köhler, A.K.; Jaarsma, T.; Tingström, P.; Nilsson, S. The Effect of Problem-Based Learning after Coronary Heart Disease—A Randomised Study in Primary Health Care (COR-PRIM). *BMC Cardiovasc. Disord.* **2020**, *20*, 370. [CrossRef]
10. Fors, A.; Ulin, K.; Cliffordson, C.; Ekman, I.; Brink, E. The Cardiac Self-Efficacy Scale, a Useful Tool with Potential to Evaluate Person-Centred Care. *Eur. J. Cardiovasc. Nurs.* **2015**, *14*, 536–543. [CrossRef]
11. Ballengee, L.A.; Bosworth, H.B.; Zullig, L.L. The Role of Accountability in Adherence Programs. *Patient Educ. Couns.* **2022**, *105*, 2635–2636. [CrossRef]
12. Shim, J.L.; Hwang, S.Y. Long-Term Effects of Nurse-Led Individualized Education on Middle-Aged Patients with Acute Coronary Synrome: A Quasi-Experimental Study. *BMC Nurs.* **2017**, *16*, 59. [CrossRef]
13. Herring, L.Y.; Dallosso, H.; Chatterjee, S.; Bodicoat, D.; Schreder, S.; Khunti, K.; Yates, T.; Seidu, S.; Hudson, I.; Davies, M.J. Physical Activity after Cardiac EventS (PACES)—A Group Education Programme with Subsequent Text-Message Support Designed to Increase Physical Activity in Individuals with Diagnosed Coronary Heart Disease: Study Protocol for a Randomised Controlled Trial. *Trials* **2018**, *19*, 537. [CrossRef] [PubMed]
14. Herdman, T.H.; Kamitsuru, S. *NANDA International Nursing Diagnoses: Definitions and Classification 2018–2020*, 11th ed.; Thieme: New York, NY, USA, 2017.
15. Butcher, H.; Bulecheck, G.; Dochterman, J.; Wagner, C.M. (Eds.) *Nursing Interventions Classification (NIC)*; Elsevier: Amsterdam, The Netherlands, 2018.
16. Gordon, M. *Manual of Nursing Diagnosis*, 11th ed.; Jones and Bartlett: Burlington, MA, USA, 2007.
17. Mohammadpour, A.; Rahmati Sharghi, N.; Khosravan, S.; Alami, A.; Akhond, M. The Effect of a Supportive Educational Intervention Developed Based on the Orem's Self-Care Theory on the Self-Care Ability of Patients with Myocardial Infarction: A Randomised Controlled Trial. *J. Clin. Nurs.* **2015**, *24*, 1686–1692. [CrossRef] [PubMed]
18. Tok Yildiz, F.; Kaşikçi, M. Impact of Training Based on Orem's Theory on Self-Care Agency and Quality of Life in Patients with Coronary Artery Disease. *J. Nurs. Res.* **2020**, *28*, e125. [CrossRef]

19. Türen, S.; Enç, N. A Comparison of Gordon's Functional Health Patterns Model and Standard Nursing Care in Symptomatic Heart Failure Patients: A Randomized Controlled Trial. *Appl. Nurs. Res.* **2020**, *53*, 151247. [CrossRef]
20. Connolly, S.B.; Kotseva, K.; Jennings, C.; Atrey, A.; Jones, J.; Brown, A.; Bassett, P.; Wood, D.A. Outcomes of an Integrated Community-Based Nurse-Led Cardiovascular Disease Prevention Programme. *Heart* **2017**, *103*, 840–847. [CrossRef]
21. Jernberg, T.; Hasvold, P.; Henriksson, M.; Hjelm, H.; Thuresson, M.; Janzon, M. Cardiovascular Risk in Post-Myocardial Infarction Patients: Nationwide Real World Data Demonstrate the Importance of a Long-Term Perspective. *Eur. Heart J.* **2015**, *36*, 1163–1170. [CrossRef]
22. Lizcano Alvarez, A.; Villar Espejo, M.T.; Duralde Rodríguez, E.; Pérez González, M.J.; Martínez Fernández, E.; Guerrero Llamas, L.; Fernádez López, L.; Ochando García, A.; Miranda Camarero, M.V.; Armero Fuster, M.; et al. *Cuaderno Del Paciente En Autocuidados Cardiosaludables*, 1st ed.; Sociedad de Enfermería Madrileña de Atención Primaria (SEMAP): Madrid, Spain, 2012; ISBN 978-84-615-5775-2.
23. Lizcano Álvarez, Á.; Villar Espejo, T.; López Köllmer, L.; Gómez Menor, C.; Ledesma Rodríguez, R.; Fernández Zarataín, G. The Efficacy of an Integrated Care Training Program for Primary Care Nurses for the Secondary Prevention of Cardiovascular Risk. *Enferm. Clin.* **2021**, *31*, 303–312. [CrossRef]
24. Des Jarlais, D.C.; Lyles, C.; Crepaz, N. Improving the Reporting Quality of Nonrandomized Evaluations of Behavioral and Public Health Interventions: The TREND Statement. *Am. J. Public. Health* **2004**, *94*, 361–366. [CrossRef]
25. WONKA International Classification Committee. *International Classification of Primary Care (ICPC-2)*, 2nd ed.; Oxford University Press: Oxford, UK, 1998; ISBN 019262802X.
26. Association, W.M. World Medical Association Declaration of Helsinki: Ethical Principles for Medical Research Involving Human Subjects. *JAMA* **2013**, *310*, 2191–2194. [CrossRef]
27. Cronbach, L.J. Coefficient Alpha and the Internal Structure of Tests. *Psychometrika* **1951**, *16*, 297–334. [CrossRef]
28. Grinstead, C.M.; Snell, J.L. *Central Limit Theorem, Introduction to Probability*, 2nd ed.; American Mathematical Society: Rhode Island, RI, USA, 1999; pp. 325–360.
29. Carmines, E.G.; Zeller, R.A. *Reliability and Validity Assessment*; Sage Publications: New York, NY, USA, 1979.
30. Kaiser, H.F. The Application of Electronic Computers to Factor Analysis. *Educ. Psychol. Meas.* **1960**, *20*, 141–151. [CrossRef]
31. Salisbury, K.R.; Ranpariya, V.K.; Feldman, S.R. Accountability in Reminder-Based Adherence Interventions: A Review. *Patient Educ. Couns.* **2022**, *105*, 2645–2652. [CrossRef] [PubMed]
32. Freeley, S.; Broughan, J.; McCombe, G.; Casey, M.; Fitzpatrick, P.; Frawley, T.; Morrisey, J.; Treanor, J.T.; Collins, T.; Cullen, W. Promoting Nurse-led Behaviour Change Interventions to Prevent Cardiovascular Disease in Disadvantaged Communities: A Scoping Review. *Health Soc. Care Community* **2022**, *30*, 2071–2095. [CrossRef] [PubMed]
33. De Bacquer, D.; Astin, F.; Kotseva, K.; Pogosova, N.; De Smedt, D.; De Backer, G.; Ryden, L.; Wood, D.; Jennings, C. Poor Adherence to Lifestyle Recommendations in Patients with Coronary Heart Disease: Results from the EUROASPIRE Surveys. *Eur. J. Prev. Cardiol.* **2022**, *29*, 383–395. [CrossRef]
34. Delimanoli, E.; Muurlink, O.; Myrianthefs, P.; Korompeli, A. Cardiac Rehabilitation After Open Heart Surgery: A Narrative Systematic Review. *J. Cardiovasc. Dev. Dis.* **2024**, *11*, 376. [CrossRef]
35. Daniel, H.; Christian, W.; Robin, H.; Lars, S.; Thomas, M. Statin Treatment after Acute Coronary Syndrome: Adherence and Reasons for Non-Adherence in a Randomized Controlled Intervention Trial. *Sci. Rep.* **2019**, *9*, 12079. [CrossRef]
36. Moreno, G.; Vicent, L.; Rosillo, N.; Delgado, J.; Del Cerro, E.P.; Bueno, H. Do Sex and Gender Aspects Influence Non-Adherence to Secondary Prevention Measures after Myocardial Infarction? *Am. J. Prev. Cardiol.* **2024**, *19*, 100713. [CrossRef]
37. Hudiyawati, D.; Rosyid, F.N.; Pratiwi, A.; Sulastri, S.; Kartinah, K. The Effect of Structured Education and Telemonitoring on Self-Care, Self-Efficacy and Quality of Life in Heart Failure Patients: A Randomized Controlled Trial. *Evid. Based Care J.* **2023**, *13*, 7–16. [CrossRef]
38. Ruiz-Bustillo, S.; Ivern, C.; Badosa, N.; Farre, N.; Marco, E.; Bruguera, J.; Cladellas, M.; Enjuanes, C.; Cainzos-Achirica, M.; Marti-Almor, J.; et al. Efficacy of a Nurse-Led Lipid-Lowering Secondary Prevention Intervention in Patients Hospitalized for Ischemic Heart Disease: A Pilot Randomized Controlled Trial. *Eur. J. Cardiovasc. Nurs.* **2019**, *18*, 366–374. [CrossRef]
39. Jepma, P.; Jorstad, H.; Peters, R.; Snaterse, M.; ter Riet, G.; Latour, C.; Minneboo, M.; Boekholdt, S.; Scholte Op Reimer, W.B. Effects of a Community-Based Lifestyle Intervention in Older Patients with Coronary Artery Disease: Results from the RESPONSE-2 Trial. *Eur. J. Prev. Cardiol.* **2019**, *26*, S97.
40. Shi, W.; Ghisi, G.L.M.; Zhang, L.; Hyun, K.; Pakosh, M.; Gallagher, R. Systematic Review, Meta-Analysis and Meta-Regression to Determine the Effects of Patient Education on Health Behaviour Change in Adults Diagnosed with Coronary Heart Disease. *J. Clin. Nurs.* **2023**, *32*, 5300–5327. [CrossRef] [PubMed]
41. Westland, H.; Trappenburg, J.C.A.; Schuurmans, M.J.; Zonneveld, M.H.; Schröder, C.D. Fidelity of Primary Care Nurses' Delivery of a Behavioural Change Intervention Enhancing Physical Activity in Patients at Risk of Cardiovascular Disease: An Observational Study. *BMJ Open* **2021**, *11*, e046551. [CrossRef]
42. Westland, H.; Schuurmans, M.J.; Bos-Touwen, I.D.; de Bruin-van Leersum, M.A.; Monninkhof, E.M.; Schröder, C.D.; de Vette, D.A.; Trappenburg, J.C.A. Effectiveness of the Nurse-Led Activate Intervention in Patients at Risk of Cardiovascular Disease in Primary Care: A Cluster-Randomised Controlled Trial. *Eur. J. Cardiovasc. Nurs.* **2020**, *19*, 721–731. [CrossRef] [PubMed]
43. Schoenthaler, A.; Rosenthal, D.M.; Butler, M.; Jacobowitz, L. Medication Adherence Improvement Similar for Shared Decision-Making Preference or Longer Patient-Provider Relationship. *J. Am. Board. Fam. Med.* **2018**, *31*, 752–760. [CrossRef] [PubMed]

44. Christensen, R.E.; Ranpariya, V.; Kammrath, L.K.; Masicampo, E.J.; Roberson, K.B.; Feldman, S.R. The Presence of Accountability in Digital Interventions Targeting Non-Adherence: A Review. *Patient Educ. Couns.* **2022**, *105*, 2637–2644. [CrossRef]
45. Ski, C.F.; Cartledge, S.; Foldager, D.; Thompson, D.R.; Fredericks, S.; Ekman, I.; Hendriks, J.M. Integrated Care in Cardiovascular Disease: A Statement of the Association of Cardiovascular Nursing and Allied Professions of the European Society of Cardiology. *Eur. J. Cardiovasc. Nurs.* **2023**, *22*, e39–e46. [CrossRef]

Journal of
Cardiovascular Development and Disease

MDPI

Review

Cardiovascular Disease Risk Factors in the Native American Population

Krista Goerger [1], Karla Abbott [2], Mark K. Larson [3] and Michael Holinstat [1,*]

[1] Department of Pharmacology, University of Michigan, Ann Arbor, MI 48109, USA; kgoerger@umich.edu
[2] Nursing Department, Augustana University, Sioux Falls, SD 57197, USA; karla.abbott@augie.edu
[3] Biology Department, Augustana University, Sioux Falls, SD 57197, USA; mark.larson@augie.edu
* Correspondence: mholinst@med.umich.edu; Tel.: +1-734-763-8824

Abstract: Native Americans are disproportionately affected by cardiovascular disease in comparison with other racial and ethnic groups in the United States. Previous research has analyzed risk factors, quantified prevalence rates, and examined outcomes of cardiovascular disease in Native Americans, yet few studies have considered the role of societal and psychological factors on the increased burden of cardiovascular disease in Native Americans. Modifiable risk factors for cardiovascular disease, including poor nutrition, reduced physical activity, obesity, and increased substance use, are exacerbated in Native American communities due to cultural and historical factors. Further, Native Americans have endured historical trauma and continue to experience additional financial and healthcare stressors, resulting in increased levels of chronic stress. Chronic activation of stress responses through the hypothalamic–pituitary–adrenal and autonomic nervous system increases inflammation and cardiovascular dysfunction resulting in an increased risk for cardiovascular disease. Therefore, it is critical to examine the connection between these stressors and the cardiovascular health disparities in Native American communities to create effective strategies to improve health outcomes.

Keywords: cardiovascular disease; Native American; American Indian; under-represented; chronic stress

1. Introduction

Cardiovascular disease (CVD) used to be rare in the Native American population and it was thought Native Americans had inherent protection from CVD [1,2]. However, studies in recent decades have shown CVD rates continue to climb [3], and it is well-established that CVD is now the leading cause of death in Native American populations [4]. While CVD poses a significant health risk for the entire U.S. population, it is important to acknowledge the increased burden the Native American population faces. Native American and Alaskan Native populations are disproportionately affected by coronary heart disease (CHD) with a prevalence rate of 12%, which is two-fold higher compared to the U.S. population [2,5,6]. In 2018, Native Americans were 10% more likely to have a stroke compared to non-Hispanic white adults [7]. In addition, overall cardiovascular events among Native American populations are 20% more fatal [8]. There has been significant research conducted to assess the prevalence of CVD among Native Americans, but few studies have considered the role cultural and psychological factors such as Westernization, long-term neglect, and mistreatment play in the increased burden of CVD. Further, it is difficult to fully understand the various CVD risk factors present in Native American populations due to the variation between communities and tribes. There are over 500 federally recognized American Indian and Alaska Native tribes with many different traditions, beliefs, and histories [9]. While these differences should not go unnoticed and more research is needed to thoroughly consider the relationship between the culture and health within each of the communities, for the purpose of the review there will be some cultural generalizations made due to the lack of scientific research available.

2. Cultural Influence on Classic Cardiovascular Risk Factors

The well-established, classical modifiable cardiovascular risk factors include, but are not limited to, eating non-nutritious food, low levels of physical activity, smoking, and drinking [10]. While these risk factors transcend all people irrespective of age, gender, or geographic origin, some of these modifiable factors are more prominent in Native American communities due to cultural and historical factors. Pinpointing how these factors are integrated into Native American communities is key to ameliorating their effects and can inform the development and improvement of culturally relevant programs to encourage healthier habits and reduce the risk for CVD.

2.1. Nutrition

Prior to Western European expansion into Native American land and assimilation into the Western European diet, Native Americans acquired their dietary needs through hunting wild game, fishing, and harvesting native plants such as corn, beans, squash, seeds, nuts, and fruits [11]. When Native Americans were relocated from their native lands to reservations, they were forced to change their diet abruptly. The traditional food they had grown accustomed to was no longer available, resulting in an increased reliance on the U.S. government for rations. In 1871, these rations typically consisted of fresh beef, bacon, flour, corn meal, coffee, salt, sugar, and rice, which discouraged the consumption of nutritionally diverse foods and promoted the consumption of high-caloric foods with few nutritional benefits [12]. Today, many Native Americans continue to depend on the dietary food sources provided by government Commodity Supplemental Food Programs [13]. Like rations, commodity food often consists of calorie-dense, processed foods such as sugar, enriched flour, vegetable shortening, canned meat, cheese, peanut butter, sugared juices, powdered milk, and corn syrup [13].

Another factor contributing to the highly processed diet is limited access to nutritious foods, as there are fewer sources of healthy food per square mile on tribal land compared to non-tribal land [14]. When interviewed, many Native Americans expressed that the expense of nutritious foods and the transportation required to access nutritious foods were significant barriers to eating healthy [14]. The overall shift in nutrient intake is evident within the Pima Indian community residing in southern Arizona. It is estimated the traditional Pima Indian diet from over 130 years ago consisted of ~70–80% carbohydrates, ~8–12% fat, and ~12–18% protein [15], while a 1996 survey indicated their diet consisted of ~48% carbohydrates, ~34–36% fat, and ~15% protein [16]. The Strong Heart Study (Phase II) conducted with participants from 13 tribes supports these findings, as their results showed similar estimates of fat intake at around ~35% [17].

Processed foods often contain high amounts of sodium, and a 2005 report demonstrated Native American participants' intake elevated sodium levels compared to national recommendations [17]. Sodium can contribute to CVD risk by increasing blood pressure or hypertension. However, a 2023 report stated Native American adults were 10% less likely to have high blood pressure [18], suggesting sodium intake and hypertension do not contribute to the increased burden of CVD in Native American populations.

Diets of highly processed food also contain high levels of saturated fat [19,20], which is linked to an increased risk of CVD [21,22]. This is due to the development of dyslipidemia, or an unfavorable lipid profile containing high levels of low-density lipoprotein cholesterol (LDL-C) and triglycerides (TG), and lower levels of beneficial high-density lipoprotein cholesterol (HDL-C) [23,24]. Unfavorable lipid profiles can result in the buildup of plaque in the major arteries, a CVD also known as atherosclerosis [25]. In 2005, Native American participants demonstrated elevated intake of cholesterol and energy from total fat compared to national recommendations [17]. Further, a recent update from the Strong Heart Family Study found more than 70% of Native American young adults and 50% of Native American teens have dyslipidemia [26]. However, other studies have found cholesterol levels are not elevated in Native American adults compared to non-Hispanic white adults or the U.S. average [18,27]. Therefore, future studies need to continue to determine the prevalence of dyslipidemia in the Native American population and the link between consumption of highly processed foods.

Consumption of processed foods also results in the inadequate consumption of fruits and vegetables, resulting in a deficiency in essential vitamins including vitamin A, vitamin C, and folate relative to national recommendations [17]. A more recent survey further supports these original findings, in which 56% and 75% of Native American adults reported low fruit and vegetable intake, respectively [28]. Studies have shown that a decreased intake of fruits and vegetables increases the risk of CVD [29,30], and while the exact mechanisms of the ability of fruits and vegetables to reduce CVD risk is unknown, it is believed to be due to their antioxidant and anti-inflammatory properties resulting in reduced blood pressure [31,32].

The transition from a traditional diet to processed foods is strongly associated with poor cardiovascular health and may play a significant role in the increased risk of CVD among Native Americans. Although this dietary shift occurred several generations ago, limited access to nutritious foods continues to affect this population. However, diet alone does not fully account for the heightened CVD burden, as research indicates relatively minimal differences in nutritional intake between Native Americans and the general U.S. population. It is important to note that nutritional studies focusing on Native Americans have been conducted independently of those examining the broader U.S. population, complicating direct comparisons.

2.2. *Physical Activity*

Engaging in physical activity has long been observed to have beneficial effects on cardiovascular health [33], yet physical inactivity is a problem in all facets of the U.S. population, including Native American communities [34]. The results of several studies report only about ~20–30% of Native American adults and children engage in physical activity [35–38], and between ~30–50% of Native Americans are physically inactive [39,40]. There is a limited body of evidence comparing physical activity rates between Native American populations and the U.S. population, but one study claimed Native Americans are more likely to be physically inactive relative to other races [40]. Further, the National Health Interview Survey from 2018 reported that 18.7% of Native Americans met federal physical activity guidelines compared to 25.8% of non-Hispanic white adults [7]. Unfortunately, most of this evidence is based on physical activity data collected using self-reported subjective measures of physical activity, which often suffer from reporting bias [41].

The sedentary lifestyle of many Native Americans can in part be attributed to Western influence. In 2000, Pima Indians residing in Mexico were found to still live a traditional lifestyle with labor-intensive, non-mechanized farming and building, while U.S. Pima Indians in Arizona utilized mechanized farming methods and participated in more activities of lower intensity. U.S. Pimas showed significantly reduced levels of physical activity compared to age-matched Mexican Pimas [42]. Mexican Pimas are also lighter and have lower body mass indexes (BMIs) than U.S. Pimas, further supporting the importance of physical activity to protect against the development of CVD and obesity [43]. Other barriers, including inadequate exercise facilities, lack of access to transportation, unsafe walking and trail conditions, shortage of time outside work, and inclement weather, deter Native Americans from attaining normal levels of physical activity to maintain cardiovascular health [44,45]. Women are also more likely to be inactive compared to men [40], and according to a focus group interview this is likely due to insufficient support from the community to be physically active, a lack of support for household and childcare responsibilities, and difficulties balancing societal expectations with physical activity [45].

While more quantitative research is needed to fully understand the prevalence and factors contributing to physical inactivity across diverse Native American communities, existing evidence suggests that low rates of exercise, limited access to resources for physical activity, and societal pressures deprioritizing its importance likely play a significant role in the elevated rates of cardiovascular disease (CVD) within these populations. Recent studies have increasingly focused on interventional strategies, particularly targeting children and youth, to promote physical activity. However, these studies are often constrained by small sample sizes and reliance on self-reported data [46]. Interventions at the group, clinic, and individual home-based levels have demonstrated improvements in physical activity levels, but further research is necessary to broaden the application of culturally centered approaches, which may better address the unique needs of Native American communities [47].

2.3. Obesity

Obesity, defined as a BMI greater than 30, is a significant risk factor for CVD and is associated with several key contributors to CVD risk. These include an increased likelihood of hypertension, elevated levels of LDL-C and TG, and reduced levels of HDL-C [48–50]. Additionally, obesity is strongly linked to increased overall cardiovascular morbidity and mortality [48]. Consistent with high rates of CVD, obesity rates in Native American communities exceed all other racial and ethnic groups [50], and in 2018 the National Health Interview Survey found that 48.1% of Native Americans were obese compared to 33.9% of non-Hispanic whites [18]. Further, in communities surveyed in 2010, more than one-third of Native American adults were found to be obese, whereas nationally, one-fifth of U.S. adults were reported to be obese [51]. Additionally, Native American children are also at a high risk for developing childhood obesity, which is a major risk factor for adult obesity [52–54]. The prevalence rate of obesity in Native American preschoolers (31.2%) was found to be higher when compared to other racial/ethnic groups, including whites (15.9%) [52]. With obesity rates increasing at younger ages, obesity continues to be embedded into the population, exacerbating the burden of CVD.

Obesity is a multifaceted disease caused by biological, socioeconomic, and environmental factors resulting in energy intake exceeding energy expenditure. Two classic causes of obesity are poor nutrition and lack of physical activity. Therefore, the increased rate of obesity in Native Americans is anticipated, as studies have shown Native Americans consume more processed foods and engage in less physical activity than the general population.

2.4. Tobacco Use

Native Americans have a long history of ceremonial tobacco use. While the purpose of tobacco use varies widely across tribes, it was traditionally primarily for religious and therapeutic purposes, and today, it is still used for burial offerings or as a gift [55]. Although tobacco has cultural origins, its shift to recreational use has become a major source of addiction for Native Americans across the nation. The 2018 SAMHSA study reports Native Americans have higher rates of cigarette use in their lifetime compared to all other racial/ethnic groups [56]. Additionally, 43.3% of Native American adults used tobacco in the past month compared to 25.4% of whites [56]. Youth and adolescents also have increased rates of tobacco use compared to the overall U.S. population [57–59].

Cigarette smoking is a major cause of CVD and about one in three deaths from CVD in the U.S. are attributed to smoking [60,61]. The exact mechanisms linking cigarette smoking to related CVDs are poorly understood, but research has shown smoking cigarettes promotes mitochondrial oxidative stress, endothelial dysfunction, procoagulant states, and reduced HDL-C [62,63]. These alterations increase blood pressure, risk for thrombosis, and inflammation [64]. To combat the high rates of tobacco use in Native American communities and other minorities, several public health programs have been put in place [65]. Prevention and/or cessation interventions enlist elders, tribal leaders, parents, or school personnel to develop a curriculum to intervene with adolescents in a school-based setting [65]. In general, the prevention programs have reduced adolescent tobacco initiation rates but have not improved cessation rates [65,66]. Instead, it was found individuals who received a diagnosis of diabetes mellitus, hypertension, or renal insufficiency were more likely to quit tobacco use [67]. There is still a need to create more effective programs to reduce cigarette use in this high-risk population, and the programs must also address the rise of e-cigarette and smokeless tobacco products, which, despite being marketed as a safer alternative to cigarettes, are both linked to adverse health effects [68,69].

2.5. Alcohol Use

Prior to European colonization, Native Americans had minimal exposure to alcohol. However, with the widespread availability of alcohol introduced by European settlers through trade, recreational alcohol use increased rapidly among Native American tribes [70]. This historical shift has contributed to the enduring perception of high alcohol misuse within Native American communities. Yet, evidence suggests that Native Americans exhibit higher rates of alcohol abstinence compared to whites [71]. For instance, the 2018 SAMHSA study reported that lifetime alcohol use, as well as alcohol use in the past month or year, was lower among Native Americans than among whites across all age groups [56].

Despite lower overall alcohol consumption, lifetime rates of alcohol dependence in some tribal groups have been reported to range from 20% to 70%, far exceeding the epidemiological prevalence of DSM-IV alcohol dependence, which is 13% in the U.S. general population [72]. Additionally, episodic heavy drinking or binge drinking appears to be more prevalent among Native Americans [56,73]. One study found that 37% of individuals from the Cheyenne River Sioux Tribe in South Dakota had consumed more than five drinks on a single occasion at least once in the past month, compared to 29% of the general South Dakota population [73]. The high rates of binge drinking are concerning as binge drinking is correlated with increased risk for several CVDs, including thrombosis, hypertension, and sudden cardiac death [74].

One promising trend within Native American communities is an increase in the number of heavy-drinking men deciding to quit drinking without treatment programs. These men reported the main motivation for quitting was health concerns [75]. Additionally, there are higher rates of alcohol abstinence among Native American females [73]. These findings suggest that alcohol use within Native American populations may be on a gradual decline. Nevertheless, the persistence of alcohol abuse and binge drinking highlights the need for continued attention, as these behaviors likely contribute to the elevated prevalence of CVD observed in Native American communities.

3. Societal Stressors as Cardiovascular Risk Factors

Many classical cardiovascular risk factors can be eliminated with proper resources to support lifestyle modifications and access to health care. However, other risk factors constructed by society and the surrounding environment also play a large role in Native American cardiovascular disparities. Native Americans have endured many traumatic events since the colonization of the Americas and continue to experience discrimination at both individual and institutional levels [76]. Enduring mistreatment and oppression today, on top of years of generational trauma and stress, can have a large impact on overall health [77,78]. These stressors can result in physiological changes that have been shown to negatively impact cardiovascular health and increase the risk for CVD [79], demonstrating the importance of considering societal stressors when discussing the current state of Native American heart health.

3.1. Historical Trauma

Multi-generational physical, psychological, and cultural trauma experienced by the Native American communities have resulted in a longer-lasting composite stressor and is called "historical trauma" [9]. Historical trauma was defined by Maria Yellow Horse Brave Heart as "cumulative trauma over both the life span and across generations results from massive cataclysmic events" [9]. Throughout the history of interactions between Western Europe and the Native American nations, there has been a continual decline in the Native American population. Due to diseases carried by American settlers to North America and armed conflict, the Native American population declined rapidly from an estimated 12 million prior to European settlement to less than 300,000 in 1990 [80]. Discussions in Native American focus groups have shown many Native Americans across all ages often have thoughts about historical losses in their community, and these thoughts are accompanied by emotional distress [76].

The passage of the Civilization Fund Act in 1819 led to the creation of Indian boarding schools, forcing children to leave their homes to attend boarding schools [81]. The mission of these schools was to integrate the children into Western American culture, and they often discouraged children from speaking their native language, practicing their native religion, or engaging in any other native traditions [81]. In addition to the forced integration policies, children were often placed in physical and psychological danger, as evidenced by the numerous reports of sexual and physical abuse, malnutrition, child labor, neglect, and death [82,83]. One Lakota study found parents who attended boarding school as children felt like inadequate parents and were overwhelmed by their role. Subsequently, the children of adults who were raised in boarding schools more often reported abuse and neglect in their own childhoods and felt unprepared to raise their own children [84].

Based on these studies, trauma experienced from the rapid decline in population, assimilation policies, and boarding schools was likely passed down through multiple generations. One study has reported that early-life intrapersonal trauma and community family dysfunction were significantly associated with an increased risk of diabetes, a major risk factor for CVD [85]. Therefore, historical trauma is still reverberating in Native American communities today and affecting overall health, including the risk for CVD.

3.2. Socioeconomic Status and Financial Strain

According to a 2022 poll from NPR and Harvard, Native Americans experience more financial strain compared to any other racial or ethnic group in the U.S. [86]. Nearly 40% of Native Americans struggle to afford food compared to 21% of white adults, and a majority (58%) of Native Americans do not have enough emergency savings to cover one month of expenses. In 2010, 23% of Native American families reported an income level below poverty as defined by the U.S. government, compared to 16% of the general U.S. population [87]. The increased poverty rates of Native Americans can be largely attributed to a lack of jobs and low wages [88], as the unemployment rate of American Indians in 2022 averaged 6.2%, more than any other racial group [89].

Both increased financial strain and low socioeconomic status have been shown to increase the risk for CVD [90,91]. This is largely because people with low socioeconomic status and increased financial strain are less likely to eat nutritious food [92,93] and are less likely to be physically active during leisure time [94]. Further, financial instability in Native Americans increases the risk of hypertension by 88% [95]. Therefore, increased financial strain in the Native American communities is exacerbating risk factors for CVD and contributing to the disproportionate burden of CVD.

3.3. Healthcare Stressors

Healthcare illiteracy is the lack of fluency with language commonly utilized in healthcare settings and influences the level of comfort patients feel when interacting with physicians and other healthcare professionals. Native American communities have high rates of healthcare illiteracy, which is associated with worse health outcomes [96]. One study reported that 48% of Native American adults have limited healthcare literacy, compared with 36% of all U.S. adults [87]. Despite the lack of research linking healthcare literacy or discrimination in the healthcare setting specifically with CVD, research has linked overall stress and anxiety with an increased risk for CVD [97].

Previous and current discrimination against Native Americans in the healthcare setting also acts as a significant barrier to receiving appropriate and timely healthcare. Much of this discrimination can be attributed to healthcare professionals not exhibiting cultural competency when working with Native American patients [98]. The ability of a healthcare worker to appropriately interact with patients from different backgrounds than their own and to respect the patient's cultural beliefs greatly impacts the quality of care a patient receives. In a sample of Native American adults with type 2 diabetes mellitus, 36% reported they had experienced microaggressions from their healthcare providers [13]. Microaggressions include negative comments about a person's background or portray stereotypes that can ultimately minimize a patient's experience which can have negative impacts on their health [99]. Experiencing microaggressions is positively correlated with a history of heart attacks [99]. Poor experiences in a healthcare setting may deter a patient from receiving care again and could contribute to worse outcomes of CVD.

4. Physiological Links Between Chronic Stress and Cardiovascular Health

High levels of chronic stress from historical, financial, and healthcare struggles are apparent in the Native American community and it has been shown that increased stress is correlated with an increased risk for CVD [79,97,100,101]. The INTERHEART study found elevated psychosocial stress over the past year was associated with an over two-fold increased risk for myocardial infarction [102]. As a population endures high levels of chronic stress, it is important to consider and understand the connection between stress and cardiovascular health. The exact mechanisms by which chronic stress affects cardiovascular physiology are not fully understood, but many studies have led to the development of several hypotheses [79]. Addressing these links could provide the ability to improve the physiological response to stress and potentially lower the rate of CVD.

4.1. Autonomic Nervous System Dysfunction

The autonomic nervous system (ANS) innervates nearly all the organs of the body and is activated within seconds after exposure to a stressor. The two balancing systems of the

ANS are the sympathetic nervous system (SNS) and the parasympathetic nervous system (PNS). The SNS is responsible for the fight-or-flight response by releasing epinephrine from the adrenal medulla and norepinephrine from the sympathetic nerve terminals [103]. The release of these catecholamines promotes optimized blood flow to muscle tissues by increasing heart rate, myocardial contractility, and vascular tone [103]. The PNS functions to inhibit the sympathetic nervous system and predominates during resting conditions.

However, chronic stress results in autonomic dysregulation characterized by sustained sympathetic overactivity and reduced parasympathetic activity. Studies have shown individuals experiencing higher levels of chronic stress have impaired autonomic regulation of cardiovascular functions leading to increased blood pressure, increased variability in heart rate, and reduced ANS sensitivity to acute stressors. Blunted reactivity of the ANS can be analyzed via salivary alpha-amylase, a marker of SNS activation, which is reduced in chronically stressed individuals following an acute mental stressor [104]. An increase in autonomic dysfunction following chronic stress is associated with increased risk for CVDs such as arrhythmias, thrombosis, acute coronary syndromes, and heart failure [105].

Few studies have been conducted assessing the ANS in the Native American population. In Pima Indians, lower SNS activity was associated with a high prevalence of obesity [106]. Further, in Native American adults, a history of alcohol use disorders was associated with low autonomic control and increased hypertension [107]. It is unclear if the autonomic dysregulation is directly caused by chronic stress or if chronic stress may be altering health behaviors such as increased overeating, reduced physical activity, and increased alcohol consumption, resulting in autonomic dysregulation. However, overall, these findings suggest that blunted reactivity of the ANS could contribute to CVD risk in Native Americans.

4.2. Hypothalamic–Pituitary–Adrenal Axis Disruption

The hypothalamic–pituitary–adrenal (HPA) axis also acts as the human body's stress response system and functions to resolve acute stressors [108]. Acute stressors are infrequent and stimulate the hypothalamus to release corticotropin-releasing hormone (CRH) and vasopressin. CRH stimulates the release of adrenocorticotropin hormone (ACTH) from the anterior pituitary which induces the release of glucocorticoids, like cortisol, from the adrenal cortex. One of the functions of cortisol is to maintain control of the HPA axis activation via negative feedback. Cortisol also regulates the production of the glucocorticoid dehydroepiandrosterone (DHEA) which reduces inflammation and protects the brain from damage due to increased cortisol levels. However, chronic stress results in frequent and prolonged activation of the HPA axis marked by hypercortisolism [104]. High levels of cortisol can lead to increased adiposity, insulin resistance, and hypertension, which are known risk factors for CVD [109].

Interestingly, ACTH and cortisol levels are comparable between Pima Indians and whites, suggesting that chronic stress does not lead to hypercortisolism in Native Americans [106,110]. Research indicates that early childhood stress can result in a blunted physiological response to acute stress [111]. This is supported by findings showing that when Pima Indians were administered acute cortisol, their SNS activity decreased—an effect opposite to that observed in whites [110]. Blunted cardiovascular responses to acute physiological stress are associated with adverse health outcomes, including an increased risk of diabetes and higher mortality rates in patients with heart failure. Additionally, it has been suggested that blunted stress reactivity may indirectly contribute to poor cardiovascular outcomes through an increase in adverse health behaviors, such as substance use and overeating, which can lead to addiction and obesity [111]. Further studies are needed to confirm these findings and establish a clearer connection between blunted stress reactivity, adverse health behaviors, and cardiovascular outcomes in the Native American population.

4.3. Systemic Low-Level Inflammation

Another key consequence of chronic stress is immune system dysregulation. Cortisol levels following chronic stress are associated with an increase in tumor necrosis factor α (TNF-α) and interleukin 6 (IL-6), markers of low-level inflammation and predictors of cardiovascular health. TNF-α induces the release of IL-6, which is a known factor that links stress and CVDs by promoting vascular damage and the development of atherosclerosis [112].

In addition, studies have shown lower socioeconomic status is inversely correlated with concentrations of other markers of chronic levels of inflammation, such as fibrinogen [113]. Fibrinogen expression can be induced by IL-6 and is an important molecule in both inflammatory and coagulation pathways, leading to an increased risk of thrombosis and acute coronary events [114–116]. The production of C-reactive protein (CRP) is also induced by IL-6 and triggers the coagulation pathway by inducing monocytes to express tissue factor [117]. Increased CRP levels can have deleterious effects on the cardiovascular system, demonstrated by the increased risk of recurrent ischemia or myocardial infarction [118,119].

CRP has been established as an independent predictor of cardiovascular events [120]. Additionally, findings from Phase II of the Strong Heart Study demonstrated that elevated levels of CRP and fibrinogen in Native Americans were associated with an increased risk of heart failure [121]. These findings suggest that systemic inflammation may play a significant role in the heightened burden of CVD observed in the Native American population.

4.4. Oxidative Stress

In vivo studies have found that chronically stressed rats showed increased levels of oxidative stress [122,123]. Oxidative stress occurs when there is an excess of free radicals, or reactive oxygen species (ROS), that the body cannot neutralize due to a shortage of antioxidants [124]. Chronic inflammatory pathways triggered by prolonged stress elevate TNF-α levels, which promote ROS production [125]. Oxidative stress contributes to platelet hyper-reactivity by exposing a pro-thrombotic environment that triggers platelet activation, which, in turn, generates additional ROS, perpetuating a cycle of oxidative stress [126]. Elevated ROS levels further amplify inflammatory pathways, leading to endothelial dysfunction, and resulting in an increased risk for CVDs such as thrombosis and atherosclerosis [124].

5. Discussion

There are a multitude of factors that influence an individual's risk for CVD. The classical and well-understood modifiable risk factors include diet, exercise, and substance use. We recognize that this review provides only a limited discussion of lipids and atherosclerotic CVD, a gap that reflects the scarcity of research on lipid-related factors in this population and underscores the need for future studies in this area. When considering modifiable factors for CVD, it is crucial to simultaneously evaluate the effect culture may have on them. In Native American communities, there are many social structures that differ from the Western culture and are necessary to consider when trying to understand the increased burden of CVD in Native American populations. These factors are deeply entwined in the culture, so cultural competency is the first step to addressing the cardiovascular disparities in the communities. With a better understanding and appreciation for cultural differences, adequate resources and programs can be created to improve food availability, wellness facilities, education, healthcare access, and programs to reduce substance use.

Other risk factors, such as historical trauma, are more difficult to modify as they are deeply rooted in Native American history and poorly understudied, but may equally contribute to Native Americans' risk for CVD. Much of this relates to the chronic stress Native Americans may experience due to systemic discrimination and burdens from previous generations. Continued studies of the Native American population are needed to assess the unique mechanisms that have led to increased incidence of CVD compared to the general population, resulting in high levels of morbidity and mortality. The sparse number of published studies has resulted in a limited understanding of the unique pressures, both physiological and environmental, that drive the pathophysiology of the cardiovascular system in the Native American population. Several cellular processes have been identified that are critical for the translation of chronic stress responses to tissue damage resulting in CVDs. Analyzing these pathways and biomarkers in Native American populations could be used to determine if the increased levels of chronic stress in Native Americans contribute to the increased burden of CVD.

Another promising area for future research is platelet reactivity, as thrombosis resulting from platelet hyper-reactivity underlies the pathophysiology of many cardiovascular diseases. Platelet reactivity can be influenced by factors such as diet, cholesterol levels, and smoking [127], and is further exacerbated by conditions like obesity, diabetes, and chronic stress [128,129]. Recent findings have demonstrated, for the first time, that platelets from Native Americans exhibit heightened reactivity compared to those from whites [130]. However, additional studies are needed to explore whether this increased platelet reactivity is associated with specific CVD risk factors within the Native American population.

Due to the historical under-representation of this population in basic and clinical studies, there remains a significant gap in our understanding of Native American health, especially in cardiovascular function. Future studies focused on delineating the underlying pathophysiology of cardiovascular health in Native Americans will aid in the targeting and development of pharmacological, societal, and environmental strategies to limit morbidity due to cardiovascular risk in the Native American population.

Author Contributions: Writing, K.G. and M.H.; editing, K.G., K.A., M.K.L. and M.H.; funding acquisition, M.K.L. All authors have read and agreed to the published version of the manuscript.

Funding: This research was funded by an Institutional Development Award (IDeA) from the National Institute of General Medical Sciences of the National Institutes of Health under grant number P20GM103443 (K.G. and M.K.L.).

Institutional Review Board Statement: Not applicable.

Informed Consent Statement: Not applicable.

Data Availability Statement: Not applicable.

Conflicts of Interest: The authors K.G., K.A., and M.K.L. declare no conflicts of interest. M.H. is a consultant and equity holder for Veralox Therapeutics and a consultant for Cereno Scientific, which has an option to license platelet inhibitory compounds from the University of Michigan. There are no conflicts with the current manuscript.

Abbreviations

BMI = body mass index, CHD = coronary heart disease, CVD = cardiovascular disease, HDL-C = high-density lipoprotein cholesterol, LDL-C = low-density lipoprotein cholesterol, TG = triglycerides.

References

1. Sievers, M.L.; Fisher, J.R. Diseases of North American Indians. In *Biocultural Aspects of Disease*; Rothschild, H.R., Ed.; FAO: Rome, Italy, 1981; pp. 191–252.
2. Howard, B.V.; Lee, E.T.; Cowan, L.D.; Fabsitz, R.R.; Howard, W.J.; Oopik, A.J.; Robbins, D.C.; Savage, P.J.; Yeh, J.L.; Welty, T.K. Coronary heart disease prevalence and its relation to risk factors in American Indians. The Strong Heart Study. *Am. J. Epidemiol.* **1995**, *142*, 254–268. [CrossRef] [PubMed]
3. Howard, B.V.; Lee, E.T.; Cowan, L.D.; Devereux, R.B.; Galloway, J.M.; Go, O.T.; Howard, W.J.; Rhoades, E.R.; Robbins, D.C.; Sievers, M.L.; et al. Rising Tide of cardiovascular disease in American Indians. The Strong Heart Study. *Circulation* **1999**, *99*, 2389–2395. [CrossRef] [PubMed]
4. Tsao, C.W.; Aday, A.W.; Almarzooq, Z.I.; Alonso, A.; Beaton, A.Z.; Bittencourt, M.S.; Boehme, A.K.; Buxton, A.E.; Carson, A.P.; Commodore-Mensah, Y.; et al. Heart Disease and Stroke Statistics-2022 Update: A Report From the American Heart Association. *Circulation* **2022**, *145*, e153–e639. [CrossRef] [PubMed]
5. Benjamin, E.J.; Muntner, P.; Alonso, A.; Bittencourt, M.S.; Callaway, C.W.; Carson, A.P.; Chamberlain, A.M.; Chang, A.R.; Cheng, S.; Das, S.R.; et al. Heart Disease and Stroke Statistics-2019 Update: A Report From the American Heart Association. *Circulation* **2019**, *139*, e56–e528. [CrossRef]
6. Breathett, K.; Sims, M.; Gross, M.; Jackson, E.A.; Jones, E.J.; Navas-Acien, A.; Taylor, H.; Thomas, K.L.; Howard, B.V.; American Heart Association Council on Epidemiology and Prevention; et al. Cardiovascular Health in American Indians and Alaska Natives: A Scientific Statement From the American Heart Association. *Circulation* **2020**, *141*, e948–e959. [CrossRef]
7. CDC. Summary Health Statistics: National Health Interview Survey: 2018. Available online: https://ftp.cdc.gov/pub/Health_Statistics/NCHS/NHIS/SHS/2018_SHS_Table_A-14.pdf (accessed on 8 January 2024).
8. Deen, J.F.; Adams, A.K.; Fretts, A.; Jolly, S.; Navas-Acien, A.; Devereux, R.B.; Buchwald, D.; Howard, B.V. Cardiovascular Disease in American Indian and Alaska Native Youth: Unique Risk Factors and Areas of Scholarly Need. *J. Am. Heart Assoc.* **2017**, *6*, e007576. [CrossRef]
9. Brave Heart, M.Y. The historical trauma response among natives and its relationship with substance abuse: A Lakota illustration. *J. Psychoact. Drugs* **2003**, *35*, 7–13. [CrossRef]
10. Fryar, C.D.; Chen, T.C.; Li, X. *Prevalence of Uncontrolled Risk Factors for Cardiovascular Disease: United States, 1999–2010*; NCHS Data Brief, No. 103; National Center for Health Statistics: Hyattsville, MD, USA, 2012; pp. 1–8.
11. Mihesuah, D.A. Decolonizing Our Diets by Recovering Our Ancestors' Gardens. *Am. Indian Q.* **2003**, *27*, 807–839. [CrossRef]
12. Wiedman, D. Native American embodiment of the chronicities of modernity: Reservation food, diabetes, and the metabolic syndrome among the Kiowa, Comanche, and Apache. *Med. Anthropol. Q.* **2012**, *26*, 595–612. [CrossRef]
13. Warne, D.; Lajimodiere, D. American Indian health disparities: Psychosocial influences. *Soc. Personal. Psychol. Compass* **2015**, *9*, 567–579. [CrossRef]
14. Chodur, G.M.; Shen, Y.; Kodish, S.; Oddo, V.M.; Antiporta, D.A.; Jock, B.; Jones-Smith, J.C. Food Environments around American Indian Reservations: A Mixed Methods Study. *PLoS ONE* **2016**, *11*, e0161132. [CrossRef] [PubMed]
15. Boyce, V.L.; Swinburn, B.A. The traditional Pima Indian diet. Composition and adaptation for use in a dietary intervention study. *Diabetes Care* **1993**, *16*, 369–371. [CrossRef] [PubMed]
16. Smith, C.J.; Nelson, R.G.; Hardy, S.A.; Manahan, E.M.; Bennett, P.H.; Knowler, W.C. Survey of the diet of Pima Indians using quantitative food frequency assessment and 24-hour recall. Diabetic Renal Disease Study. *J. Am. Diet. Assoc.* **1996**, *96*, 778–784. [CrossRef] [PubMed]
17. Stang, J.; Zephier, E.M.; Story, M.; Himes, J.H.; Yeh, J.L.; Welty, T.; Howard, B.V. Dietary intakes of nutrients thought to modify cardiovascular risk from three groups of American Indians: The Strong Heart Dietary Study, Phase II. *J. Am. Diet. Assoc.* **2005**, *105*, 1895–1903. [CrossRef]
18. National Center for Health Statistics. NHIS Adult Summary Health Statistics. 2023. Available online: https://wwwn.cdc.gov/NHISDataQueryTool/SHS_adult/index.html (accessed on 1 January 2025).
19. Weaver, C.M.; Dwyer, J.; Fulgoni, V.L.r.; King, J.C.; Leveille, G.A.; MacDonald, R.S.; Ordovas, J.; Schnakenberg, D. Processed foods: Contributions to nutrition. *Am. J. Clin. Nutr.* **2014**, *99*, 1525–1542. [CrossRef]
20. Steele, E.M.; Batis, C.; Cediel, G.; Louzada, M.L.D.C.; Khandpur, N.; Machado, P.; Moubarac, J.C.; Rauber, F.; Jedlicki, M.R.; Levy, R.B.; et al. The burden of excessive saturated fatty acid intake attributed to ultra-processed food consumption: A study conducted with nationally representative cross-sectional studies from eight countries. *J. Nutr. Sci.* **2021**, *10*, e43. [CrossRef]
21. Ma, Y.; Li, Y.; Chiriboga, D.E.; Olendzki, B.C.; Hebert, J.R.; Li, W.; Leung, K.; Hafner, A.R.; Ockene, I.S. Association between carbohydrate intake and serum lipids. *J. Am. Coll. Nutr.* **2006**, *25*, 155–163. [CrossRef]
22. Guasch-Ferré, M.; Babio, N.; Martínez-González, M.A.; Corella, D.; Ros, E.; Martín-Peláez, S.; Estruch, R.; Arós, F.; Gómez-Gracia, E.; Fiol, M.; et al. Dietary fat intake and risk of cardiovascular disease and all-cause mortality in a population at high risk of cardiovascular disease. *Am. J. Clin. Nutr.* **2015**, *102*, 1563–1573. [CrossRef]

23. Wilson, P.W.; D'Agostino, R.B.; Levy, D.; Belanger, A.M.; Silbershatz, H.; Kannel, W.B. Prediction of coronary heart disease using risk factor categories. *Circulation* **1998**, *97*, 1837–1847. [CrossRef]
24. Boullart, A.C.; de Graaf, J.; Stalenhoef, A.F. Serum triglycerides and risk of cardiovascular disease. *Biochim. Biophys. Acta* **2012**, *1821*, 867–875. [CrossRef]
25. Jellinger, P.S.; Smith, D.A.; Mehta, A.E.; Ganda, O.; Handelsman, Y.; Rodbard, H.W.; Shepherd, M.D.; Seibel, J.A.; AACE Task Force for Management of Dyslipidemia and Prevention of Atherosclerosis; AACE Task Force for the Management of Dyslipidemia and Prevention of Atherosclerosis Writing Committee. American Association of Clinical Endocrinologists' Guidelines for Management of Dyslipidemia and Prevention of Atherosclerosis. *Endocr. Pract.* **2012**, *18* (Suppl. 1), 1–78. [CrossRef]
26. Reese, J.A.; Roman, M.J.; Deen, J.F.; Ali, T.; Cole, S.A.; Devereux, R.B.; Fretts, A.M.; Howard, W.J.; Lee, E.T.; Malloy, K.; et al. Dyslipidemia in American Indian Adolescents and Young Adults: Strong Heart Family Study. *J. Am. Heart Assoc.* **2024**, *13*, e031741. [CrossRef] [PubMed]
27. Howard, B.V.; Robbins, D.C.; Sievers, M.L.; Lee, E.T.; Rhoades, D.; Devereux, R.B.; Cowan, L.D.; Gray, R.S.; Welty, T.K.; Go, O.T.; et al. LDL cholesterol as a strong predictor of coronary heart disease in diabetic individuals with insulin resistance and low LDL: The Strong Heart Study. *Arter. Thromb. Vasc. Biol.* **2000**, *20*, 830–835. [CrossRef] [PubMed]
28. Jernigan, V.B.B.; Wetherill, M.; Hearod, J.; Jacob, T.; Salvatore, A.L.; Cannady, T.; Grammar, M.; Standridge, J.; Fox, J.; Spiegel, J.; et al. Cardiovascular Disease Risk Factors and Health Outcomes Among American Indians in Oklahoma: The THRIVE Study. *J. Racial Ethn. Health Disparities* **2017**, *4*, 1061–1068. [CrossRef] [PubMed]
29. Wang, J.; Liu, F.; Li, J.; Huang, K.; Yang, X.; Chen, J.; Liu, X.; Cao, J.; Chen, S.; Shen, C.; et al. Fruit and vegetable consumption, cardiovascular disease, and all-cause mortality in China. *Sci. China Life Sci.* **2022**, *65*, 119–128. [CrossRef]
30. Hu, F.B.; Rimm, E.B.; Stampfer, M.J.; Ascherio, A.; Spiegelman, D.; Willett, W.C. Prospective study of major dietary patterns and risk of coronary heart disease in men. *J. Clin. Nutr.* **2000**, *72*, 912–921. [CrossRef]
31. Alissa, E.M.; Ferns, G.A. Dietary fruits and vegetables and cardiovascular diseases risk. *Crit. Rev. Food Sci. Nutr.* **2017**, *57*, 1950–1962. [CrossRef]
32. Pallazola, V.A.; Davis, D.M.; Whelton, S.P.; Cardoso, R.; Latina, J.M.; Michos, E.D.; Sarkar, S.; Blumenthal, R.S.; Arnett, D.K.; Stone, N.J.; et al. A Clinician's Guide to Healthy Eating for Cardiovascular Disease Prevention. *Mayo Clin. Proc. Innov. Qual. Outcomes* **2019**, *3*, 251–267. [CrossRef]
33. Dempsey, P.C.; Rowlands, A.V.; Strain, T.; Zaccardi, F.; Dawkins, N.; Razieh, C.; Davies, M.J.; Khunti, K.K.; Edwardson, C.L.; Wijndaele, K.; et al. Physical activity volume, intensity, and incident cardiovascular disease. *Eur. Heart. J.* **2022**, *43*, 4789–4800. [CrossRef]
34. Lavie, C.J.; Ozemek, C.; Carbone, S.; Katzmarzyk, P.T.; Blair, S.N. Sedentary Behavior, Exercise, and Cardiovascular Health. *Circ. Res.* **2019**, *124*, 799–815. [CrossRef]
35. Barnes, P.M.; Adams, P.F.; Powell-Griner, E. *Health Characteristics of the American Indian or Alaska Native Adult Population: United States, 2004–2008*; National Health Statistics Reports; No. 20; National Center for Health Statistics: Hyattsville, MD, USA, 2010; pp. 1–22.
36. Johnson, N.B.; Hayes, L.D.; Brown, K.; Hoo, E.C.; Ethier, K.A.; Centers for Disease Control and Prevention (CDC). CDC National Health Report: Leading causes of morbidity and mortality and associated behavioral risk and protective factors—United States, 2005–2013. *MMWR Suppl.* **2014**, *63*, 3–27.
37. Foulds, H.J.; Warburton, D.E.; Bredin, S.S. A systematic review of physical activity levels in Native American populations in Canada and the United States in the last 50 years. *Obes. Rev.* **2013**, *14*, 593–603. [CrossRef] [PubMed]
38. Dennison, M.E.; Sisson, S.B.; Lora, K.; Stephens, L.D.; Copeland, K.C.; Caudillo, C. Assessment of Body Mass Index, Sugar Sweetened Beverage Intake and Time Spent in Physical Activity of American Indian Children in Oklahoma. *J. Community Heal.* **2015**, *40*, 808–814. [CrossRef] [PubMed]
39. Schoenborn, C.A.; Adams, P.F.; Barnes, P.M.; Vickerie, J.L.; Schiller, J.S. *Health Behaviors of Adults: United States, 1999–2001*; Vital and health statistics. Series 10, Data from the National Health Survey; No. 219; National Center for Health Statistics: Hyattsville, MD, USA, 2004; pp. 1–79.
40. Jernigan, V.B.; Duran, B.; Ahn, D.; Winkleby, M. Changing patterns in health behaviors and risk factors related to cardiovascular disease among American Indians and Alaska Natives. *Am. J. Public Health* **2010**, *100*, 677–683. [CrossRef]
41. Sember, V.; Meh, K.; Sorić, M.; Starc, G.; Rocha, P.; Jurak, G. Validity and Reliability of International Physical Activity Questionnaires for Adults across EU Countries: Systematic Review and Meta Analysis. *Int. J. Environ. Res. Public Health* **2020**, *17*, 7161. [CrossRef] [PubMed]
42. Esparza, J.; Fox, C.; Harper, I.T.; Bennett, P.H.; Schulz, L.O.; Valencia, M.E.; Ravussin, E. Daily energy expenditure in Mexican and USA Pima indians: Low physical activity as a possible cause of obesity. *Int. J. Obes.* **2000**, *24*, 55–59. [CrossRef] [PubMed]
43. Ravussin, E.; Valencia, M.E.; Esparza, J.; Bennett, P.H.; Schulz, L.O. Effects of a traditional lifestyle on obesity in Pima Indians. *Diabetes Care* **1994**, *17*, 1067–1074. [CrossRef]
44. Jahns, L.; McDonald, L.R.; Wadsworth, A.; Morin, C.; Liu, Y. Barriers and facilitators to being physically active on a rural U.S. Northern Plains American Indian reservation. *Int. J. Environ. Res. Public Health* **2014**, *11*, 12053–12063. [CrossRef]

45. Thompson, J.L.; Allen, P.; Cunningham-Sabo, L.; Yazzie, D.A.; Curtis, M.; Davis, S.M. Environmental, policy, and cultural factors related to physical activity in sedentary American Indian women. *Women Health* **2002**, *36*, 59–74. [CrossRef]
46. Kokenge, M.C.; Ruppar, T.M.; Buchholz, S. Physical Activity Interventions Among American Indian and Alaska Native Persons: A Systematic Review. *Am. J. Health Promot.* **2022**, *36*, 1350–1370. [CrossRef]
47. Pedersen, M.; Harris, K.J.; Brown, B.; Anderson, K.; Lewis, J.P. A Systematic Review of Interventions to Increase Physical Activity Among American Indian and Alaska Native Older Adults. *Gerontologist* **2022**, *62*, e328–e339. [CrossRef]
48. Powell-Wiley, T.M.; Poirier, P.; Burke, L.E.; Després, J.P.; Gordon-Larsen, P.; Lavie, C.J.; Lear, S.A.; Ndumele, C.E.; Neeland, I.J.; Sanders, P.; et al. Obesity and Cardiovascular Disease: A Scientific Statement From the American Heart Association. *Circulation* **2021**, *143*, e984–e1010. [CrossRef] [PubMed]
49. Hubert, H.B.; Feinleib, M.; McNamara, P.M.; Castelli, W.P. Obesity as an independent risk factor for cardiovascular disease: A 26-year follow-up of participants in the Framingham Heart Study. *Circulation* **1983**, *67*, 968–977. [CrossRef] [PubMed]
50. Adakai, M.; Sandoval-Rosario, M.; Xu, F.; Aseret-Manygoats, T.; Allison, M.; Greenlund, K.J.; Barbour, K.E. Health Disparities Among American Indians/Alaska Natives—Arizona, 2017. *MMWR Morb. Mortal. Wkly. Rep.* **2018**, *67*, 1314–1318. [CrossRef]
51. Liao, Y.; Tucker, P.; Okoro, C.A.; Giles, W.H.; Mokdad, A.H.; Harris, V.B. REACH 2010 Surveillance for Health Status in Minority Communities—United States, 2001–2002. *Morb. Mortal. Wkly. Rep.* **2004**, *53*, 1–36.
52. Anderson, S.E.; Whitaker, R.C. Prevalence of obesity among US preschool children in different racial and ethnic groups. *Arch. Pediatr. Adolesc. Med.* **2009**, *163*, 344–348. [CrossRef]
53. Willows, N.D.; Johnson, M.S.; Ball, G.D. Prevalence estimates of overweight and obesity in Cree preschool children in northern Quebec according to international and US reference criteria. *Am. J. Public Health* **2007**, *97*, 311–316. [CrossRef]
54. Hearst, M.O.; N Laska, M.; Himes, J.H.; Butterbrodt, M.; Sinaiko, A.; Iron Cloud, R.; Tobacco, M.; Story, M. The co-occurrence of obesity, elevated blood pressure, and acanthosis nigricans among American Indian school children: Identifying individual heritage and environment-level correlates. *Am. J. Hum. Biol.* **2011**, *23*, 346–352. [CrossRef]
55. Eichner, J.E.; Wang, W.; Zhang, Y.; Lee, E.T.; Welty, T.K. Tobacco use and cardiovascular disease among American Indians: The strong heart study. *Int. J. Environ. Res. Public Health* **2010**, *7*, 3816–3830. [CrossRef]
56. SAMHSA. *2018 National Survey on Drug Use and Health: Detailed Tables*; Substance Abuse and Mental Health Services Administration (SAMHSA): Rockville, MD, USA, 2019.
57. Unger, J.B.; Sussman, S.; Begay, C.; Moerner, L.; Soto, C. Spirituality, Ethnic Identity, and Substance Use among American Indian/Alaska Native Adolescents in California. *Subst. Use Misuse* **2020**, *55*, 1194–1198. [CrossRef]
58. Odani, S.; Armour, B.S.; Agaku, I.T. Racial/Ethnic Disparities in Tobacco Product Use Among Middle and High School Students—United States, 2014-2017. *MMWR Morb. Mortal. Wkly. Rep.* **2018**, *67*, 952–957. [CrossRef]
59. Stanley, L.R.; Swaim, R.C. Latent Classes of Substance Use Among American Indian and White Students Living on or Near Reservations, 2009–2013. *Public Health Rep.* **2018**, *133*, 432–441. [CrossRef] [PubMed]
60. Centers for Disease Control and Prevention; National Center for Chronic Disease Prevention and Health Promotion; Office on Smoking and Health. *How Tobacco Smoke Causes Disease: The Biology and Behavioral Basis for Smoking-Attributable Disease: A Report of the Surgeon General*; Centers for Disease Control and Prevention: Atlanta, GA, USA, 2010.
61. CDC. Smoking-attributable mortality, years of potential life lost, and productivity losses--United States, 2000–2004. *MMWR Morb. Mortal. Wkly. Rep.* **2008**, *57*, 1226–1228.
62. Dikalov, S.; Itani, H.; Richmond, B.; Vergeade, A.; Rahman, S.M.J.; Boutaud, O.; Blackwell, T.; Massion, P.P.; Harrison, D.G.; Dikalova, A. Tobacco smoking induces cardiovascular mitochondrial oxidative stress, promotes endothelial dysfunction, and enhances hypertension. *Am. J. Physiol. Heart Circ. Physiol.* **2019**, *316*, H639–H646. [CrossRef] [PubMed]
63. Messner, B.; Bernhard, D. Smoking and cardiovascular disease: Mechanisms of endothelial dysfunction and early atherogenesis. *Arterioscler. Thromb. Vasc. Biol.* **2014**, *34*, 509–515. [CrossRef]
64. Ambrose, J.A.; Barua, R.S. The pathophysiology of cigarette smoking and cardiovascular disease: An update. *J. Am. Coll. Cardiol.* **2004**, *43*, 1731–1737. [CrossRef]
65. Kong, G.; Singh, N.; Krishnan-Sarin, S. A review of culturally targeted/tailored tobacco prevention and cessation interventions for minority adolescents. *Nicotine Tob. Res.* **2012**, *14*, 1394–1406. [CrossRef]
66. Horn, K.; McGloin, T.; Dino, G.; Manzo, K.; McCracken, L.; Shorty, L.; Lowry-Chavis, L.; Noerachmanto, N. Quit and reduction rates for a pilot study of the American Indian Not On Tobacco (N-O-T) program. *Prev. Chronic Dis.* **2005**, *2*, A13.
67. Hoffman, L.; Ganz, O.; Delahanty, J.; Jones, C.; Homsi, G.; Nonnemaker, J. Tobacco Product Use Health Equity Among Non-Hispanic American Indian Alaska Native Youth in 29 States, 2007–2013. *Am. J. Prev. Med.* **2019**, *57*, e43–e50. [CrossRef]
68. Khorrami, A.; Khorrami, M.A.; Gheriani, H. Vaping-induced acute epiglottitis: A case report. *Int. J. Emerg. Med.* **2023**, *16*, 56. [CrossRef]
69. Zhao, S.; Zhang, X.; Wang, J.; Lin, J.; Cao, D.; Zhu, M. Carcinogenic and non-carcinogenic health risk assessment of organic compounds and heavy metals in electronic cigarettes. *Sci. Rep.* **2023**, *13*, 16046. [CrossRef]
70. Beauvais, F. American Indians and alcohol. *Alcohol Health Res. World* **1998**, *22*, 253–259.

71. Cunningham, J.K.; Solomon, T.A.; Muramoto, M.L. Alcohol use among Native Americans compared to whites: Examining the veracity of the 'Native American elevated alcohol consumption' belief. *Drug Alcohol Depend.* **2016**, *160*, 65–75. [CrossRef] [PubMed]
72. Ehlers, C.L.; Gizer, I.R. Evidence for a genetic component for substance dependence in Native Americans. *Am. J. Psychiatry* **2013**, *170*, 154–164. [CrossRef] [PubMed]
73. May, P.A.; Sandefur, G.D.; Rindfuss, R.R.; Cohen, B. *Changing Numbers, Changing Needs: American Indian Demography and Public Health*; National Academies Press (US): Washington, DC, USA, 1996.
74. Piano, M.R.; Mazzuco, A.; Kang, M.; Phillips, S.A. Cardiovascular Consequences of Binge Drinking: An Integrative Review with Implications for Advocacy, Policy, and Research. *Alcohol. Clin. Exp. Res.* **2017**, *41*, 487–496. [CrossRef] [PubMed]
75. Kunitz, S.J.; Levy, J.E. *Drinking Careers: A Twenty-Five-Year Study of Three Navajo Populations*; Yale University Press: New Haven, CT, USA, 1994. [CrossRef]
76. Whitbeck, L.B.; Adams, G.W.; Hoyt, D.R.; Chen, X. Conceptualizing and measuring historical trauma among American Indian people. *Am. J. Community Psychol.* **2004**, *33*, 119–130. [CrossRef] [PubMed]
77. Yaribeygi, H.; Panahi, Y.; Sahraei, H.; Johnston, T.P.; Sahebkar, A. The impact of stress on body function: A review. *EXCLI J.* **2017**, *16*, 1057–1072. [CrossRef]
78. Severson, E.; Olson, J.K.; Hyde, A.; Brémault-Phillips, S.; Spiers, J.; King, S.; Bick, J.; Lipschutz, R.; Verstraeten, B.S.E.; Olson, D.M. Experiencing Trauma During or Before Pregnancy: Qualitative Secondary Analysis After Two Disasters. *Matern. Child Health J.* **2023**, *27*, 944–953. [CrossRef]
79. Kivimäki, M.; Steptoe, A. Effects of stress on the development and progression of cardiovascular disease. *Nat. Rev. Cardiol.* **2018**, *15*, 215–229. [CrossRef]
80. Fixico, D.L. When Native Americans Were Slaughtered in the Name of 'Civilization'. In *HISTORY*; A&E Television Networks: New York, NY, USA, 2018.
81. Wong, A. The Schools That Tried—But Failed—To Make Native Americans Obsolete. *The Atlantic*, 5 March 2019.
82. Charbonneau-Dahlen, B.K.; Lowe, J.; Morris, S.L. Giving voice to historical trauma through storytelling: The impact of boarding school experience on American Indians. *J. Aggress. Maltreatment Trauma* **2016**, *25*, 598–617. [CrossRef]
83. Running Bear, U.; Croy, C.D.; Kaufman, C.E.; Thayer, Z.M.; Manson, S.M.; Team, A.-S. The relationship of five boarding school experiences and physical health status among Northern Plains Tribes. *Qual. Life Res. Int. J. Qual. Life Asp. Treat. Care Rehabil.* **2018**, *27*, 153–157. [CrossRef]
84. Brave Heart, M.Y.H. Oyate Ptayela: Rebuilding the Lakota nation through addressing historical trauma among Lakota parents. *J. Hum. Behav. Soc. Environ.* **1999**, *2*, 109–126. [CrossRef]
85. Jiang, L.; Beals, J.; Whitesell, N.R.; Roubideaux, Y.; Manson, S.M. Stress burden and diabetes in two American Indian reservation communities. *Diabetes Care* **2008**, *31*, 427–429. [CrossRef] [PubMed]
86. National Public Radio; The Robert Wood Johnson Foundation; Harvard University T.H. Chan School of Public Health. *Personal Experiences of U.S. Racial/Ethnic Minorities in Today's Difficult Times*; Harvard University: Cambridge, MA, USA, 2022.
87. Sardu, C.; De Lucia, C.; Wallner, M.; Santulli, G. Diabetes Mellitus and Its Cardiovascular Complications: New Insights into an Old Disease. *J. Diabetes Res.* **2019**, *2019*, 1905194. [CrossRef] [PubMed]
88. Redbird, B. *Islands of Labor: Reservation Labor Markets and American Indian Well-Being*; Chief Evaluation Office, U.S. Department of Labor: Washington, DC, USA, 2021; pp. 1–50.
89. Bureau of Labor Statistics Reports. *Labor Force Characteristics by Race and Ethnicity, 2022*; U.S. Bureau of Labor Statistics: Washington, DC, USA, 2023.
90. Bhatnagar, A. Environmental determinants of cardiovascular disease. *Circ. Res.* **2017**, *121*, 162–180. [CrossRef]
91. Carlsson, A.C.; Starrin, B.; Gigante, B.; Leander, K.; Hellenius, M.L.; de Faire, U. Financial stress in late adulthood and diverse risks of incident cardiovascular disease and all-cause mortality in women and men. *BMC Public Health* **2014**, *14*, 17. [CrossRef]
92. Lallukka, T.; Laaksonen, M.; Rahkonen, O.; Roos, E.; Lahelma, E. Multiple socio-economic circumstances and healthy food habits. *Eur. J. Clin. Nutr.* **2007**, *61*, 701–710. [CrossRef]
93. Darmon, N.; Drewnowski, A. Does social class predict diet quality? *Am. J. Clin. Nutr.* **2008**, *87*, 1107–1117. [CrossRef]
94. Beenackers, M.A.; Kamphuis, C.B.; Giskes, K.; Brug, J.; Kunst, A.E.; Burdorf, A.; van Lenthe, F.J. Socioeconomic inequalities in occupational, leisure-time, and transport related physical activity among European adults: A systematic review. *Int. J. Behav. Nutr. Phys. Act.* **2012**, *9*, 116. [CrossRef]
95. Zamora-Kapoor, A.; Hebert, L.E.; Montañez, M.; Buchwald, D.; Sinclair, K. Risk Factors in Adolescence for the Development of Elevated Blood Pressure and Hypertension in American Indian and Alaskan Native Adults. *J. Immigr. Minor. Health* **2021**, *23*, 717–724. [CrossRef]
96. Magnani, J.W.; Mujahid, M.S.; Aronow, H.D.; Cené, C.W.; Dickson, V.V.; Havranek, E.; Morgenstern, L.B.; Paasche-Orlow, M.K.; Pollak, A.; Willey, J.Z.; et al. Health Literacy and Cardiovascular Disease: Fundamental Relevance to Primary and Secondary Prevention: A Scientific Statement From the American Heart Association. *Circulation* **2018**, *138*, e48–e74. [CrossRef]
97. Kivimäki, M.; Kawachi, I. Work Stress as a Risk Factor for Cardiovascular Disease. *Curr. Cardiol. Rep.* **2015**, *17*, 630. [CrossRef] [PubMed]

98. Rainie, S.; Jorgensen, M.; Cornell, S.; Arsenault, J. The Changing Landscape of Health Care Provision to American Indian Nations. *Am. Indian Cult. Res. J.* **2015**, *39*, 1–24. [CrossRef]
99. Walls, M.L.; Gonzalez, J.; Gladney, T.; Onello, E. Unconscious biases: Racial microaggressions in American Indian health care. *J. Am. Board Fam. Med.* **2015**, *28*, 231–239. [CrossRef] [PubMed]
100. Barthle, P. Heart-Focused Anxiety: An Evolutionary Concept Analysis. *ANS Adv. Nurs. Sci.* **2022**, *45*, 69–85. [CrossRef]
101. Booth, J.; Connelly, L.; Lawrence, M.; Chalmers, C.; Joice, S.; Becker, C.; Dougall, N. Evidence of perceived psychosocial stress as a risk factor for stroke in adults: A meta-analysis. *BMC Neurol.* **2015**, *15*, 1–12. [CrossRef]
102. Rosengren, A.; Hawken, S.; Ounpuu, S.; Sliwa, K.; Zubaid, M.; Almahmeed, W.A.; Blackett, K.N.; Sitthi-amorn, C.; Sato, H.; Yusuf, S.; et al. Association of psychosocial risk factors with risk of acute myocardial infarction in 11,119 cases and 13,648 controls from 52 countries (the INTERHEART study): Case-control study. *Lancet* **2004**, *364*, 953–962. [CrossRef]
103. Khemani, P.; Mehdirad, A.A. Cardiovascular Disorders Mediated by Autonomic Nervous System Dysfunction. *Cardiol. Rev.* **2020**, *28*, 65–72. [CrossRef]
104. Teixeira, R.R.; Díaz, M.M.; Santos, T.V.; Bernardes, J.T.; Peixoto, L.G.; Bocanegra, O.L.; Neto, M.B.; Espindola, F.S. Chronic stress induces a hyporeactivity of the autonomic nervous system in response to acute mental stressor and impairs cognitive performance in business executives. *PLoS ONE* **2015**, *10*, e0119025. [CrossRef]
105. Hadaya, J.; Ardell, J.L. Autonomic Modulation for Cardiovascular Disease. *Front. Physiol.* **2020**, *11*, 617459. [CrossRef]
106. Tataranni, P.A.; Cizza, G.; Snitker, S.; Gucciardo, F.; Lotsikas, A.; Chrousos, G.P.; Ravussin, E. Hypothalamic-pituitary-adrenal axis and sympathetic nervous system activities in Pima Indians and Caucasians. *Metabolism* **1999**, *48*, 395–399. [CrossRef]
107. Criado, J.R.; Gilder, D.A.; Kalafut, M.A.; Ehlers, C.L. Cardiovascular disease risks in adult Native and Mexican Americans with a history of alcohol use disorders: Association with cardiovascular autonomic control. *Clin. Auton. Res.* **2016**, *26*, 87–95. [CrossRef] [PubMed]
108. Guilliams, T.G.; Edwards, L. Chronic stress and the hpa axis: Clinical assessment and therapeutic considerations. *Standard* **2010**, *9*, 1–12.
109. Brotman, D.J.; Golden, S.H.; Wittstein, I.S. The cardiovascular toll of stress. *Lancet* **2007**, *370*, 1089–1100. [CrossRef] [PubMed]
110. Vozarova, B.; Weyer, C.; Snitker, S.; Gautier, J.F.; Cizza, G.; Chrousos, G.; Ravussin, E.; Tataranni, P.A. Effect of cortisol on muscle sympathetic nerve activity in Pima Indians and Caucasians. *J. Clin. Endocrinol. Metab.* **2003**, *88*, 3218–3226. [CrossRef] [PubMed]
111. John-Henderson, N.A.; Gruman, H.E.; Counts, C.J.; Ginty, A.T. American Indian young adults display diminished cardiovascular and cortisol responses to acute psychological stress. *Psychoneuroendocrinology* **2020**, *114*, 104583. [CrossRef]
112. Yudkin, J.S.; Kumari, M.; Humphries, S.E.; Mohamed-Ali, V. Inflammation, obesity, stress and coronary heart disease: Is interleukin-6 the link? *Atherosclerosis* **2000**, *148*, 209–214. [CrossRef]
113. Kelly, S.; Hertzman, C.; Daniels, M. Searching for the biological pathways between stress and health. *Annu. Rev. Public Health* **1997**, *18*, 437–462. [CrossRef]
114. Cronjé, H.T.; Nienaber-Rousseau, C.; Zandberg, L.; de Lange, Z.; Green, F.R.; Pieters, M. Fibrinogen and clot-related phenotypes determined by fibrinogen polymorphisms: Independent and IL-6-interactive associations. *PLoS ONE* **2017**, *12*, e0187712. [CrossRef]
115. Luc, G.; Bard, J.M.; Juhan-Vague, I.; Ferrieres, J.; Evans, A.; Amouyel, P.; Arveiler, D.; Fruchart, J.C.; Ducimetiere, P.; Group, P.S. C-Reactive Protein, Interleukin-6, and Fibrinogen as Predictors of Coronary Heart Disease. *Arterioscler. Thromb. Vasc. Biol.* **2003**, *23*, 1255–1261. [CrossRef]
116. Jousilahti, P.; Salomaa, V.; Rasi, V.; Vahtera, E.; Palosuo, T. Association of markers of systemic inflammation, C reactive protein, serum amyloid A, and fibrinogen, with socioeconomic status. *J. Epidemiol. Community Health* **2003**, *57*, 730–733. [CrossRef]
117. Sproston, N.R.; Ashworth, J.J. Role of C-Reactive Protein at Sites of Inflammation and Infection. *Front. Immunol.* **2018**, *9*, 754. [CrossRef] [PubMed]
118. Lainampetch, J.; Panprathip, P.; Phosat, C.; Chumpathat, N.; Prangthip, P.; Soonthornworasiri, N.; Puduang, S.; Wechjakwen, N.; Kwanbunjan, K. Association of Tumor Necrosis Factor Alpha, Interleukin 6, and C-Reactive Protein with the Risk of Developing Type 2 Diabetes: A Retrospective Cohort Study of Rural Thais. *J. Diabetes Res.* **2019**, *2019*, 9051929. [CrossRef] [PubMed]
119. Tohgi, H.; Konno, S.; Takahashi, S.; Koizumi, D.; Kondo, R.; Takahashi, H. Activated coagulation/fibrinolysis system and platelet function in acute thrombotic stroke patients with increased C-reactive protein levels. *Thromb. Res.* **2000**, *100*, 373–379. [CrossRef] [PubMed]
120. Ridker, P.M.; Cushman, M.; Stampfer, M.J.; Tracy, R.P.; Hennekens, C.H. Inflammation, aspirin, and the risk of cardiovascular disease in apparently healthy men. *N. Engl. J. Med.* **1997**, *336*, 973–979. [CrossRef]
121. Barac, A.; Wang, H.; Shara, N.M.; de Simone, G.; Carter, E.A.; Umans, J.G.; Best, L.G.; Yeh, J.; Dixon, D.B.; Devereux, R.B.; et al. Markers of inflammation, metabolic risk factors, and incident heart failure in American Indians: The Strong Heart Study. *J. Clin. Hypertens* **2012**, *14*, 13–19. [CrossRef]
122. Dong, T.; Cheng, Y.W.; Yang, F.; Sun, P.W.; Zhu, C.J.; Zhu, L.; Zhang, G.X. Chronic Stress Facilitates the Development of Deep Venous Thrombosis. *Oxidative Med. Cell. Longev.* **2015**, *2015*, 384535. [CrossRef]
123. Møller, P.; Wallin, H.; Knudsen, L.E. Oxidative stress associated with exercise, psychological stress and life-style factors. *Chem.-Biol. Interact.* **1996**, *102*, 17–36. [CrossRef]
124. Madamanchi, N.R.; Vendrov, A.; Runge, M.S. Oxidative Stress and Vascular Disease. *Arterioscler. Thromb. Vasc. Biol.* **2005**, *25*, 29–38. [CrossRef]

125. Federico, A.; Morgillo, F.; Tuccillo, C.; Ciardiello, F.; Loguercio, C. Chronic inflammation and oxidative stress in human carcinogenesis. *Int. J. Cancer* **2007**, *121*, 2381–2386. [CrossRef]
126. Masselli, E.; Pozzi, G.; Vaccarezza, M.; Mirandola, P.; Galli, D.; Vitale, M.; Carubbi, C.; Gobbi, G. ROS in Platelet Biology: Functional Aspects and Methodological Insights. *Int. J. Mol. Sci.* **2020**, *21*, 4866. [CrossRef]
127. Ghahremanfard, F.; Semnani, V.; Ghorbani, R.; Malek, F.; Behzadfar, A.; Zahmatkesh, M. Effects of cigarette smoking on morphological features of platelets in healthy men. *Saudi Med. J.* **2015**, *36*, 847–850. [CrossRef] [PubMed]
128. Ferroni, P.; Basili, S.; Falco, A.; Davì, G. Platelet activation in type 2 diabetes mellitus. *J. Thromb. Haemost.* **2004**, *2*, 1282–1291. [CrossRef] [PubMed]
129. Koudouovoh-Tripp, P.; Hüfner, K.; Egeter, J.; Kandler, C.; Giesinger, J.M.; Sopper, S.; Humpel, C.; Sperner-Unterweger, B. Stress Enhances Proinflammatory Platelet Activity: The Impact of Acute and Chronic Mental Stress. *J. Neuroimmune Pharmacol.* **2021**, *16*, 500–512. [CrossRef]
130. Goerger, K.; Caldwell, M.; Biermann, G.; Besh, F.; Flickema, T.; Patel, P.; Abbott, K.; Holinstat, M.; Larson, M.K. Observational Analyses of Ex Vivo Native American Platelet Responses. *Int. J. Mol. Sci.* **2024**, *25*, 11990. [CrossRef] [PubMed]

Journal of
Cardiovascular Development and Disease

MDPI

Review

Pre-Workout Supplements and Their Effects on Cardiovascular Health: An Integrative Review

Yanesko Fernandes Bella [1], Samantha Rodrigues Silva Cupido [1], Pedro Augusto Querido Inacio [2], Marcelo Luiz Peixoto Sobral [3] and Rodolfo P. Vieira [2,*]

1 Department of Medicine, School of Medicine, University Center of the Americas (FAM), São Paulo 01304-001, SP, Brazil; yanesko@hotmail.com (Y.F.B.); samantharscupido@gmail.com (S.R.S.C.)
2 Laboratory of Pulmonary and Exercise Immunology (LABPEI), Evangelical University of Goias (Unievangelica), Anápolis 75083-515, GO, Brazil; pedroqinacio@gmail.com
3 Department of Cardiovascular and Thoracic Surgery, Heart Institute, University of São Paulo (USP), São Paulo 05508-220, SP, Brazil; mlpsobral@uol.com.br
* Correspondence: rodrelena@yahoo.com.br; Tel.: +55-62-99391-2112

Abstract: Introduction: Dietary supplements have become a popular aid for improving training performance. Pre-workout supplements contain a mixture of ingredients used to boost physical performance, with some components having been associated with the promotion of cardiovascular health. However, there is insufficient scientific literature on the effects of pre-workout supplements, and the studies often have conflicting results. Objective: The aim of this review was to analyze the impact of multi-ingredient pre-workout supplements on cardiovascular health, in order to identify the main adverse effects and the roles of the most common substances in these supplements. Methodology: A systematic search was carried out in the Web of Science and PubMed databases by three independent researchers between January 2010 and August 2024. The inclusion criteria were available articles published in English. Articles that did not evaluate cardiovascular outcomes and the use of pre-workout supplements were excluded. Results: The 24 studies analyzed demonstrated an overall increase in supplement intake. Pre-workout supplements were associated with improved physical performance and possible cardiovascular changes, with these effects being classified as adverse or cardioprotective. This discrepancy in the results may be due to the different dosages and populations investigated (including active and non-active participants, and healthy participants or those with a history of cardiovascular diseases), as well as other factors that correlate with deleterious cardiac conditions. Conclusions: Multi-ingredient pre-workout supplements may offer physical and cardiovascular benefits, including increased energy, focus, endurance, and strength during exercise, as well as having potential positive impacts on blood pressure and triglyceride, low-density lipoprotein (LDL), and homocysteine levels. However, due to the conflicting results of the analyzed studies, additional studies are necessary to fill in the knowledge gaps and establish clearer guidelines for the safe and effective use of these supplements.

Keywords: heart disease risk factors; dietary supplements; performance-enhancing substances; illicit drugs

1. Introduction

A dietary supplement is defined as nutrient, food component, or non-food compound that is consumed with the purpose of achieving specific benefits for performance and/or health [1]. Supplements can be classified as contributing to muscle mass gain or weight loss, improving sports and cognitive performance, or offering convenience (foods in the form of bars or energy drinks) [2,3].

Pre-workout supplements are consumed before physical exercise and often contain a combination of ingredients including caffeine, creatine, and arginine, among others. These supplements are used with the intention of increasing the availability of energy substrates, reducing fatigue, and creating conditions that favor physical performance, endurance, strength, and muscle mass gain [4]. Pre-workout supplement intake can be classified as acute when used for a short period or chronic when its use exceeds 8–12 weeks or is continuous [5].

In addition to their benefits for physical performance, pre-workout supplements have also been studied for their influence on cardiovascular health. Pre-workout supplements often include compounds that can affect the cardiovascular system. These effects can be negative, such as causing increased blood pressure, or positive, such as improving cardiac activity, reducing total cholesterol levels, having anti-inflammatory and antioxidant effects, regulating blood pressure, and improving blood flow [6–12].

Due to this duality of positive and negative effects, this integrative review analyzed the impact of pre-workout supplements on cardiovascular health in order to clarify their effects and advise users regarding their safety, particularly possible effects on the user's hemodynamic levels.

2. Methods

This integrative literature review analyzed scientific studies investigating the use of pre-workout supplements and their relationship with the cardiovascular system. In order to provide greater transparency and clarity about the methods of this review, we used the systematic review protocol from the "Preferred Reporting Items for Systematic Reviews and Meta-Analyses" [13].

2.1. Search Strategy

The search was performed in the PubMed and Web of Science databases. The search was conducted by two independent researchers (YFB and SRSC); disagreements on the entry or exclusion of articles were resolved by a third researcher (RPV). Additionally, the reference lists of reviews were examined to identify other relevant studies. The search covered English-language articles published in the last thirteen years, from January 2010 to August 2023.

The descriptors extracted from the "Health Sciences Descriptors" (DeCS/MeSH) and keywords were combined using the Boolean operators OR and AND as follows: ("pre workout" OR "ergogenic aids" OR "supplements pre workout") AND ("adverse effects" AND "arrhythmias" AND "ischaemic heart disease" AND "heart health" AND "heart disease").

A second search was conducted to broaden the scope to include more recent articles and to extend the search locations. One of the other researchers (PAQI) independently performed this search. The search used the previously discussed strategies, incorporating newly published research articles and case reports from 2024.

2.2. Inclusion and Exclusion Criteria

Original clinical studies conducted in humans, reviews, systematic reviews, and meta-analyses were considered for inclusion. The PICOTS framework model was used to determine the inclusion and exclusion criteria. (1) Population: clinical studies in humans, of any sex, age, or level of physical conditioning (athletes or non-athletes). We did not limit the age range, in order to guarantee a greater entry of possible studies within the scope of the review. (2) Intervention: studies that evaluated the effects of multi-ingredient pre-workout supplements (MIPWs) and possible adverse cardiovascular effects as the primary outcomes. (3) Comparator: studies that used a control drink or placebo were included. (4) Outcome: studies that included the effects of MIPWs (including drink or food supplements that are commonly marketed as products to be consumed before engaging in any form of training and are characterized by a mix of nutrients that can promote positive effects on exercise performance) on cardiovascular outcomes as the primary outcome and changes in physical performance as secondary outcomes. (5) Time: intervention studies with acute or chronic effects were included in this review. The exclusion criteria included articles that were not published in journals in English, studies without complete abstracts available, studies that were not available, and studies in pre-print that have not gone through a double-blind review process. This approach guarantees a greater scope for the findings and maintains the methodological quality of the articles indexed in the body of this review. Studies that were not available in full were requested by the researchers directly from the corresponding authors through ResearchGate, a platform that connects researchers and allows them to share their research.

3. Results

A total of 406 studies were found through the electronic and manual searches. Due to duplication, 149 studies were removed from the list. After reviewing the titles and abstracts, 224 articles were excluded, leaving 33 for the full-text analysis. Of these, two were excluded due to the inability to locate the full text, and nine did not evaluate cardiovascular markers. The results of the remaining 24 articles were synthesized into a narrative form for this integrative review. The second search found two articles that were later included (Figure 1).

3.1. *Cardiovascular Outcomes*

Among the 24 articles included, only 4 studied cardiovascular complications and hemodynamic changes, and the remaining 20 investigations on acute or chronic MIPW consumption did not find deleterious changes in cardiovascular parameters, such as systolic or diastolic blood pressure, arrhythmias, cardiac events, or adverse events. The outcomes are listed in Tables 1 and 2.

3.2. *Synephrine*

Of the 24 articles, only 4 used an MIPW containing synephrine. In the Section 4, we will present the rationale for using this type of product and its cardiovascular effects.

3.3. *Caffeine*

Caffeine antagonizes adenosine receptors, allowing for the release of catecholamines, which alter cardiovascular responses. Its effects are augmented when co-administered with isopropylnorsynephrine or other by-products. Caffeine is one of the most common components of pre-workout supplements. Of the 24 articles, 22 reported the use of MIPWs containing caffeine, with the dosage ranging from 100 to 400 mg. For more information, see Tables 1 and 2.

3.4. *Other MIPW Ingredients—Creatine, Beta-Alanine, Nitric Oxide*

Pre-workout supplements also commonly contain creatine and beta-alanine. Of the studies included in this review, 7 investigations used MIPWs with creatine or creatine monohydrate, 16 studies used MIPWs with the non-essential amino acid beta-alanine, and 4 studies used MIPWs containing nitric oxide. Some studies also added vitamin complexes from the B1 family to the MIPW, as well as other compounds (see Tables 1 and 2).

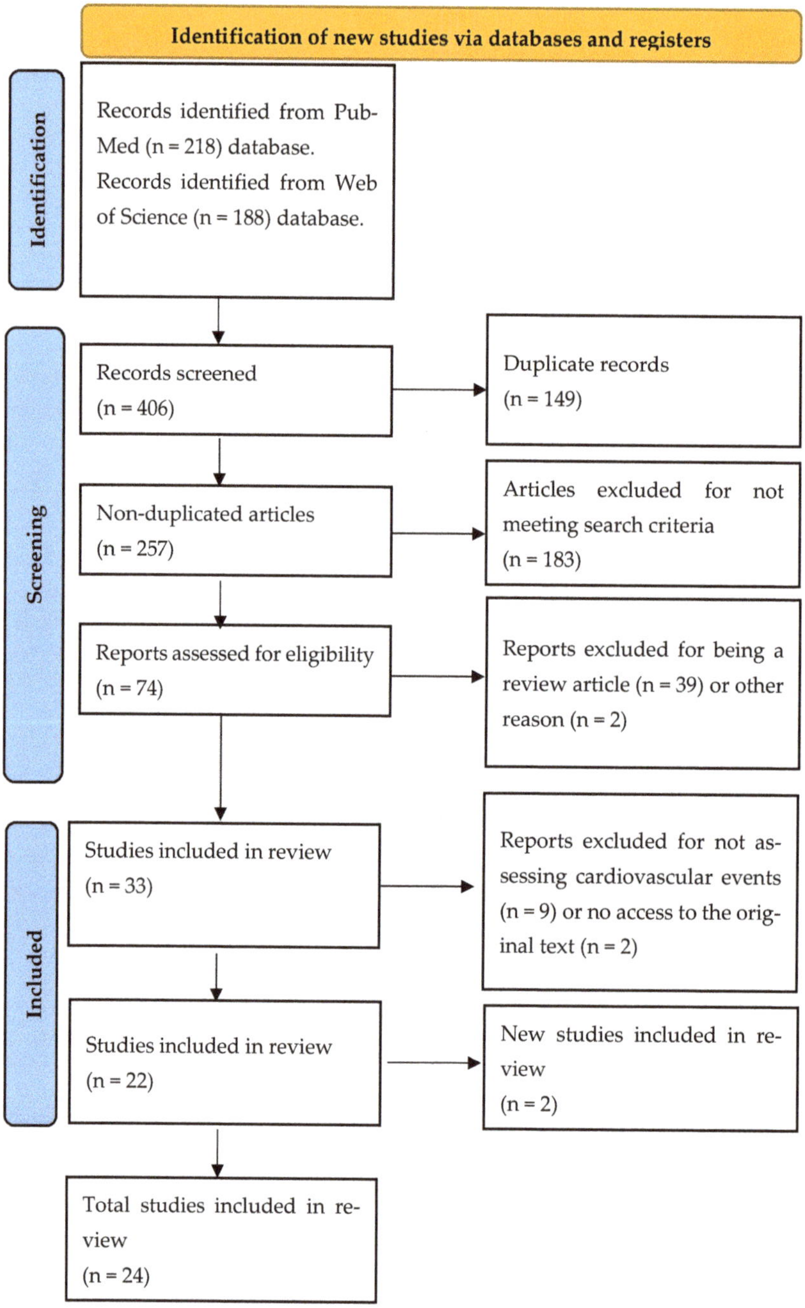

Figure 1. Flowchart describing the inclusion and exclusion of articles in this review according to the PRISMA protocol.

Table 1. Summary of results of case report and research articles.

Author/Year	Study Type	Participants	Supplement (Ingredients)	Cardiovascular and Other Reported Adverse Outcomes
De Jonge et al., 2023 [14].	Case Report	35 patients (16 man and 16 women) Age: 16–57 Healthy, trained and untrained	MIPW (synephrine: 12 to 100 mg)	Chest pains and palpitations Cardiac arrhythmia and ischemia Cerebrovascular diseases
Rodrigues Guerra et al., 2023 [15].	Case Report	1 woman Age: 35 No activity level reported	MIPW (caffeine and nitric oxide—doses not disclosed)	Tachycardia and elevated troponin levels Subclinical hyperthyroidism
Wang S.S.Y., 2020 [16].	Case Report	1 woman Age: 33 Healthy	Alpha Lean-7® (caffeine, synephrine, green tea extract, and betaine) (200 mg caffeine)	Chest tightness Dyspnea and presyncope
Pilegaard et al., 2022 [17]	Observational study	63 male gym-goers Age: 15–35 Trained	MIPW (several proteins, caffeine, and green tea) (caffeine dose varied from 5 to 1323 mg per day)	Pre-workout supplements were responsible for 53% of the adverse effects reported Main cardiovascular symptom reported was palpitations Insomnia, tremors, and headaches
Knapik et al., 2022 [18]	Observational study on adverse effects in dietary supplement users in the US military service	2005 US military service members Trained and healthy	C4 Extreme® C4 original® (caffeine, beta-alanine, and creatine) Caffeine intake: 218 ± 2 and 167 ± 3 mg/day for men and women	Palpitations and/or increased heart rate (11%) Numbness and tingling (13%), diarrhea (5%), insomnia (5.5%), nausea/vomiting (3.5%), and tremors and seizures (1.5%)
Jagim et al., 2019 [19]	Interviews with MIPW users to assess their customs, habits, and safe usage of MIPWs	872 interviewees (636 men and 233 women) Age: 27.7 ± 8	MIPW (beta-alanine (87%; 2.0 ± 0.8 g), caffeine (86%; 254.0 ± 79.5 mg), citrulline (71%; 4.0 ± 2.5 g), tyrosine (63%; 348.0 ± 305.7 mg), taurine (51%; 1.3 ± 0.6 g), and creatine (49%; 2.1 ± 1.0 g))	Accelerated heartbeat/palpitations (23.4%) Nausea (26.6%), skin reactions (34.3%), and dizziness (14.7%)
Altaf et al., 2024 [20]	Case report	36-year-old male with hypertension and a history of renal stones Trained but not healthy	MIPW (creatine, caffeine, nitric oxide, and blast complex composed of arginine, alpha-ketoglutarate, citrulline malate, L-arginine HCL, beta-alanine, and L-norvaline) (3000 mg caffeine, creatine, and nitric oxide)	No cardiac arrhythmia, ischemia, or adverse cardiovascular events were reported, but rhabdomyolysis associated with the use of MIPWs was reported

MIPW: multi-ingredient pre-workout supplement.

Table 2. Summary of the results of selected clinical studies.

Author/Year	Objective of the Study	Participants	Supplement (Ingredients)	Cardiovascular and Other Reported Adverse Outcomes	Ergogenic Effects
Cameron et al., 2018 [21]	Investigation of the effect (safety and performance) of the acute consumption of pre-workouts in women undergoing resistance training	30 recreationally active women: 15 given MIPW vs. 15 given placebo Age: 21.5 ± 1.7	MusclePharm, Fitmiss™ Ignite™ (caffeine, beta-alanine, beet root, L tyrosine—doses not disclosed)	Increased diastolic blood pleasure	Increased muscular resistance, anaerobic capacity, and increased perception of focus.
Erickson et al., 2020 [22]	Evaluation of the effect of acute pre-workout intake during moderate-intensity treadmill running	12 women: 6 given MIPW vs. 6 given placebo Age: 25 ± 9 No activity level reported	Cellucor Bryan TX® (caffeine (150 mg), beta-alanine (1.6 g), explosive energy blend, L-dopa, carnitine and vitamin mix)	Increased diastolic blood pleasure in supplemented group	There was no improvement in performance markers, but there was an increase in the feeling of effort.
Kedia et al., 2014 [23]	Assessment of the effect of supplements on performance and body composition during supervised resistance exercises	40 men and women: 22 given MIPW vs. 18 given placebo Age: 26 ± 5 No activity level reported	MIPW (creatine, betaine, and Dendrobium extract—doses not disclosed)	Increase in systolic and diastolic blood pressure and heart rate in the MIPW group (acute effect). These differences were not noted after six weeks. No changes in clinical and laboratory parameters (hemodynamic, biochemical, and liver enzyme parameters) in both groups	There was an improvement in the subjective feeling of focus and resistance to fatigue, but no improvement in global markers of muscle performance and body composition.
Curtis et al., 2023 [24]	Evaluation of the effect of multi-ingredient supplements on physical and mental performance	14 well-trained men and women: 7 given MIPW vs. 7 given placebo Age: 19.9 ± 1	MIPW (caffeine (250 mg), beta-alanine (2.5 g), and creatine (5 g))	Heart rate and blood pressure did not changed with supplementation	Significant improvements in attention, reaction time and measures of vigor and fatigue in the supplemented group.
Fye et al., 2021 [25]	Evaluation of the effect of multi-ingredient supplements on NCAA division athletes during a running test	11 athletes (6 men and 5 women) Age: 20 ± 2	Perform Elit™ (beet root, caffeine (150 mg), beta-alanine (3200 mg))	No difference in heart rate was observed	There was an increase in time until fatigue and lactate levels in the supplemented group.
Blake et al., 2020 [26]	Assessment of the effect of pre-workouts on blood flow and heart rate compared to the a single ingredient (caffeine) during resistance exercises	12 well-trained men: 4 given MIPW vs. 4 given pure caffeine vs. 4 given placebo Age: 22.7 ± 4	Iron Pump™ (caffeine, nitric oxide blend, vitamins) and caffeine pill (Bitartarato de colina, L-tirosina, cafeína anidra, vinpocetina (2.051 mg))	There was no change in heart rate or blood pressure No change in blood flow markers	There was no difference in perceived effort between the two groups. There was no improvement in performance in either group.

Table 2. *Cont.*

Author/Year	Objective of the Study	Participants	Supplement (Ingredients)	Cardiovascular and Other Reported Adverse Outcomes	Ergogenic Effects
Schwarz et al., 2019 [27]	Evaluation of the safety and effectiveness of using the supplement in resistance exercises for 4 weeks	16 recreationally trained men: 8 given MIPW vs. 8 given placebo Age: 22.5 ± 3	Bang® Master Blaster® Pre-Workouts (caffeine (350 mg), beta-alanine (2400 mg), creatine (5000 mg), betaine (2500 mg))	Hemodynamic parameters and other blood health markers did not change after taking the supplement	Increased lean mass and greater adaptation to the use of maximum strength in resistance exercises.
Nelson et al., 2019 [28]	Investigation of the effect and safety of consuming pre-workouts in women undergoing resistance training over a seven-week period	19 recreationally active women: 10 given MIPW vs. 9 given placebo Age: 18–30	Muscle Pharm, Fitmiss™ Ignite™ (5700 mg of caffeine, beta-alanine, beet root, and L tyrosine blend)	No changes in blood pressure, heart rate, or lipid profile	No effect of supplementation on performance was observed.
Jung et al., 2017 [29]	Assessment of the effects of acute intake of supplements with and without synephrine on perception of readiness, cognitive function, and performance and health markers	50 recreationally active men and women: 25 given MIPW + synephrine vs. 25 given placebo	MIPW (beta-alanine (3 g), creatine nitrate as a salt (2 g), arginine alpha-ketoglutarate (2 g), N-acetyl-L-tyrosine (300 mg), caffeine (284 mg), Mucuna pruiriens extract standardized for 15% L-Dopa (15 mg), ascorbic acid (500 mg), niacin (60 mg), folic acid (50 mg), and methylcobalamin (70 mg) with 2 g of maltodextrin and flavoring) or a PWS with Citrus aurantium extract and synephrine (20 mg) (PWS + S)	No differences were observed in heart rate, blood pressure, electroencephalogram, and overall blood biochemical profile.	There was an improvement in the perceptions of readiness for performance and cognitive function. The effects on muscular endurance and aerobic capacity were limited or nonexistent in the groups supplemented with and without synephrine.
Jung et al., 2017 [30]	Assessment of the effects of chronic intake (8 weeks) of supplements with and without synephrine on perceived readiness, cognitive function, and performance and health markers	80 well-trained men: 27 given MIPW vs. 26 given supplement + synephrine vs. 27 given placebo Age: 22.0 ± 3	MIPW (beta-alanine (3 g), creatine nitrate as a salt (2 g), arginine alpha-ketoglutarate (2 g), N-acetyl-L-tyrosine (300 mg), caffeine (284 mg), Mucuna pruiriens extract standardized for 15% L-Dopa (15 mg), ascorbic acid (500 mg), niacin (60 mg), folic acid (50 mg), and methylcobalamin (70 mg)) or an MIPW supplemented with Citrus aurantium extract containing 20 mg of synephrine	No adverse effects reported	Increased cognitive function and performance during resistance exercises; no additional benefit from adding synephrine.

Table 2. *Cont.*

Author/Year	Objective of the Study	Participants	Supplement (Ingredients)	Cardiovascular and Other Reported Adverse Outcomes	Ergogenic Effects
Collins et al., 2017 [31]	Evaluation of the effects of pre-workouts on performance and recovery in muscular endurance training	25 well-trained men and women Age: 23.9 ± 4	"Ready to drink" (caffeine (200 mg), β-alanine (2.1 g), arginine nitrate (1.3 g), niacin (65 mg), folic acid (325 mcg), and vitamin B12 (45 mg))	No adverse effects were reported	No differences were observed between the groups.
Vogel et al., 2015 [32]	Assessment of the safety of pre-workout supplement consumption for 28 days	34 recreationally active adult women: 18 given MIPW vs. 10 given placebo Age: 27.1 ± 5	MIPW (1 g of carbohydrate, 23 mg of calcium, and 5700 mg of a proprietary blend consisting of beta-alanine, choline bitartrate, L-tyrosine, glycine, taurine, L-carnitine, beetroot extract, hawthorn berry powder, agmatine sulfate, caffeine anhydrous, and huperzine)	Hemodynamic and biochemical markers and vital signs did not change after taking the supplement	Not evaluated.
Joy et al., 2015 [33]	Assessment of the safety of chronic use (28 days) of a pre-workout supplement	44 men and women: 14 given one dose of MIPW vs 18 given two doses of MIPW versus 12 given placebo Age: 27 ± 5	Iron Pump™ (L-arginine, nitric oxide, and caffeine—doses not disclosed)	No changes in laboratory parameters (cardiac, kidney, and liver function markers) were observed	Not evaluated.
Martin et al., 2017 [34]	Investigation of the effect of pre-training on blood flow and hyperemia during resistance training	30 recreationally active men and women: 15 given MIPW vs. 15 given placebo Age: 22.1 ± 1.3	Reckless™ (L-arginine, L-citrulline, creatine, L-norvaline, elevATP®, and Spectra™ (β-alanine (1600 mg) caffeine (300 mg), and creatine monohydrate (1500 mg)))	No adverse effects were reported	No differences were observed between the groups.
Kendall et al., 2014 [35]	Investigation of the safety and effectiveness of taking pre-workouts for 28 days	17 recreationally trained men: 9 given MIPW vs. 8 given placebo Age: 21 ± 4	MIPW (BCAAs (6 g), creatine (5 g), β-alanine (4 g), citrulline malate (1.5 g), and caffeine (300 mg))	No change in heart rate or blood pressure Normal liver and kidney markers in both groups	Decrease in the percentage of body fat, increase in lean mass, decrease in maximum oxygen consumption, and increase in the number of repetitions in the leg press with supplementation.

Table 2. *Cont.*

Author/Year	Objective of the Study	Participants	Supplement (Ingredients)	Cardiovascular and Other Reported Adverse Outcomes	Ergogenic Effects
Smith et al., 2010 [36]	Evaluation of the effect of pre-workouts combined with three weeks of high-intensity interval training (HIIT) on aerobic and anaerobic performance	24 recreational athletes: 13 given MIPW + HIIT vs. 11 given HIIT control Age: 21.1 ± 1.9	Game Time® (proprietary blend: 2100 milligrams of Cordyceps sinensis, arginine AKG, Kre-Alkalyn, Citrulline AKG, *Eleutherococcus senticosus*, taurine, leucine, *Rhodiola rosea*, sodium chloride, valine, isoleucine, caffeine, and whey protein concentrate)	No adverse effects were reported	There was an increase in training volume and critical speed in the supplemented group. There was no difference in the performance markers and body composition between the groups.
Martos-Arregui et al., 2024 [37]	Investigation of the acute effects of caffeine and beta-alanine administered prior to four supersets of bench presses and bench pulls on mechanical, metabolic, cardiovascular, and perceptual variables	21 young resistance-trained males Age: 23.5 ± 4.5	Caffeine alone (200 mg), beta-alanine alone (3 g), or their combination (200 mg caffeine and 3 g beta-alanine)	No adverse effects were reported	Supplement did not significantly affect any mechanical variables. Heart rate was consistent across the different groups. There was no difference in performance between the groups.

MIPW: multi-ingredient pre-workout supplement.

3.5. Risk Factors, Age, Training Level, and Other Factors

Some risk factors that may contribute to adverse cardiovascular outcomes were reported in some studies, including smoking, alcohol consumption, a high body mass index, high blood pressure, and a family history of cardiovascular disease. In one case report, no pre-reported risk factors for the patient were highlighted [15]. Similarly, in another reported case, the patient had no history of cardiovascular risks. However, the study found that she was highly sensitive to caffeine, which explained her condition [16]. In contrast to these results, a case study reported a patient with a history of hypertension, smoking, and alcohol consumption, and was suffering hospital complications, which were correlated with the use of MIPW beverages [20]. The remaining articles included participants who were physically active or who were already engaged in training sessions and did not have any previous cardiovascular complications. In the 24 articles, the majority of the investigated population was young adults with an average age of between 18 and 35 years.

3.6. Dose and Time of Use

Most articles used MIPWs with varying doses of the ingredients, with the dose of caffeine—the most common ingredient—ranging between 100 and 300 mg. One article investigated the amounts of several ingredients used in MIPW drinks and found that the amounts of beta-alanine and caffeine were below or at the lower limit of the recommended doses for efficacy [19], while the doses of beta-alanine varied between 1 and 3 g, the creatine content was approximately 5 g, and the synephrine doses ranged between 10 and 200 mg. Some studies did not provide the doses for each ingredient. The amount of time between consuming the MIPW and engaging in any type of exercise in the studies ranged between 30 and 40 min.

4. Discussion

MIPWs contain a blend of ingredients designed to elicit an optimized effect on acute exercise performance and subsequent training adaptations [5,38]. These supplements typically contain ingredients such as synephrine, caffeine, creatine, beta-alanine, taurine, and nitric oxide boosters [1,4,5,14]. Some of these components are commonly associated with adverse cardiovascular effects anecdotally and, due to the increasing use of MIPW drinks, this review sought to discuss and present the current knowledge on the safety and efficacy of the use of these products and their effects on cardiovascular outcomes. Our findings corroborated the safety of MIPWs. Cardiovascular events such as palpitations and hemodynamic changes were only reported in cases with other factors affecting cardiovascular health, which could not be controlled for and prevents us from making conclusions based on these results. The following discussion explains the most common ingredients used in MIPWs.

4.1. Creatine

It is common to add ingredients such as creatine and beta-alanine to pre-workout supplements, especially in products that are marketed as drinks to be ingested before some activity or workout. Creatine, commonly used by bodybuilders and recreational practitioners in the gym, increases the creatine phosphate reserves in muscle tissue, increasing the energy reserves for short-term tasks and creating maximum and explosive strength. Creatine monohydrate, a non-essential energy compound synthesized by combining three amino acids (arginine, glycine, and methionine), is also found in various pre-workout supplements and is used to maintain high-energy phosphate levels during exercise. It has been shown that creatine monohydrate provides beneficial effects in physical activities, including increasing the overall average power and muscle mass development during training, and extending the time to exhaustion [39].

Creatine in safe doses (up to 5 g/day) has been shown to have considerable beneficial effects for the cardiovascular system. Creatine plays a crucial role in the production and storage of adenosine triphosphate (ATP), indirectly contributing to the maintenance of optimal cardiac function as ATP is an essential energy molecule for several bodily functions, including cardiac activity. In addition, studies suggest that creatine supplementation may have a protective effect on cardiac muscle tissue. This is due to its antioxidant properties, which help to mitigate the effects of oxidative stress, a process associated with several heart diseases, such as myocardial infarction and heart failure [7,39,40]. Our results support the use of creatine in MIPW products as it is safe and does not have hemodynamic effects. It is worth noting that, although this is not the topic of this review, it has been suggested that the use of creatine should be chronic and continuous, as its acute intake does not seem to increase adenosine triphosphate reserves. This same scenario also occurs with beta-alanine, which is discussed below.

4.2. *β-Alanine*

Beta-alanine, a non-essential amino acid, is often used as a pre-workout supplement due to its crucial role in carnosine synthesis. Carnosine is a dipeptide that acts as an intracellular pH buffer, regulating the acid–base balance in muscle cells during exercise. Thus, beta-alanine can significantly contribute to improved endurance, allowing for athletes to optimize their performance and support more intense workloads for prolonged periods [6]. Like creatine, carnosine also has anti-inflammatory and antioxidant properties; thus, beta-alanine supplementation could indirectly contribute to cardiovascular system health [10]. β-alanine in MIPW formulas does not seem to generate adverse effects on the cardiovascular system. A recent meta-analysis, based on 12 randomized clinical trials in humans, concluded that betaine supplementation, when used at doses below 4 g/day, has a positive cardiovascular effect through reducing homocysteine concentrations [6].

A study conducted in animals supplemented with β-alanine and subsequently subjected to 45 min of left coronary artery trunk occlusion showed a 57% reduction in infarct size compared to the control area. Although this effect was attributed to taurine depletion induced by the high beta-alanine intake, the possible role of carnosine and N-acetylcarnosine was not evaluated in this study [10]. These findings corroborate the safe and possibly effective use of β-alanine in MIPWs. As previously mentioned, it has been suggested that it should be used chronically. This should be investigated in future work or randomized clinical trials. However, the use of β-alanine is commonly accompanied by symptoms of paresthesia, which could make it difficult to blind clinical study participants to the presence/absence of this compound.

4.3. *Caffeine*

Caffeine, an alkaloid present in plants, is one of the most widely used stimulants worldwide and is known to increase energy, focus, and endurance, playing a significant role in improving physical performance. As a component of various pre-workouts, its ergogenic effect has been observed across a broad spectrum of sports modalities [14,17]. The mechanism of action of caffeine mainly occurs in the central nervous system, where it antagonizes adenosine receptors, a crucial neurotransmitter involved in sleep regulation and the promotion of tiredness and drowsiness. Additionally, it increases the activity of excitatory neurotransmitters such as dopamine and norepinephrine, resulting in greater alertness and vigilance [17].

In 2017, it was demonstrated that moderate caffeine intake (400–600 mg/day) is associated with a reduced risk of cardiovascular disease and can be considered a protective factor in healthy adults. Furthermore, caffeine consumption has not been consistently associated with changes in heart rate, cardiac output, electrocardiogram parameters, or heart rate variability [12]. Its combination with other ingredients, such as beta-alanine, which is common in MIPW drinks, does not appear to acutely affect heart rate parameters when consumed within the recommended dosages [37].

4.4. Synephrine

With the withdrawal of ephedrine from the market, the use of supplements containing synephrine, mainly obtained from bitter orange peel (*Citrus aurantium*), has become popular. Synephrine is an alternative adrenergic alkaloid to ephedrine, which indirectly potentiates the release of norepinephrine. Synephrine increases energy expenditure due to its lipolytic effect and may improve sports performance [41].

There was a comprehensive review of 30 case reports analyzing 35 patients presenting medical symptoms such as chest pain, palpitations, syncope, dizziness, and myalgia related to the use of synephrine-containing supplements for performance enhancement, with a primary emphasis on weight loss motivation. It was concluded that the use of pre-workout supplements containing synephrine may be associated with severe adverse health events, especially those related to the cardiovascular system. Synephrine, due to its similarity to ephedrine, may trigger increased blood pressure, an accelerated heart rate, arrhythmias, and stroke, especially when combined with caffeine [14], tested caffeine, synephrine, and other ingredients, including guarana, an herb containing a high dose of caffeine, yohimbine (an indoline alkaloid), deterenol combined with theophylline, and beta-phenylethylamine. Jung reported the use of isopropylnorsynephrine by a female patient through the consumption of an MIPW (which also included caffeine at 200 mg per capsule) [29]. However, it is relevant to note that synephrine appears to only manifest significant cardiovascular effects at doses exceeding 100 mg, and some studies have suggested that isolated synephrine consumption may not raise blood pressure [42–44].

4.5. Nitric Oxide and Other Ingredients

Nitric oxide is a powerful vasodilator and is important in scenarios that involve high energy expenditure and cardiovascular demands. It helps relax blood vessels, thus improving blood flow and regulating blood pressure, positively impacting cardiovascular health. It is synthesized from nitrate, which can be found in specific foods. Its effects include relaxation of blood vessels, regulation of blood pressure, and a possible improvement in exercise performance in specific populations [45]. These factors have led to the use of this compound in MIPW drinks (Table 1). In one study, a favorable effect was observed on blood lipid profiles, with a reduction in triglyceride levels and an increase in high-density lipoprotein (HDL) cholesterol levels, which are associated with a lower risk of cardiovascular diseases [7].

Taurine, or 2-aminoethanesulfonic acid, is a common component in energy drinks. Its biological mechanisms are based on its ability to conjugate bile acids, modulate Ca++ homeostasis, regulate blood pressure, and act as an antioxidant and anti-inflammatory agent [9]. In addition, taurine is essential for maintaining normal cardiac contractile function [46]. Despite elevated serum cholesterol levels in some individuals taking taurine at high concentrations, it is associated with protection against coronary heart diseases and has been used as a treatment for these conditions in Japan since 1985 [47].

Betaine (trimethylglycine) is a methylated amino acid that was first isolated from sugar beet. It has ergogenic effects in doses ranging from 500 to 9000 mg/day and can promote reductions in adiposity and/or increases in muscle mass [48]. Interestingly, betaine can also help reduce fatigue and muscle damage. It is believed to have anti-inflammatory properties, which can aid in post-workout recovery by attenuating the stress and inflammation induced by intense physical activity [48,49].

A systematic review and meta-analysis published in 2022 highlighted the significantly positive effect of betaine supplementation on total cholesterol, low-density lipoprotein (LDL) cholesterol, homocysteine, dimethylglycine, and methionine concentrations [6]. Additionally, it was observed that betaine supplementation did not negatively influence blood pressure and the serum concentrations of triglycerides, high-density lipoprotein (HDL) cholesterol, fasting glucose, C-reactive protein, and liver enzymes (alanine aminotransferase, aspartate aminotransferase, and gamma-glutamyl transferase) [6]. These parameters, when elevated, are associated with a higher risk of cardiovascular diseases.

Some pre-workout supplements have been developed to increase nitric oxide (NO) production, with the expectation that they will improve physical training performance, mainly endurance. L-citrulline and L-arginine are amino acids often found in supplements marketed as nitric oxide boosters [50]. L-citrulline is a non-essential amino acid with antioxidant properties, and is used in the urea cycle as a precursor of L-arginine which, in turn, is a precursor amino acid of nitric oxide, a substance known for its role in vasodilation and regulation of blood flow, suggesting a possible interconnection between the consumption of these supplements and the promotion of cardiovascular health [8]. Nitric oxide plays a significant role in protecting against the onset and progression of cardiovascular diseases. Its major cardioprotective roles include the regulation of blood pressure and basal vascular tone, prevention of platelet aggregation and leukocyte adhesion to the endothelium, and regulation of myocardial contractility [11].

4.6. Adverse Cardiovascular Outcomes

A study with 32 men and women aged between 16 and 57 years showed that the use of MIPWs causes cardiovascular anomalies. The main symptoms were chest pain (n = 11), palpitations (n = 4), syncope (n = 6), dizziness (n = 6), and myalgia (n = 4). The most common diagnoses were ischemic heart disease (n = 10), cardiac arrhythmias (n = 4), and cerebrovascular disease (n = 2), which were mainly observed after the use of pre-workouts containing synephrine [14]. Consistent with these findings, a study conducted with 63 men who regularly exercise showed that the most common adverse effects of MIPW consumption were insomnia, tremors, headache, palpitations, skin itching, and a burning sensation [17]. A more recent case study [20] reported the admission of a middle-aged man to an emergency care center with a diagnosis of rhabdomyolysis. This condition was associated with the recurrent use of an MIPW drink over the past two months containing caffeine, creatine, and nitric oxide. The study concluded that the patient exhibited electrolyte imbalances, as well as kidney and liver damage. However, no evidence of ischemia or cardiovascular injuries was observed. This review focused on cardiovascular effects, and it is notable that none were reported in this case, apart from the patient's pre-existing hypertension, which did not appear to be exacerbated by the MIPW. The adverse effects found in the analyzed studies include a small amount of evidence from case studies, where the patients already had factors that may aggravate cardiovascular complications, such as sensitivity to caffeine, a sedentary lifestyle, a family history of cardiac complications, and a history of smoking and/or alcoholism.

4.7. Motivations for Using Multi-Ingredient Pre-Workout Supplements

In 2016, it was estimated that the dietary supplement industry generated an economic impact of USD 122 billion, with USD 278 billion projected for 2021. Currently, the global economic impact of the dietary supplement market is expected to expand by approximately 9% annually, potentially reaching USD 327.420.1 million by the year 2030 [51].

According to the "National Health and Nutrition Examination Survey" taken by the American population, approximately 50% of adults regularly consume one or more dietary supplements. Similarly, a survey conducted in 2022 by the Council for Responsible Nutrition found that 75% of respondents use nutritional supplements, with 39% reporting the use of supplements for sports purposes [52,53]. An IOC consensus statement: dietary supplements involving elite athletes highlighted that the consumption of pre-workout supplements is more prevalent in this group compared to recreational athletes, and it was observed that this pattern did not vary significantly between genders [1].

A study with 12 adult men who used pre-workout supplements acutely evaluated the resistance, strength, and power of their upper and lower limbs using cycle ergometry. There was a 9% increase in the total exercise volume and a 14% increase in the lower limb volume compared to the placebo group. These results indicate the potential use of pre-workouts to improve endurance exercise volume [54].

Another study evaluated the effects of MIPW intake in 12 physically active men in the context of a high-intensity interval exercise protocol. Pre-workout supplement intake was found to improve aerobic and anaerobic energy; compared to placebo, there was a significant increase in the number of efforts made (MIPW (41 $\pm$ 10) vs. placebo (36 $\pm$ 12), $p = 0.0220$) and in the time to exhaustion (MIPW (20.1 $\pm$ 6 min) vs. placebo (17 $\pm$ 5 min), $p = 0.0226$) [55].

The consumption of MIPWs by recreationally trained middle-aged adults for five days was shown to increase endurance and promote fat oxidation during low-intensity exercise [56]. In contrast, an analysis of acute pre-workout supplement consumption in 12 adult men during upper limb resistance training did not show improvements in performance or blood flow [22].

On the other hand, in another study, in twelve adult women using MIPW acutely and performing three treadmill running sets at 90% of their ventilatory threshold, no performance benefits related to energy metabolism were observed, but there was a reduction in effort perception [22]. In agreement with this, a study using chronic pre-workout supplements for seven weeks and involving a resistance-training program in active women found that the supplements were not effective in improving body composition and training adaptation. It is important to note that no negative hematological or metabolic changes were recorded in these women.

These findings show the rationale for the popularity of the use of these multi-ingredient beverages among amateur practitioners, recreational trainers, and those who engage in some type of training, even if there may be adverse effects (see Table 1).

4.8. Limitations and Future Research

This review, despite its extensive body of included articles, is not without limitations. First, only two databases were used. We recognize that this approach may have missed some relevant studies. However, we chose this approach to easily find articles that were peer-reviewed and published in English. Future research should perform a more comprehensive search. Second, despite adopting a systematic process, this was an integrative narrative review and did not use statistical methods or calculate effect sizes, which are commonly performed in meta-analyses. Finally, although the PICOTS framework was used to determine the inclusion and exclusion criteria applied in our searches, future review articles may benefit from quality analyses using tools such as the PEDRO scale [57], Black and Downs [58] scale, and risk of bias assessment tools. This review summarizes the important findings from studies on MIPWs' effects on cardiovascular health and can be used as a resource for systematic and meta-analyses in the future. However, our findings should not be extrapolated to other populations that were not included in the scope of this investigation, such as the elderly, children, or high-performance athletes; investigations into these populations could be the focus of future research.

4.9. Practical Applications

Our findings corroborate that MIPW products are safe when taken in the doses recommended by the manufacturers. People already engaged in physical activities can safely take products containing caffeine, beta-alanine, synephrine, taurine, arginine, creatine, and other commonly used MIPW ingredients without significant or deleterious effects. In addition, these compounds may have a positive effect on the cardiovascular system. However, people with a history of complications from cardiovascular diseases, with a sedentary lifestyle, and/or who smoke or consume alcohol should consult doctors and specialists before taking any products.

5. Conclusions

MIPWs are formulated to enhance physical performance, but can also have direct effects on cardiovascular health. The most common components in these supplements, such as caffeine, creatine, beta-alanine, betaine, taurine, and nitric oxide boosters, have been associated with potential benefits for cardiovascular health.

The reviewed studies showed that pre-workout supplements may provide improvements in cardiovascular health, including reductions in triglyceride, low-density lipoprotein (LDL), and homocysteine levels, regulation of blood pressure and basal vascular tone, prevention of platelet aggregation and leukocyte adhesion to the endothelium, and regulation of myocardial contractility. These findings suggest that the use of pre-workout supplements may have positive impacts on heart and blood vessel health; however, MIPWs should be used with caution, as any abuse of MIPWs may result in the opposite effects.

Author Contributions: Each author contributed to the development of the manuscript. Y.F.B. contributed to the research, conception, analysis, interpretation of data, and writing the paper. S.R.S.C. contributed to the intellectual content of the review. P.A.Q.I. contributed to the final review and translation of the manuscript into English. R.P.V. contributed to the final manuscript review as well as the approach to the subject. M.L.P.S. contributed to the conception, final approval of the manuscript version, and guidance of the work. All authors approved the final version and agreed to be accountable for all aspects of the work, ensuring that any issues related to the integrity or accuracy of any part of it are properly investigated and resolved. All authors have read and agreed to the published version of the manuscript.

Funding: This research received no external funding.

Institutional Review Board Statement: Not applicable.

Informed Consent Statement: Not applicable.

Data Availability Statement: No new data were created or analyzed in this study. Data sharing is not applicable.

Conflicts of Interest: The authors declare that there are no conflicts of interest.

References

1. Maughan, R.J.; Burke, L.M.; Dvorak, J.; Larson-Meyer, D.E.; Peeling, P.; Phillips, S.M.; Rawson, E.S.; Walsh, N.P.; Garthe, I.; Geyer, H.; et al. IOC consensus statement: Dietary supplements and the high-performance athlete. *Br. J. Sports Med.* **2018**, *52*, 439–455. [CrossRef]
2. Mietus-Snyder, M.L.; Shigenaga, M.K.; Suh, J.H.; Shenvi, S.V.; Lal, A.; McHugh, T.; Olson, D.; Lilienstein, J.; Krauss, R.M.; Gildengoren, G.; et al. A nutrient-dense, high-fiber, fruit-based supplement bar increases HDL cholesterol, particularly large HDL, lowers homocysteine, and raises glutathione in a 2-wk trial. *FASEB J.* **2012**, *26*, 3515–3527. [CrossRef] [PubMed]
3. Jovanov, P.; Sakač, M.; Jurdana, M.; Pražnikar, Z.J.; Kenig, S.; Hadnađev, M.; Jakus, T.; Petelin, A.; Škrobot, D.; Marić, A. High-Protein Bar as a Meal Replacement in Elite Sports Nutrition: A Pilot Study. *Foods* **2021**, *10*, 2628. [CrossRef] [PubMed]
4. Spradley, B.D.; Crowley, K.R.; Tai, C.Y.; Kendall, K.L.; Fukuda, D.H.; Esposito, E.N.; Moon, S.E.; Moon, J.R. Ingesting a pre-workout supplement containing caffeine, B-vitamins, amino acids, creatine, and beta-alanine before exercise delays fatigue while improving reaction time and muscular endurance. *Nutr. Metab.* **2012**, *9*, 28. [CrossRef]
5. Harty, P.S.; Zabriskie, H.A.; Erickson, J.L.; Molling, P.E.; Kerksick, C.M.; Jagim, A.R. Multi-ingredient pre-workout supplements, safety implications, and performance outcomes: A brief review. *J. Int. Soc. Sports Nutr.* **2018**, *15*, 41. [CrossRef]
6. Ashtary-Larky, D.; Bagheri, R.; Ghanavati, M.; Asbaghi, O.; Tinsley, G.M.; Mombaini, D.; Kooti, W.; Kashkooli, S.; Wong, A. Effects of betaine supplementation on cardiovascular markers: A systematic review and Meta-analysis. *Crit. Rev. Food Sci. Nutr.* **2022**, *62*, 6516–6533. [CrossRef]
7. Balestrino, M. Role of Creatine in the Heart: Health and Disease. *Nutrients* **2021**, *13*, 1215. [CrossRef]
8. Bloomer, R.J.; Farney, T.M.; Trepanowski, J.F.; McCarthy, C.G.; Canale, R.E.; Schilling, B.K. Comparison of pre-workout nitric oxide stimulating dietary supplements on skeletal muscle oxygen saturation, blood nitrate/nitrite, lipid peroxidation, and upper body exercise performance in resistance trained men. *J. Int. Soc. Sports Nutr.* **2010**, *7*, 16. [CrossRef]
9. Jong, C.J.; Sandal, P.; Schaffer, S.W. The Role of Taurine in Mitochondria Health: More Than Just an Antioxidant. *Molecules* **2021**, *26*, 4913. [CrossRef]
10. McCarty, M.F.; DiNicolantonio, J.J. beta-Alanine and orotate as supplements for cardiac protection. *Open Heart* **2014**, *1*, e000119. [CrossRef]
11. Naseem, K.M. The role of nitric oxide in cardiovascular diseases. *Mol. Asp. Med.* **2005**, *26*, 33–65. [CrossRef]
12. Turnbull, D.; Rodricks, J.V.; Mariano, G.F.; Chowdhury, F. Caffeine and cardiovascular health. *Regul. Toxicol. Pharmacol.* **2017**, *89*, 165–185. [CrossRef]
13. Page, M.J.; McKenzie, J.E.; Bossuyt, P.M.; Boutron, I.; Hoffmann, T.C.; Mulrow, C.D.; Shamseer, L.; Tetzlaff, J.M.; Akl, E.A.; Brennan, S.E.; et al. The PRISMA 2020 statement: An updated guideline for reporting systematic reviews. *BMJ* **2021**, *372*, n71. [CrossRef]
14. De Jonge, M.L.L.; Kieviet, L.C.; Sierts, M.; Egberink, L.B.; van der Heyden, M.A.G. Review of Case Reports on Adverse Events Related to Pre-workout Supplements Containing Synephrine. *Cardiovasc. Toxicol.* **2023**, *23*, 1–9. [CrossRef]
15. Rodriguez Guerra, M.A.; Urena Neme, A.P.; Shaban, M.; Matos Noboa, C.; Trinh, T. Pre-workout Induced Demand Ischemia. *Cureus* **2023**, *15*, e33694. [CrossRef]
16. Wang, S.S.Y. Pre-Workout Supplement Induced Cardiac Ischaemia in a Young Female. *J. Sports Sci.* **2020**, *38*, 187–191. [CrossRef]
17. Pilegaard, K.; Uldall, A.S.M.; Ravn-Haren, G. Intake of Food Supplements, Caffeine, Green Tea and Protein Products among Young Danish Men Training in Commercial Gyms for Increasing Muscle Mass. *Foods* **2022**, *11*, 4003. [CrossRef]
18. Knapik, J.J.; Trone, D.W.; Steelman, R.A.; Farina, E.K.; Lieberman, H.R. Adverse Effects Associated with Multiple Categories of Dietary Supplements: The Military Dietary Supplement Use Study. *J. Acad. Nutr. Diet.* **2022**, *122*, 1851–1863. [CrossRef] [PubMed]
19. Jagim, A.R.; Camic, C.L.; Harty, P.S. Common Habits, Adverse Events, and Opinions Regarding Pre-Workout Supplement Use Among Regular Consumers. *Nutrients* **2019**, *11*, 855. [CrossRef]
20. Altaf, F.; Bhatt, V.; Venkatram, S.; Diaz-Fuentes, G. Crushing Muscles: A Case Study on Rhabdomyolysis, Renal Failure, and Compartment Syndrome Triggered by Pre-Workout Supplement Abuse. *Cureus* **2024**, *16*, e58775. [CrossRef]
21. Cameron, M.; Camic, C.L.; Doberstein, S.; Erickson, J.L.; Jagim, A.R. The acute effects of a multi-ingredient pre-workout supplement on resting energy expenditure and exercise performance in recreationally active females. *J. Int. Soc. Sports Nutr.* **2018**, *15*, 1. [CrossRef] [PubMed] [PubMed Central]
22. Erickson, J.R.; Camic, C.L.; Jagim, A.R.; Pellersels, P.M.; Wright, G.A.; Henert, S.E.; Foster, C. Effects of One Versus Two Doses of a Multi-Ingredient Pre-Workout Supplement on Metabolic Factors and Perceived Exertion during Moderate-Intensity Running in Females. *Sports* **2020**, *8*, 52. [CrossRef] [PubMed]
23. Kedia, A.W.; Hofheins, J.E.; Habowski, S.M.; Ferrando, A.A.; Gothard, M.D.; Lopez, H.L. Effects of a pre-workout supplement on lean mass, muscular performance, subjective workout experience and biomarkers of safety. *Int. J. Med. Sci.* **2014**, *11*, 116–126. [CrossRef] [PubMed] [PubMed Central]
24. Curtis, J.; Evans, C.; Mekhail, V.; Czartoryski, P.; Santana, J.C.; Antonio, J. The Effects of a Pre-workout Supplement on Measures of Alertness, Mood, and Lower-Extremity Power. *Cureus* **2022**, *14*, e24877. [CrossRef] [PubMed] [PubMed Central]

25. Fye, H.; Pass, C.; Dickman, K.; Bredahl, E.; Eckerson, J.; Siedlik, J. The Effect of a Multi-Ingredient Pre-Workout Supplement on Time to Fatigue in NCAA Division I Cross-Country Athletes. *Nutrients* **2021**, *13*, 1823. [CrossRef]
26. Blake, M.S.; Johnson, N.R.; Trautman, K.A.; Grier, J.W.; Stastny, S.N.; Hackney, K.J. Neither a Multi-Ingredient Pre-Workout Supplement nor Caffeine Were Effective at Improving Markers of Blood Flow or Upper-Body Resistance Exercise Performance. *Int. J. Exerc. Sci.* **2020**, *13*, 167–182. [CrossRef]
27. Schwarz, N.A.; McKinley-Barnard, S.K.; Blahnik, Z.J. Effect of Bang(R) Pre-Workout Master Blaster(R) combined with four weeks of resistance training on lean body mass, maximal strength, mircoRNA expression, and serum IGF-1 in men: A randomized, double-blind, placebo-controlled trial. *J. Int. Soc. Sports Nutr.* **2019**, *16*, 54. [CrossRef]
28. Nelson, A.; Camic, C.L.; Foster, C.; Zajac, B.; Hoecherl, K.; Erickson, J.; Jagim, A.R. Supplementation with a Multi-ingredient Pre-workout Supplement does not Augment Resistance Training Adaptations in Females. *Int. J. Exerc. Sci.* **2019**, *12*, 187–202. [CrossRef] [PubMed] [PubMed Central]
29. Jung, Y.P.; Earnest, C.P.; Koozehchian, M.; Galvan, E.; Dalton, R.; Walker, D.; Rasmussen, C.; Murano, P.S.; Greenwood, M.; Kreider, R.B. Effects of acute ingestion of a pre-workout dietary supplement with and without p-synephrine on resting energy expenditure, cognitive function and exercise performance. *J. Int. Soc. Sports Nutr.* **2017**, *14*, 3. [CrossRef]
30. Jung, Y.P.; Earnest, C.P.; Koozehchian, M.; Cho, M.; Barringer, N.; Walker, D.; Rasmussen, C.; Greenwood, M.; Murano, P.S.; Kreider, R.B. Effects of ingesting a pre-workout dietary supplement with and without synephrine for 8 weeks on training adaptations in resistance-trained males. *J. Int. Soc. Sports Nutr.* **2017**, *14*, 1. [CrossRef]
31. Collins, P.B.; Earnest, C.P.; Dalton, R.L.; Sowinski, R.J.; Grubic, T.J.; Favot, C.J.; Coletta, A.M.; Rasmussen, C.; Greenwood, M.; Kreider, R.B. Short-Term Effects of a Ready-to-Drink Pre-Workout Beverage on Exercise Performance and Recovery. *Nutrients* **2017**, *9*, 823. [CrossRef] [PubMed] [PubMed Central]
32. Vogel, R.M.; Joy, J.M.; Falcone, P.H.; Mosman, M.M.; Kim, M.P.; Moon, J.R. Safety of a dose-escalated pre-workout supplement in recreationally active females. *J. Int. Soc. Sports Nutr.* **2015**, *12*, 12. [CrossRef] [PubMed] [PubMed Central]
33. Joy, J.M.; Mosman, M.M.; Falcone, P.H.; Tai, C.Y.; Carson, L.R.; Kimber, D.; Choate, D.; Vogel, R.M.; Hughes, C.M.; Kim, M.P.; et al. Safety of 28 days consumption of a pre-workout supplement. *J. Int. Soc. Sports Nutr.* **2014**, *11* (Suppl S1), P30. [CrossRef] [PubMed Central]
34. Martin, J.S.; Mumford, P.W.; Haun, C.T.; Luera, M.J.; Muddle, T.W.D.; Colquhoun, R.J.; Feeney, M.P.; Mackey, C.S.; Roberson, P.A.; Young, K.C.; et al. Effects of a pre-workout supplement on hyperemia following leg extension resistance exercise to failure with different resistance loads. *J. Int. Soc. Sports Nutr.* **2017**, *14*, 38. [CrossRef] [PubMed]
35. Kendall, K.L.; Moon, J.R.; Fairman, C.M.; Spradley, B.D.; Tai, C.Y.; Falcone, P.H.; Carson, L.R.; Mosman, M.M.; Joy, J.M.; Kim, M.P.; et al. Ingesting a preworkout supplement containing caffeine, creatine, β-alanine, amino acids, and B vitamins for 28 days is both safe and efficacious in recreationally active men. *Nutr. Res.* **2014**, *34*, 442–449. [CrossRef] [PubMed]
36. Smith, A.E.; Fukuda, D.H.; Kendall, K.L.; Stout, J.R. The effects of a pre-workout supplement containing caffeine, creatine, and amino acids during three weeks of high-intensity exercise on aerobic and anaerobic performance. *J. Int. Soc. Sports Nutr.* **2010**, *7*, 10. [CrossRef] [PubMed] [PubMed Central]
37. Martos-Arregui, A.; Li, Z.; Miras-Moreno, S.; Marcos-Frutos, D.; Jimenez-Martinez, P.; Alix-Fages, C.; Janicijevic, D.; Garcia-Ramos, A. Comparative effects of caffeine, beta-alanine, and their combination on mechanical, physiological, and perceptual responses to upper-body superset resistance training. *Eur. J. Appl. Physiol.* **2024**, *125*, 837–850. [CrossRef]
38. Vicente-Salar, N.; Fuster-Munoz, E.; Martinez-Rodriguez, A. Nutritional Ergogenic Aids in Combat Sports: A Systematic Review and Meta-Analysis. *Nutrients* **2022**, *14*, 2588. [CrossRef]
39. Bemben, M.G.; Lamont, H.S. Creatine supplementation and exercise performance: Recent findings. *Sports Med.* **2005**, *35*, 107–125. [CrossRef]
40. Butts, J.; Jacobs, B.; Silvis, M. Creatine Use in Sports. *Sports Health* **2018**, *10*, 31–34. [CrossRef]
41. Gutierrez-Hellin, J.; Del Coso, J. Acute p-synephrine ingestion increases fat oxidation rate during exercise. *Br. J. Clin. Pharmacol.* **2016**, *82*, 362–368. [CrossRef] [PubMed]
42. Schmitt, G.C.; Arbo, M.D.; Lorensi, A.L.; Jacques, A.L.B.; Nascimento, S.N.d.; Mariotti, K.d.C.; Garcia, S.C.; Dallegrave, E.; Leal, M.B.; Limberger, R.P. Gender differences in biochemical markers and oxidative stress of rats after 28 days oral exposure to a mixture used for weight loss containing p-synephrine, ephedrine, salicin, and caffeine. *Braz. J. Pharm. Sci.* **2016**, *52*, 59–68.
43. Shara, M.; Stohs, S.J.; Smadi, M.M. Safety evaluation of p-synephrine following 15 days of oral administration to healthy subjects: A clinical study. *Phytother. Res.* **2018**, *32*, 125–131. [CrossRef] [PubMed]
44. Keisler, B.D.; Armsey, T.D., 2nd. Caffeine as an ergogenic aid. *Curr. Sports Med. Rep.* **2006**, *5*, 215–219. [CrossRef]
45. Gonzalez, A.M.; Townsend, J.R.; Pinzone, A.G.; Hoffman, J.R. Supplementation with Nitric Oxide Precursors for Strength Performance: A Review of the Current Literature. *Nutrients* **2023**, *15*, 660. [CrossRef]
46. Schaffer, S.W.; Kramer, J.; Chovan, J.P. Regulation of calcium homeostasis in the heart by taurine. *Fed. Proc.* **1980**, *39*, 2691–2694.
47. Tzang, C.-C.; Lin, W.-C.; Lin, L.-H.; Lin, T.-Y.; Chang, K.-V.; Wu, W.-T.; Özçakar, L. Insights into the cardiovascular benefits of taurine: A systematic review and meta-analysis. *Nutr. J.* **2024**, *23*, 93. [CrossRef]

48. Cholewa, J.M.; Wyszczelska-Rokiel, M.; Glowacki, R.; Jakubowski, H.; Matthews, T.; Wood, R.; Craig, S.A.; Paolone, V. Effects of betaine on body composition, performance, and homocysteine thiolactone. *J. Inter. Soc. Sports Nutr.* **2013**, *10*, 39. [CrossRef]
49. Xu, J.; Zizheng, N.; Xinyi, Q.; Jianyun, Z.; Han, S. Effects of betaine supplementation on inflammatory markers: A systematic review and meta-analysis of randomised controlled trials. *Inter. J. Food Sci. Nutr.* **2023**, *74*, 721–729. [CrossRef]
50. Theodorou, A.A.; Zinelis, P.T.; Malliou, V.J.; Chatzinikolaou, P.N.; Margaritelis, N.V.; Mandalidis, D.; Geladas, N.D.; Paschalis, V. Acute L-Citrulline Supplementation Increases Nitric Oxide Bioavailability but Not Inspiratory Muscle Oxygenation and Respiratory Performance. *Nutrients* **2021**, *13*, 3311. [CrossRef]
51. ReportLinker. Dietary Supplements Market Size, Share & Trends Analysis Report by Ingredient, by Form, by Application, by End User, by Distribution Channel, by Region and Segment Forecasts, 2020–2027. 2020. Available online: https://www.globenewswire.com/news-release/2020/03/05/1995948/0/en/Dietary-Supplements-Market-Size-Share-Trends-Analysis-Report-by-Ingredient-By-Form-By-Application-By-End-User-By-Distribution-Channel-By-Region-And-Segment-Forecasts-2020-2027.html (accessed on 18 March 2025).
52. National Center for Health Statistics. National Health and Nutrition Examination Survey: Dietary Supplement Use Among U.S. Adults. Available online: https://blogs.cdc.gov/nchs/2021/02/25/5492/ (accessed on 18 March 2025).
53. Council for Responsible Nutrition. 2022 CRN Consumer Survey on Dietary Supplements. Available online: https://www.crnusa.org/resources/2022-crn-consumer-survey-dietary-supplements (accessed on 18 March 2025).
54. Bergstrom, H.C.; Byrd, M.T.; Wallace, B.J.; Clasey, J.L. Examination of a Multi-ingredient Preworkout Supplement on Total Volume of Resistance Exercise and Subsequent Strength and Power Performance. *J. Strength. Cond. Res.* **2018**, *32*, 1479–1490. [CrossRef] [PubMed]
55. Figueiredo, C.; Santos, L.F.; Eduardo, R.F.; François, B.; Rodrigo, L.; Padilha, C.S. Multi-ingredient pre-workout supplementation changes energy system contribution and improves performance during high-intensity intermittent exercise in physically active individuals: A double-blind and placebo controlled study. *J. Inter. Soc. Sports Nutr.* **2020**, *17*, 30. [CrossRef]
56. Puente-Fernandez, J.; Seijo, M.; Larumbe-Zabala, E.; Jimenez, A.; Liguori, G.; Rossato, C.J.L.; Mayo, X.; Naclerio, F. Effects of Multi-Ingredient Preworkout Supplementation across a Five-Day Resistance and Endurance Training Microcycle in Middle-Aged Adults. *Nutrients* **2020**, *12*, 3778. [CrossRef] [PubMed]
57. Cashin, A.G.; McAuley, J.H. Clinimetrics: Physiotherapy Evidence Database (PEDro) Scale. *J. Physiother.* **2020**, *66*, 59. [CrossRef]
58. Downs, S.H.; Black, N. The feasibility of creating a checklist for the assessment of the methodological quality both of randomised and non-randomised studies of health care interventions. *J. Epidemiol. Community Health* **1998**, *52*, 377–384. [CrossRef]

MDPI AG
Grosspeteranlage 5
4052 Basel
Switzerland
Tel.: +41 61 683 77 34

Journal of Cardiovascular Development and Disease Editorial Office
E-mail: jcdd@mdpi.com
www.mdpi.com/journal/jcdd

www.ingramcontent.com/pod-product-compliance
Lightning Source LLC
Chambersburg PA
CBHW061627210926
51850CB00009B/2463